WOMEN'S SEXUALITY ACROSS THE LIFE SPAN

WOMEN'S SEXUALITY ACROSS THE LIFE SPAN

Challenging Myths, Creating Meanings

JUDITH C. DANILUK

Foreword by Sandra R. Leiblum

THE GUILFORD PRESS
New York London

For my mother—
In loving memory of her kindness,
support, and unwavering belief
in her children

A Division of Guilford Publications, Inc.
72 Spring Street, New York, NY 10012
www.guilford.com

Paperback edition 2003

Printed in the United States of America

This book is printed on acid-free paper.

Last digit is print number: 9 8 7 6 5 4 3 2

Library of Congress Cataloging-in-Publication Data

Daniluk, Judith C.
Women's sexuality across the life span: challenging myths, creating meanings / Judith C. Daniluk.
p. cm.
Includes bibliographical references and index.
ISBN 1-57230-350-6 (hc.) ISBN 1-57230-911-3 (pbk.)
1. Women—Sexual behavior. I. Title.
HQ29.D255 1998
306.7′082—dc21 98-22508
CIP

ACKNOWLEDGMENTS

Each woman's sexuality is both an individual and a shared construction. So, too, was this book. During its years of gestation, several people were instrumental in shaping the manuscript. I am indebted to the many women I have worked with who have allowed me to share their stories as they struggled to construct a more self-defined and agentic sexuality. In particular, I would like to thank the members of my first sexuality research group, who inspired the writing of this book, and whose words and experiences are reflected throughout these pages. Sally Halliday worked tirelessly to gather articles and resources. My dear friend, confidante, and co-conspirator Michele Phillips provided insightful comments on several chapters of this book, and has been tremendously influential in shaping my ideas about women's sexuality and sexual development over the last 17 years. My thanks go out to Esther Rothblum, who first reviewed the book proposal and generously provided suggestions, references, and resource material. I am grateful to the two anonymous reviewers who waded through the first, unpolished draft of this book. Their astute and formative feedback proved critical to improving the quality, content, and flow of the text. I am most indebted to my editor, Barbara Watkins, who, like a midwife, has been steadfast in her support during the long and protracted process of birthing this book. Her gift is being able to provide critical and transformative feedback in a kind and nurturing manner. Most importantly, I am grateful to my son, Andrew, who generously gave up so much of our time together so that Mom could "work on her book," and who has added so much depth and richness to my life. Finally, I am indebted to my life partner, David, whose supportive feedback and comments throughout my process of envisioning and writing this book were invaluable. His belief in my ability to complete this project sustained me during periods of tremendous self-doubt. I thank him also for providing a safe and loving context within which I have been free to explore and nurture my sexuality.

FOREWORD

Throughout history, any discussion of female sexuality has been characterized by contradictions and paradox. On the one hand, women are viewed as vulnerable, inhibited, modest maidens requiring tender nurturing and loving words, if their sexuality is to be ignited. On the other hand, they are portrayed as tempting teases with limitless sexual appetites and unsavory motives from whom men must be protected. Still another version of female sexuality casts women as obliging, dutiful lovers—not passionate but receptive—particularly when they want to fulfill their presumed biological "mandate" of maternity. While it is certainly true that women can play any or all of these roles, given the right experiences, expectations, and encouragement, it is not true that any of these accurately reflects the true measure of women and their sexuality.

In fact, female sexuality is a complex entity, fueled by biological inheritance and social conditioning and constraints. At virtually every stage of female development, girls and women receive confusing, and at times, contradictory messages concerning their bodies, their behavior, and their sexuality. As Judith Daniluk points out, during early childhood, girl children display a healthy curiosity and pleasure in their naked bodies. They like to look and they like to touch—all parts of their anatomy. Yet, normal interest and sensory pleasure are often discouraged by parents and other authority figures as being immodest or inappropriate and girls internalize both the negative overt and covert messages they receive. Often, they come to feel that an active interest in their sexual self is somehow shameful or dirty. Such feelings are reinforced by the lack of a positive language naming and describing female genitals and sexual feelings.

The discrepant messages girl children receive continue into puberty and adolescence. Menstruation as a marker of womanhood is viewed as a "hygienic crisis" and it is the rare woman who joyfully celebrates the transition from girlhood to womanhood with positive ritual and unambivalent feelings. While the bodily changes that occur during puberty are exciting and attention-getting, they are also the signals for parents and others to provide admonitory messages about pregnancy and unwanted sexual solicitations. The first genital "debut" with a partner is often marked by a myriad of feelings—not all of which are positive. Often, young women recall their first intercourse as a negative experience, feeling that neither they nor their partner was adequately prepared or fully present—either because of the location or the circumstances under which it was conducted. The reality that women are responsible for contraception and the consequences of an unplanned pregnancy inhibits sexual spontaneity and easy descent into bodily pleasures—the conscious mind is often monitoring the what, where, whom, and why of sexual exchange.

Lesbian women are not exempt from the concerns and worries of heterosexual women. Feeling aroused by or passionately loving toward another woman is seen as unconventional and by some as unacceptable, and adolescent girls are often confused by the intensity and unexpected nature of their feelings. There are few adults to whom they can turn for guidance and reassurance.

And so it goes, on through adult development. The pregnant woman is susceptible to more touch than she invites as her body is tenanted by a third party and her physical shape balloons and expands in both comfortable and uncomfortable ways. While motherhood is almost universally experienced as a positive experience, the decision to remain childless is not equally applauded and women experiencing problems conceiving or opting not to have children are often made to feel defensive or defective. The midlife woman is rendered invisible by the media and the elderly woman is stripped of her sexuality both by her children and by societal agents, though passion and sexual interest may continue to percolate internally.

It is not surprising, then, that so many women report sexual difficulties. As the recent *Sex in America* survey (Michael, Gagnon, Laumann, & Kolata, 1994) noted, one in three women complains of sexual disinterest and one in five says that sex provides little pleasure. Trouble reaching orgasm consistently is a common female complaint, although rare in men. Overall, women report many more sexual difficulties than do men, stemming not only from socialization practices that inhibit female sexuality, but from the realities of abuses of power, sexual molestation, gynecological difficulties, and interpersonal conflicts.

The paradox is that women are so resilient and so invulnerable in so many other areas of their lives. Capable of tackling multiple tasks, such as domestic chores and meeting the needs of dependent children, elderly parents, and demanding partners, women are exceptionally capable both physically and psychologically. Yet their sexual expressiveness and pleasure is easily squelched and socially defined in ways that deny the reality of women's bodies and spirit.

In *Women's Sexuality across the Life Span: Challenging Myths, Creating Meanings*, Daniluk focuses on normal sexual development and suggests that the problems women face are due in large part to the sexual meanings they construct and under which they operate. She argues that these constructions are frequently negative or contradictory and deprive women of the pleasure and gratification they are fully capable of realizing in their sexual lives. And, most importantly, she demonstrates how these sexual meanings can be challenged and changed. Most chapters in this remarkable and thoughtful book conclude with a series of exercises that counselors, educators, and clinicians can use to stimulate new ways for girls and women to think about their bodies, their experiences, and their sexuality.

This is a positive approach to female sexuality—one that emphasizes agency, activity, and choice. It is empowering. It recognizes that women of all ages are sexual creatures, that same-gender sex is as privileged and deserving of attention as heterosexual sex, and that women need not be constrained or constricted by their biology. Daniluk exposes both obvious and subtle gender stereotypes and provides an alternative vision of women and their sexuality—one that makes them active decision makers in their own lives. She not only tells us what is wrong or harmful about the ways in which women are raised, but instructs us about how things can be different. Daniluk is to be congratulated for her vision and recommendations—if taken seriously, they will go a long way toward liberating and extending women's experience of themselves and their sexuality.

SANDRA R. LEIBLUM, PHD

REFERENCE

Michael, R., Gagnon, J., Laumann, E., & Kolata, G. (1994). *Sex in America: A definitive survey*. Boston: Little, Brown.

PREFACE

Over 50 years after Freud penned the question: What does a woman want? We appear no closer to knowing the answer when it comes to women's sexuality. Despite the plethora of "how to" books and articles (e.g., Barbach, 1975, 1984, 1988; Loulan, 1984, 1987; Masters & Johnson, 1966), women's sexuality is still very much an enigma. So why write another book on women's sexuality? It is because this book is not about achieving the most satisfying orgasms, or dealing with problems commonly characterized in the sex therapy literature as "sexual dysfunctions" (e.g., "vaginismus," "preorgasmia"). Rather, this book attempts to expand the literature's traditional focus beyond the functioning of the genitals—to gain some understanding of how sexuality is more broadly defined, lived, and experienced by women at each distinct stage in their lives. It is an attempt to address the multifaceted and complex nature of women's sexuality from a developmental perspective, one that enhances our understanding of how women's sexuality is shaped, changed, and expressed throughout life, based on their unique biopsychosocial realities. It is a book about the interaction between women and their worlds—their internal environments, in the form of their changing bodies and evolving sexual selves, and their external environments, in terms of the social context within which women live and make sense of these changes.

I use an interactionist theoretical perspective throughout this book because I believe that with its focus on co-constructed meanings, it is a useful and empowering framework for understanding the development and experience of sexuality for women (Gagnon, 1977, 1985; Gagnon & Simon, 1973; Mead, 1934; Parker & Gagnon, 1995; Plummer, 1975, 1982; Weeks, 1985). The book is based on the belief that women's sexuality is a powerful source of energy and pleasure, but the paradoxical way women's sexuality is constructed in our society makes it difficult for most women to feel at home in their bodies and comfortable with their sexuality. Attention is turned to the highly ambiguous and conflictual messages girls and women receive regarding their sexuality and sexual expression that frequently leave them feeling alienated from their bodies and disconnected from their needs and desires. I concur with Lewis (1980) that "there is much in female sexuality that is truly unique, . . . but inhibitions, stereotypes, and false premises must be disposed of before this uniqueness can be fully discerned" (p. 36). The goal of this book is to help women expand definitions of their sexuality beyond these limiting constructions and to begin to discover and create a more self-defined and affirming sexuality, one that takes on new meanings and qualities in the context of emergent relationships and developmental changes throughout life.

Any woman may find the material in this book of interest. It is, however, directed primarily to professional counselors, social workers, educators, or nurse practitioners who assist girls and women in responding to the biological, psychological, and social transitions that occur throughout their lives. Detailed information on dealing with the sexual concerns specific to certain groups of women (e.g., survivors of sexual victimization; bisexual women; lesbian women; women with disabilities) is beyond the scope of this book. There is considerable literature available by authors more qualified than I to respond to the unique needs of these women. Their work is referred to where applicable throughout the book.

Rather, I present in this book a comprehensive review of the available literature on women's sexuality, using a developmental framework. Within each section, I review theory and research about women's biological and psychological development. Each of the book's major parts represents a stage of the life cycle from childhood to later life. A qualification at this point is necessary. Much of the available literature is based on the experiences of white, European American women, which limits its generalizability. Wherever possible, I attempt to include literature on diverse groups of women. I then turn my attention to context, in discussing the often contradictory messages women receive from significant others and from their cultures about sexuality in three primary areas: reproductive health, body image, and sexual expression. The role of women's sexual and reproductive organs and processes in shaping their experiences of themselves as sexual persons is important and I have tried to acknowledge this, but without assuming a biologically essentialist position. Living comfortably within their changing bodies is also central to women's "embodied sexuality." So, too, are the various relationships within which girls and women express their sexual needs and desires. I discuss how messages about these aspects of women's experiences can contribute to the creation of problematic sexual meanings and be damaging to women's sexual self-constructions. Examples of exercises and interventions are provided that can be used by counselors and educators to help girls and women begin to challenge these messages and create more affirming sexual meanings. In addition to examining the work of other theorists and researchers, I have given voice throughout the pages of this book to the experiences and struggles of clients, research and workshop participants (Daniluk, 1991b, 1993, 1996; Daniluk, Taylor, & Pattinson, 1996), students, colleagues, and women friends.

The book begins in Chapter 1 with a discussion of the various ways sex and sexuality may be defined and constructed, and attempts to expand our understanding of sexual possibilities. Emphasis is placed on the centrality of meaning in women's sexual development and sexual self-conceptions. The chapter concludes with a discussion of how sexual meanings are constructed, why they can be problematic, and how they may be challenged and changed.

The remainder of the book is divided into three developmental time periods: childhood and adolescence; young adulthood; and middle adulthood and later life. The emphasis in Part II (Chapters 2 through 6) is on childhood and adolescence. Chapter 2 addresses the development of sexuality and sexual awareness for children from infancy to approximately 12 years of age. Particular emphasis is placed on the behaviors and experiences that constitute "normal" sexual exploration and development for children. The responses of children's caretakers to these behaviors and the meanings children derive from others' reactions to their developing sexuality are also explored. Chapters 3, 4, 5, and 6 deal with the developmental period of adolescence (ages 13–19). In Chapter 3, attention is paid to girls' biological and psychological development. Common biological transitions are identified and examined against the backdrop of the girls' developing cognitive capacities and interactional abilities. Chapters 4, 5, and 6 focus on the messages that girls receive from significant others and from their cultures as they make the transition from girl to woman during adolescence. Particular attention is paid to the impact of these often contradictory messages on girls' perceptions and experiences of their developing bodies and on their evolving sexual self-constructions.

Part III (Chapters 7 through 10) focuses on the period of young adulthood (ages 20–39), the time in women's lives when they are engaged in making critical sexual choices and commitments to various roles and relationships. Chapter 7 involves a discussion of the typical biological changes and psychological issues that characterize this period of development for women. In Chapters 8, 9, and 10, attention is paid to the interaction between women and their worlds relative to reproductive decision making, roles, and losses; physical changes and transitions; and intimate relationships.

Part IV (Chapters 11 through 15) is devoted to woman's sexuality and sexual self-conceptions during the middle (ages 40–65) and later (over 65) years of life. Chapter 11 addresses normative biological changes and psychological issues. Chapters 12, 13, and 14 focus on negotiating the menopause; adapting to the aging process; and dealing with the needs, desires, and expectations of midlife women in their intimate relationships. Chapter 15 is dedicated to addressing the way sexuality is defined, lived, and expressed by women in later life.

In 10 of the chapters that follow Chapter 4, I provide recommendations to help girls and women explore their sexual feelings and self-perceptions, challenge the contradictory messages and meanings they hold about their embodied sexuality, and begin to redefine their sexuality based on their own needs and desires. These suggested activities can be found under the headings "Challenge and Change: Creating New Meanings" and are directed at helping girls and women develop a sense of sexual agency and entitlement. Although far from being exhaustive, the exercises in these chapters present a starting point for counselors and educators alike to facilitate the construction of more personally empowering sexual meanings. Most lend themselves to individual and group work, and some can be easily adapted for work with couples. I expect that readers will bring their own theoretical perspectives and experiences to bear in determining the usefulness and applicability of these exercises in their work with girls and women.

In some ways, these goals of helping women to become the subjects and authors of their own sexuality may seem naive. Certainly, the only way to really know the full nature and breadth of women's sexuality is to liberate women from the constraints of oppressive patriarchy, a macrogoal that is fundamental to all feminist practice, my own included. As clinicians and educators, however, we cannot expect the women with whom we work to wait for the overthrow of patriarchy before finding ways to live more comfortably and freely within their bodies and within the world. While we work for social change, I believe we also have an obligation to assist the women with whom we now work to embrace and celebrate that aspect of self that is distinctly female, their sexuality. My hope is that this book will be of assistance to mental health professionals and educators in this regard. As Tiefer (1987) said: "Scholarship that challenges the prevailing empiricist, medical model of sexuality . . . confronts more than merely a prevailing theory. It will inevitably have political impact" (p. 90). Ideally, my hope is that at some level this book will have such an impact.

JUDITH C. DANILUK, PHD

CONTENTS

I

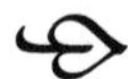

THE ENIGMA OF WOMEN'S SEXUALITY

I

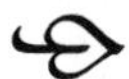

THE ENIGMA OF WOMEN'S SEXUALITY

1

OPENING PANDORA'S BOX

I know no woman—virgin, mother, lesbian, married, celibate—whether she earns her keep as a housewife, a cocktail waitress, or a scanner of brain waves—for whom her body is not a fundamental problem: its clouded meanings, its fertility, its desire, its so-called frigidity, its bloody speech, its silences, its changes and mutilations, its rapes and ripenings. There is for the first time today a possibility of converting our physicality into both knowledge and power.

—ADRIENNE RICH, *Of Woman Born*

EVERYONE KNOWS WHAT SEX IS, DON'T THEY?

In a book about women's sexuality, it is important at the outset to define the subject matter. We might expect this to be self-evident. After all, "sex" is everywhere. We need only turn on the television or pick up a magazine to be bombarded with highly provocative "sexual" images of scantily clad women. In our consumerist culture, it is common knowledge that sex sells. Whether it is blue jeans, automobiles, or beer, the promotion of most products is accompanied by female body parts: breasts, thighs, or buttocks (Faludi, 1991; Wolf, 1991). It is impossible even to buy groceries without coming face-to-face with this month's *Cosmo* queen, usually a waif-like creature with large breasts and doe eyes, accompanied by a caption that promises the secrets to a better "sex life."

But what is sex anyway? In its most essentialist sense, the word "sex" is used to refer to the anatomical characteristics that serve to differentiate between women and men. In this definition, sex depends on the genitals with which we are born. "It's a boy" or "It's a girl" are the words that first herald our entrance into the world. The expectations of the significant people in our lives are based on this basic anatomical fact. This sex assignment shapes our experience of ourselves throughout life. Our identification with the characteristics commonly associated with our biological femaleness or maleness is referred to as our "sexual identity." How we think and feel about this aspect of ourselves is a reflection of our sexual self-esteem (Andersen & Cyranowski, 1994; Unger & Crawford, 1992).

But clearly, sex and sexuality involve more than just anatomical characteristics, do they not? On a more personal level, we often think of an individual possessing varying degrees of sex appeal, allure, or desire. Based on attitude, style, body language, and behavior, we make interpretations about how "sexual" or "sensual" particular individuals are—interpretations that may have little to do with how individuals actually experience themselves. This would appear to suggest that sexuality is something individuals possess to greater or lesser degrees, a characteristic that we are born with or develop as we progress throughout life. So sex is about body parts and attitudes.

But it is also about relationships is it not? In popular notions of sexual contact between two (or more) people, sex takes on a sense of being a commodity to be given by a woman or taken by a man as the case may be. This notion is reflected in locker-room comments such as "I had her," in rock song lyrics such as "I want your sex," and in the lines of romance novels where the heroine "gives herself" to the hero after having expended an appropriate amount of energy in resisting his pursuits.

So sex is usually viewed as an activity engaged in by at least two individuals. Even then, there are distinctions made between "having sex" and "making love," depending on the purpose and intentions of the people involved and on the level of emotional intensity, mutuality, trust, and intimacy that characterizes the encounter. The underlying assumption is that there is genital contact, with successful sex presumably resulting in the physiological release of orgasm. Based on who a woman expresses her sexuality with, how frequently, or whether, indeed, she selects to express this aspect of herself with anyone, assumptions are made about her sexual orientation or preference, and her sexual appetite. Judgments are also made about her normality and morality.

What is common in most of these popular conceptions is that sexuality is located in the body and involves genital contact between "lovers." Despite the erotic sensitivity of the various parts of the human body to touch and stimulation (e.g., ears, back, thighs, feet), sexual expression and behavior is focused on the genitals. According to this conception, all other erotic and sensual encounters, including masturbation, somehow do not quite count as having sex, even though they may be pleasurable and may even culminate in the physiological release of orgasm. A woman is considered to have become "sexually active" only when penis penetrates vagina. All other behaviors and experiences, however erotic or stimulating, are considered secondary or preemptive to the main event of intercourse. The inference is that sexuality is located in the genitals, and that status as sexually "active" is conferred upon a woman by a male partner. This means that the only role for a woman in determining how her sexuality is to be defined and expressed is based on whether and when she chooses to submit to or resist becoming sexually active by engaging in intercourse.

This is a phallocentric, goal-oriented conceptualization of sexuality. It can be seen in many religious practices (female circumcision to ensure virginity, grounds for annulment of a Christian marriage, etc.), in our current laws (e.g., the legal definitions of rape and virginity), in our sex-education programs (e.g., the emphasis of many of these programs is on contraception and the prevention of sexually transmitted diseases), and in our social and cultural norms. This is reflected in the sexual accounting surveys that have been conducted over the years to measure the changing sexual pulse of North American men and women (e.g., Hite, 1981, 1987; Kinsey, Pomeroy, & Martin, 1948; Kinsey, Pomeroy, Martin, & Gebhard, 1953). The physiological focus of Masters and Johnson (1966) on sexual desire and the sexual response cycle also reflects this emphasis on genital sexuality. Much of the sex therapy literature is based on this popular assumption. This means that only problems related to a woman's desire or ability to engage in intercourse or to achieve orgasm would be defined as "sexual" concerns (hypoactive sexual desire, vaginismus, nonorgasmia, etc.). And yet this definition seems woefully inadequate to account for the range and breadth of experiences that might be characterized as sexual. Sexuality must involve more than just intercourse.

In her essay "Are We Having Sex Now or What?", Greta Christina (1992) speaks with wry humor about the dilemma inherent in these narrow and proscriptive definitions of sex. She contemplates how to fit the wide range of encounters that are highly erotic and satisfying into the narrowly circumscribed cultural definitions of having "had sex."

> When I first started having sex with other people, I used to like to count them. I wanted to keep track of how many there had been. It was a source or some kind of pride, or identity. . . . It kept getting harder, though. I began to question what counted as sex and what didn't. There was that time with Gene, for instance. . . . He gave me a backrub, and we talked and touched and confided and hugged, and then we started kissing, and then we snuggled up a little closer, and then we started fondling each other, and then all heck broke loose, and we rolled around on the bed groping and rubbing and grabbing and smooching and pushing and pressing and squeezing. He never did actually get it in. . . . We never even got our clothes off . . . [but boy] it was some night. One of the best really. But for a long time I didn't count it as one of the times I'd had sex. He never got inside, so it didn't count. . . . Later, I'd start to wonder: Why doesn't Gene count? Does he not count because he never got inside? Then I started having sex with women, and boy, did that ever shoot holes in the system. . . . The problem was, as I kept doing more kinds of sexual things, the line between sex and not-sex kept getting more hazy and indistinct. (pp. 25–26)

Although genitals indeed appear to be significant in anatomically distinguishing between women and men, their importance in defining women's sexuality seems less certain (Janeway, 1980; Rich, 1980; Snitow, 1980; Snitow, Stansell, & Thompson, 1983; Ussher, 1989, 1992a; Vance, 1992). For example, a woman may feel very sexual while pregnant and yet not be engaging in intercourse. Another may be celibate and yet experience herself, and be experienced by others, as highly sexual. Still another may be engaging in intercourse regularly but not experience herself or the interaction as being sexual at all. Two women who have committed themselves to each other in an intimate relationship may experience themselves and their relationship as sexual and yet never engage in genital contact, as in the case of Boston marriages (Rothblum & Brehony, 1993). An exclusive emphasis on genital sexuality then, seems too narrow a focus to encompass the many experiences that a woman may perceive as sexual.

IF IT'S NOT JUST INTERCOURSE, WHAT IS IT?

If women's sexuality is not just about what we do with our genitals and with whom, what is it? What constitutes a sexual encounter? What differentiates a sexual from a nonsexual experience? How much of a woman's body is relevant, and what aspects of behavior and experiencing are to be included in such a discussion? Does sexuality take on different meanings based on the developmental life stage of the woman, or is sexuality a relatively stable component of human experience? Must a discussion of sexuality include intimacy, or are there encounters that are sexual but devoid of intimacy, or highly intimate but not sexual? Does sexuality express itself only in relational terms, or is it also an intrapersonal experience? The questions are numerous, and the answers remain elusive.

Depending on one's vantage point (medical, religious, psychological, etc.), it would appear that sexuality may be defined and circumscribed by a woman's physiology and reproductive capacity, by the relationships and activities she engages in, by her feelings, attitudes and self perceptions, or by particular organs and body parts. Based on the perspective taken, women's sexuality may be viewed as static or as fluid, as noun or as verb. Defining and circumscribing women's sexuality for the purpose of this book, then, present a dilemma. This difficulty is underscored by Webster (1988) when she says,

> I'm not sure if I used to know what "sexuality" meant and forgot, or whether the meanings of the word have become so varied that nobody knows what anyone is talking about. Or have the norms which informed the meanings been so radically shaken that new meanings must be identified and put into language that reflect new realities? Maybe we

never really knew what it meant, and some of us just pretended that we did. (p. 296)

So what would constitute a more accurate and expanded vision of women's sexuality? When I asked the women who participated in my research on women's sexuality (Daniluk, 1993) to complete a collage of their sexual histories, the images that they selected included a wide range of activities and experiences. Sexuality for these women was clearly not limited to their genitals or to their relationships with men.

Several writers have attempted to provide more inclusive definitions of women's sexuality by emphasizing the physical expression of interpersonal intimacy (Laws, 1980), as well as the more relational components of women's sexuality (Jordan, 1987; Kitzinger, 1985). For example, Kasl (1989) broadens the traditional definition of women's sexuality to include "how we live in our bodies . . . being alive to our senses . . . taking pleasure in stroking velvet, smelling bread baking, walking barefoot in the sand, and gazing with wonder at a beautiful sunset" (p. 5). Adrienne Rich (1980) suggests that sexuality is "unconfined to any single part of the body or solely to the body itself" (p. 650). She proposes that women's sexuality is "an energy not only diffuse but, . . . omnipresent in the sharing of joy, whether physical, emotional, or psychic, and in the sharing of work" (1980, p. 81). From the perspective of these writers, there would appear to be no limit to the experiences that a woman may perceive as sexual. At any point in time, sexuality may be highly personal or interactive; it may be profoundly physical, relational, emotional or spiritual, and it may include a woman's body, mind, or soul.

Taking these definitions into consideration, whether an experience is defined as sexual or not seems to have less to do with which part of a woman's body is involved in the experience, who else, if anyone, participates, or where the interaction takes place. Rather, it has more to do with whether or not a woman *defines* the experience as sexual. What appears to be most important is the *meaning* of the experience to the particular woman in question. This would help explain why the same body part (e.g., breast, clitoris, tongue) might mean different things to different women. For example, the meaning and significance of breasts may be very different for a woman who makes her living in the sex trade than for a lactating mother. For the sex-trade worker, breasts may be an economic necessity but within the context of her work have little to do with sex or intimacy. The lactating mother, on the other hand, may find the experience of breast-feeding highly erotic and sensual. Whether the ability to breast-feed is experienced as an economic necessity, however, will depend on whether she can afford to bottle-feed her child.

It follows from this that whether a woman experiences an encounter as sexual or not is very dependent on the meaning she ascribes to the encounter. This meaning will vary based on the situation, her expectations of herself and others, her particular life circumstances, and her respective beliefs, needs, and desires. The same body part or encounter will necessarily have different meanings for different women based on each woman's unique history, and on the contextual, situational, and relational realities of her life.

The picture becomes even more complex when viewed from an outside perspective. Whether others interpret and perceive the body parts and behavior of a woman as being sexual depends on *their* particular vantage point and set of beliefs about the meaning of the experience. For example, the client of the sex-trade worker may experience her breasts as highly sexual and erotic but have no such feeling toward the breasts of the lactating mother. On the other hand, others may find the experience of watching a woman breast-feed her child to be highly erotic. Similarly, when overlaid with religious beliefs, the behavior of the sex-trade worker may be judged by others as sexually licentious and immoral, while they may consider the behavior of the lactating mother to epitomize moral fortitude. Clearly, there may be differences between the sexual perceptions of any individual woman and those of the people with whom she interacts. Indeed, these differences help to explain some of the ways sexuality becomes problematic for women. More will be said about this interaction later in the chapter.

In the meantime, returning to the task of defining women's sexuality, it seems, then, that there is no one sexuality. Women are not a homogeneous group, and there appears to be no unified experience of "sexuality" for women. Rather, a diverse array of sexualities exist. They begin with the physical potentialities of the body and evolve in interaction with the changing contextual realities of each woman's life. This means that there are many forms of sexuality. Each is shaped in a particular historical context and "differentiated along lines of class, generations, geography, religion, nationality, ethnic and racial grouping" (Weeks, 1985, p. 178). Personal history, physical capacity, age, and life stage also play important roles in how she defines her sexuality and experiences herself as a sexual person.

To understand how women define and experience their sexuality, and how their unique sexualities are shaped, changed and expressed throughout life, it is necessary to focus on their internal environments, their changing bodies and evolving sense of themselves as sexual people. In the chapters that follow, the research and literature on women's biological and psychological development at each stage of the life course, from childhood and adolescence, through to later life, are reviewed for this purpose.

To appreciate how sexuality is lived and experienced by women throughout life, or the problems women commonly experience related to sexuality, however, it is not enough to attend to women's internal worlds. In fact, much damage has been done in assuming that the source of sexual difficulties and concerns resides within the bodies or psyches of individual women (Ehrenreich & English, 1978; Kitzinger, 1985; Tiefer, 1995; Ussher, 1989). Rather, we must also attend to the external context within which these changes take place. It is this social context that helps to give *meaning* to women's experiences of their changing bodies and relationships, and shapes their evolving sense of themselves as sexual people.

Kegan (1982) suggests that the most fundamental thing we do with what happens to us is to make sense of it. We possess strong needs to create shape, form, and meaning in our sense of ourselves and our lives. Kaschak (1988) concurs that "the essence of human experience and the unifying element of all the various spheres of experience are the various meanings that are attributed to events" (p. 112). Our sexual selves and sexual lives appear to be no exception. It is the contention of other authors (e.g., Bartky, 1990; Foucault, 1978; Gagnon & Simon, 1982; Parker & Gagnon, 1995; Plummer, 1975, 1982; Ussher, 1989; Weeks, 1985) and of this book that the creation of sexual meanings is of fundamental importance in any woman's experience of her sexuality and perception of herself as a sexual person. Disempowering sexual meanings are implicated in many of the problems women experience related to sexuality. Correspondingly, the negotiation of more affirming and empowering sexual meanings is central to developing and maintaining a sense of sexual agency throughout life.

THE MEANING OF SEXUAL MEANINGS

Because sexual meanings are so significant in shaping each woman's sexual self-perceptions, and in the problems experienced by women, it is important to examine what sexual meanings are. In the most basic sense, sexual meanings involve the way we construe the sexual world. They are cognitive constructions; mental representations that reflect our understanding of what is sexual. Sexual meanings are relative, not fixed. They reflect the quality of being both a noun and a verb. As a noun, meanings "contain the elements of constructs, word systems, cognitive schemata, matrices of belief, orienting mechanisms, patterns of significance" (Baird-Carlsen, 1988, p. 23). As a verb, they are dynamic. They involve "process, movement, growth, personal intending . . . the forming and reforming of intention and significance" (p. 23). And they are never neutral. They always reflect a particular set of assumptions, beliefs, or values.

Contrary to the notion of sexuality as a noun, suggesting a fixed capacity or state of being, it seems more accurate and empowering to view women's sexuality as *process* (Caplan, 1987; Gagnon & Simon, 1982; Miller & Fowlkes, 1980; Plummer, 1975; Reid & Deaux, 1996; Weeks, 1985). This process is *emergent* and *transformative,* shaped by each woman's unique history but taking on new qualities and meanings in the context of new and varied roles, experiences, and relationships.

This would suggest that as human beings, we have infinite capacities to express our sexuality. Similarly, sexual meanings do not reside within particular body parts or activities, or within the psyche of women (Plummer, 1975). Breasts and vaginas are not inherently sexual, although sexual meanings are commonly attributed to these aspects of a woman's anatomy in our culture. As such, these body parts come to be imbued with sexual meaning for both women and men. In some cases, they may become a source of eroticism and in others, a source of shame. Underscoring the variance of meanings that can arise in the sexual arena, Gagnon and Simon (1982) suggest that "a sexual performance that is to end in orgasm can be as narrowly experienced as tension release or as complexly as the ritual expiation of sin" (p. 220). As Fillion (1996) notes, sexual meanings and motivations are indeed wide ranging:

> Sex can be motivated by excitement or boredom, physical need or affection, desire or duty, loneliness or complacency. It can be a bid for power or an egalitarian exchange, a purely mechanical release of tension or a highly emotional fusion, a way to wear oneself out for sleep or a way to revitalize oneself. Sex can be granted as a reward or inducement, an altruistic offering or a favour; it can also be an act of selfishness, insecurity, or narcissism. Sex can express almost anything and mean almost anything. (p. 41)

Sexual meanings are both social and individual constructions. They are highly dynamic products of the interaction and shared understanding of individuals within particular cultures (Baird-Carlsen, 1988; Kaschak, 1992). Sexual meanings are implicitly and explicitly embedded in the communication between women and the individuals who compose their worlds. They are constantly being created, negotiated, and modified through the process of interaction between people (Gagnon & Simon, 1973; Plummer, 1975).

In this sense, meanings are not static. They are highly negotiable. As women live out the changes in their bodies and relationships throughout life, they take in a host of messages from significant others (family, friends, lovers, etc.) and from their culture, about the meaning of these experiences relative to their sexuality. These messages both *form* and *inform* their understandings and self-conceptions. In this way, all of women's experiences are imbued with cultural and social meanings, some of which may be empowering while others are problematic. This being said, the next step is to ask *how* these meanings are constructed and negotiated?

THE CONSTRUCTION OF SEXUAL MEANINGS

At the most basic level, sexual meanings are created by each woman in *interaction* with her world (Gagnon & Simon, 1982; Plummer, 1975). This involves a process of attempting to make sense of the biological and psychological changes that characterize her development throughout life, and to incorporate these into her understanding of herself as a woman and as a sexual person. The meaning ascribed to sexuality or particular aspects of sexual behavior for any woman will vary based on each woman's unique interactional history and experiences of her body. As a woman lives with the physical changes of puberty, menstruation, and menopause, or undergoes events such as hysterectomy or sexual violence, the meanings she ascribes to these experiences will be based on her psychological development, her values, and the beliefs she has come to hold about herself as a sexual person. These will also be a product of the meanings available to her within her external world.

Sexual meanings are not entirely an individual construction. Rather, they are subject to certain *cultural* and *interactive* constraints. As women, we are born into a "pre-existing 'sexual world' with its own laws, norms, values, [and] meanings" (Plummer, 1975, p. 40). Every social situation is bounded by implicit rules and meanings that are *situationally constructed* (Plummer, 1975). In this way, over time and with continued reinforcement of these rules and meanings, we come to perceive certain situations and experiences as absolute sexual truths, based on our location within the social context. For example, we may uncritically assume that a concept such as heterosexuality relates to a permanent, *natural* human experience or function, when, in fact, heterosexuality is quite relative in the realm of experiences that one might construe as sexual (Gergen, 1985; Kitzinger, 1987).

Intercourse is another example of this. Despite the range of possible activities that could be construed as sexual, penile vaginal penetration is the one activity that has come to define a woman's sexual status in our culture. The concept of "virginity" is of particular significance in the construction and endurance of these meanings. These meanings may also differ based on the age, sex, and so on of the individual in question. For example, in a culture that lacks rituals to mark the transition from childhood to adulthood, having finally "scored" (penetrated a vagina) is often the event that marks the change in status from boy to man. This event is imbued with meaning and is characterized in many media portrayals as a cause for great celebration. Ironically, the girl who allows her vagina to be penetrated is viewed as having "lost" or "given up" something quite precious—her virginity. The same event has dramatically different cultural meanings, depending on the sex of the player involved. The power of this particular sexual meaning was reinforced for me when working with a woman who had not engaged in vaginal intercourse and as such did not perceive herself as being "sexually active," even though she had been having anal intercourse for several years. A recent decision by a Canadian judge to reduce the sentence of a father who had repeatedly sodomized his young daughter on the basis of his having "spared her virginity" also underscores the pervasiveness of this penis–vagina conception of sexuality.

This is only part of the picture, however. Another layer of meaning is generated by the particular subcultures that individuals inhabit. Based on a woman's membership in particular groups, the meaning of her sexuality will to some extent be derived from the shared beliefs of her religious, ethnic, or social communities (e.g., Fundamentalist Christian, Muslim, homosexual). For example, for a woman born into a family that strictly adheres to a fundamentalist, anti-woman religious doctrine, the meanings available to her to make sense of her bodily experiences and her sexuality will be severely limited.

Experiences commonly perceived to be related to women's sexuality also vary considerably in their meanings and connotations over the life span and across cultures. For example, the experience of menstruation will have a different meaning for a woman depending upon (1) her stage of development (adolescent, young adult, older adult), (2) her ethnic or cultural group (e.g., Native Indian, Asian, Mexican), (3) her religion (e.g., Muslim, Christian), (4) her age cohort (e.g., 50s, 60s, 80s), and (5) whether she is trying to conceive or avoid a pregnancy (Buckley & Gottlieb, 1988; Delaney, Lupton, & Toth, 1988; Golub, 1992; Martin, 1987). On an even broader societal level, the significance accorded to menstruation by any individual or social group will be relative to the importance attributed to fertility within the particular society within which they live (Bartky, 1990; Ussher, 1989). This would of course be true for the myriad of other experiences that shape a woman's sense of herself as a sexual person.

Historical context is also important in the construction of meaning. The meanings ascribed to sexual expression for women in North America have changed considerably over the years in response to shifting social and economic realities. In the late 1800s and early 1900s, the primary purpose of sex for women was viewed as procreation. As such, women were to uphold the moral standards of purity and were to "tolerate" sexual intercourse for the express purpose of satisfying the needs of their male partners and conceiving children (Ehrenreich & English, 1978). With the advent of more reliable birth control, and with the changing economic realities of women's employment outside the home, however, the cultural meaning of sex for women has shifted to a more performance- and pleasure-oriented ethos. In this way, the meaning of the same act has changed from procreation and forbearance to ecstasy and the achievement of multiple orgasms (Ehrenreich, Hess, & Jacobs, 1986). These changes have expanded the possible meanings available to any woman in understanding and expressing her sexuality—sex for love, sex for procreation, sex for pleasure, sex for comfort, sex for intimacy and connection, sex for profit, sex as currency in interpersonal relationships, and so on (Ogden, 1994; Sprinkle, 1996; Tiefer, 1996).

It is important to note as well that sexual meanings are communicated within cultures and environments, both overtly and covertly. Beliefs related to particular behaviors and bodily experiences may be quite apparent, as in the case of the sanctioning of heterosexuality. In the sexual arena in most cultures, however, silence and secrecy characterize much of the communication regarding sexuality. Meanings are often communicated even more subtly, and perhaps more powerfully, through what is only implied. What is *not* said about women's sexuality and sexual experiences, then, is as important in shaping their beliefs and self-perceptions as what is said (Foucault, 1978; Plummer, 1975). Societal messages overtly and covertly sanction particular types of sexual expression (e.g., heterosexuality, intercourse) and repudiate others (e.g., bisexuality, marital infidelity). The messages women receive from significant others and within their cultures regarding their bodies, reproductive functioning, and intimate relationships are especially important in their sexual self-constructions. These messages are explored in the chapters that follow and help to explain how sexuality may become problematic for women.

The messages and meanings available to women within their worlds and the way these are communicated, then, are critical to understanding any woman's experience of her sexuality. Cultures inevitably shape our beliefs and perceptions. We are all products of our environments. However, women are not passive recipients of their cultures. These messages are taken in and accepted to varying degrees by women, in their construction of sexual meanings. They are co-constructed by each woman in interaction with her environment. We turn now to a more detailed discussion of this process.

The Person–Environment Interaction

Women turn to their external worlds in an attempt to make sense of internal experiences. Their interpretations of the way their bodies, desires, and actions are defined and valued within their culture necessarily shape their experience and understanding of their sexuality. For example, if the focus of a woman's sexual desire is another woman, how she understands and makes sense of this desire will, to a degree, be based on the way other's in her world define her erotic focus. A woman's choice of available meanings to understand her desires will be somewhat constrained by the meanings available to her in her particular social context. In this sense, women's sexual meanings are environmentally constructed.

Indeed, there is no shortage of environmental input regarding the meaning of experiences unique to women, such as menstruation, pregnancy, or menopause, or meanings related to women's sexual appearance or expression. Women are continually bombarded with messages from significant others (e.g., parents, friends, lovers) and from the culture at large (media, schools, medical professionals, etc.) regarding their sexual needs and natures. But as indicated earlier, sexual meanings are co-constructions. They are individually created by women based on their unique histories, life circumstances, and particular contexts. This is why the same event or experience does not have the same meaning for all women.

This helps to explain why not all of the messages of significant others and of the culture will be taken in by all women, in the construction of their own *personal meanings*. In fact, several factors seem to be implicated in the degree to which any woman accepts the messages and meanings promoted in her social world in constructing an understanding of herself as a sexual person. These include the persistence of the messages, her investment in the opinions and beliefs of the messenger, her values, the source of the messages, her age and life stage, and her current sexual self-construction.

Whether a woman accepts the messages communicated to her about her sexuality and sexual experiences or not depends on the persistence of these messages, and on her investment in the beliefs and opinions of these "others." The opinions and values of someone with whom a woman is highly invested in an intimate relationship will likely be more influential in how she experiences and make sense of the focus of her erotic desire than the opinions of a stranger. If these values are consistently reinforced by others, however, as in the case of heterosexuality, there is a greater likelihood that the woman will accept them as valid, irrespective of the closeness of these relationships (Markus & Cross, 1993).

Also, some judgments and meanings are valued much more highly over others, particularly those that reflect the individual's own values and current self-perceptions. For example, a young woman who knows that smoking is compromising her health may refuse to quit because she would "rather die of lung cancer than be fat." She apparently has accepted the messages communicated by significant others and by her culture about weight and feminine value, and has judged herself as needing to meet these standards—whatever the long-term cost to her health. This young woman values the opinions and beliefs of others (e.g., friends, lovers, media) regarding her bodily acceptability over the messages of those who are opposed to her smoking (e.g., parents, medical professionals).

The individuals and institutions that are most influential in shaping any woman's sexual meanings and sexual self-perceptions differ based on her age and life stage, and the roles she assumes (Gagnon & Simon, 1982; Laws, 1980). In childhood, caretakers, family members, and the media (storybooks, videos, television, etc.) are particularly influential in the construction of sexual meanings and the shaping of sexual self-perceptions. In adolescence, peers and media appear to be more influential. Girlfriends in particular are an especially salient influence at this stage of development. The beliefs and values of a girl's selected group of friends strongly shape the way the young girl makes sense of her sexuality. Her choice of friendship group both *influences* and *reflects* the girl's perceptions of her sexual self or the self she aspires to become. In adulthood, a woman's social roles (e.g., mother, spouse, lover, prostitute) and significant relationships are important sources of information and validation in the creation of sexual meanings and self-constructions.

A woman's current sexual self-constructions also seem to be important in her acceptance or rejection of cultural meanings. For example, the clinical and popular literature would suggest that body-image dissatisfaction is highly problematic for a large number of women. Not all women, however, experience their bodies as problematic. There appear to be differences in the degree to which individual women accept and incorporate societal messages reinforcing a thin body ideal. Some women, in fact, actively resist these messages, refusing to alter their self-conceptions or their bodies based on the beliefs and values of others. Such resistance can be seen in gender bending, body piercing, and tattooing. It can be seen in the larger woman's refusal to wear clothing that masks her size.

It would appear that rejection of cultural messages and meanings, whether these meanings are positive or negative, is more likely when the messages being communicated are inconsistent with the woman's sexual self-perceptions. The more affirmative a woman's sexual self-perceptions are, the more likely it is that she will be able to reject cultural messages that challenge or are inconsistent with these self-perceptions. The notion of the sexual self is important, then, in understanding the way women interpret the messages of our cultures and the degree of influence these messages have in the construction of sexual meanings. As such, it may be helpful at this time to more fully explore the concept of the sexual self.

The Sexual Self

The sexual self is a fluid, complex entity consisting of various forms of self-relevant knowledge. Sometimes referred to as a sexual self-schema (Andersen & Cyranowski, 1995), these are the beliefs and perceptions that a woman holds about the sexual aspects of herself. These beliefs function as a "point of origin for information—judgements, decisions, inferences, predictions, and behaviors—about the current and future sexual self" (p. 1079).

The sexual self is a rather complex construction that involves physical and biological capacities, cognitive and emotional development, and evolving needs and desires. It is influenced by past history, present circumstances, and expectations and hopes regarding the future (Foucault, 1978; Gagnon & Simon, 1982; Parker & Gagnon, 1995; Plummer, 1975, 1982; Weeks, 1985). It is a product of the private and the public, the personal and the political, the individual and her context.

As women experience various events or situations that they define as sexual, they come to view themselves as a particular kind of "sexual" person, or "nonsexual" person, as the case may be. This is expressed in such identifying characteristics as sexual preference, styles of speech, and modes of dress (Plummer, 1982). We might say that women develop a "worldview" of their sexuality. They become attached to the sexual values of certain groups of people (e.g., Fundamentalist Christians, heterosexuals, lesbians) and reject the values of others. As they repeatedly encounter particular sexual situations over time, they build up particular ways of responding that reflect their characteristic sense of themselves as sexual people (Plummer, 1975).

It may be useful to view the sexual self as a hypothesis that each woman holds about herself (Kuhn, 1964). This hypothesis changes and evolves over time as women negotiate the various relationships and transitions that characterize their lives. In interaction with the significant individuals in their environment, women learn in childhood what they are expected by others to be, and they continue to develop a working conception of who they are as a sexual person and who they ought to be throughout childhood, adolescence, and adult life (Plummer, 1982). Based on this notion, if women continue to receive information that reinforces the validity of their current sexual self-perceptions, it is more likely that they will come to accept the hypothesis as a true reflection of who they are. Contrary feedback will challenge these perceptions. For example, a woman may receive messages from her body, significant people in her life, or from her culture that serve to confirm the hypothesis she holds about herself as a sexual person (e.g., attractive, fertile). This will strengthen her sexual self-perceptions. Or she may receive information that disconfirms or challenges these self-perceptions (unattractive, infertile, etc.). This information, if not rejected, must be incorporated into her understanding of herself as a sexual person. Developmental transitions such as childbirth or divorce, or particular life events such as sexual assault, hysterectomy, or infertility may challenge a woman's self conceptions, forcing her to renegotiate her experience of herself as a woman and a sexual person (Mead, 1934). Much of the work of counseling and therapy is focused on this renegotiation process.

According to Kaschak (1988), "It is the meaning implicit or explicit in any experience that becomes inextricably embedded in the developing self and is basic to the formation of the self-concept" (p. 113). Sexual self-conceptions then, are themselves meaningful in reflecting the way a woman defines and experiences herself as a sexual person. They are also important in the creation of meaning. The meaning any woman makes of her sexuality at any stage in her life will be a product of the messages of her body and of her environment, interpreted through the lenses of the values, beliefs, and sexual self-perceptions she has come to hold.

PROBLEMATIC MEANINGS

So how do sexual meanings become problematic? As women progress through life, they experience a number of normative and nonnormative changes and events related to their bodies, reproductive health, and intimate relationships that they attempt to make sense of (e.g., menstruation, divorce, mastectomy, motherhood). These changes need to be incorporated into their understanding of who they are as women and as sexual people. They need to be incorporated into their sexual self-structures. These events and experiences are sometimes difficult and developmentally formative. They are not, however, necessarily problematic in and of themselves. The difficulty comes in attempting to make sense of these experiences, based on the meanings and messages available within the culture, and on how these meanings are communicated.

On an individual level, the messages available to women to make sense of their experiences may be contradictory and, as such, difficult to reconcile. For example, a young girl often receives mixed messages from others and from her culture regarding the meaning of menstruation. On the one hand, menstruation is commonly viewed as the hallmark of a girl's initiation into womanhood—something to be celebrated. On the other hand, the girl receives messages suggesting that menstruation is something dirty or shameful, which should be hidden. How, then, is the young girl to make sense of this experience in understanding her sexuality? How is she to incorporate this bodily experience into her sexual self-structure in a way that affirms, rather than disconfirms her sexuality and sense of agency?

Interpretations may also be problematic because so many messages and meanings related to women's sexuality are implicit rather than explicit. Turning again to the example of menstruation, considerable secrecy surrounds women's menstrual cycle and monthly bleeding in most cultures of the world. This sends a powerful message to women and men that menstruation is at best a mysterious phenomena and at worst a shameful one (Golub, 1992; Kitzinger, 1985; Martin, 1987). The same can be said for masturbation and a host of other experiences that are deemed to be "sexual." Interpretations are therefore required to determine the covert meaning of these messages. How each woman interprets the messages being communicated, and the accuracy of her interpretations, will have a great deal to do with her current sexual self perceptions and worldview.

Sometimes, problems arise because the language used to communicate these messages about women's bodies and experiences is demeaning, insufficient, or inadequate. The popular language used to describe the "sexual" parts of women's bodies include tits, ass, pussy, and so on. Sexual natures are commonly described with words such as frigid, tease, whore, nympho, dyke, and so on. Women turn to their social worlds to understand their sexuality. The messages they receive and the way these messages are communicated play an important role in how they make sense of their experiences. It follows then, that when there is a lack of appropriate language to define a particular type of experience, such as menstruation, childbirth, or menopause, or when the language is demeaning or pathologizing, the experience will be invalidated. This may result in women disregarding or diminishing the significance of the unique biological and social realities of their lives. Under these circumstances, potential difficulties in the development of sexual agency become readily apparent.

Meanings reinforced by a woman's family, culture, or religious group may also become problematic, even if the woman does not share the same perceptions or values. For example, while a woman may find masturbation to be personally acceptable, she may still experience guilt or shame when involved in this form of self-pleasuring based on her perceptions of how others perceive this behavior. Similarly, a woman may believe that there is nothing inherently wrong with having multiple sexual partners. If she feels guilt about her behavior, this may be engendered by her perceptions of the contrary values of significant others and society at large (Blumer, 1969; Plummer, 1975).

On an interpersonal level, problems can occur in women's negotiation of their sexuality and intimate relationships when their partners hold different meanings and expectations about the same experience. The dinner invitation is an excellent, albeit stereotypical example of this. To the woman, an invitation to dinner may mean an opportunity to get to know someone better and share a meal. To her male partner, however, the dinner invitation may be viewed as a prelude to sexual intercourse. Based on the differing meanings both individuals bring to this situation, a different and sometimes discrepant set of expectations will be set up. The meanings of the encounter need to be renegotiated to the satisfaction of both people. Otherwise a win–lose situation occurs, with one person's meanings taking precedence over the other's. In this way, power is implicated in the negotiation and imposition of sexual meanings. With the current social arrangement between the sexes, women are often seriously disadvantaged in this regard.

Disempowering messages and meanings can profoundly shape women's sexual self conceptions and their understanding and experience of their sexuality. Women may feel alienated from their bodies, which all too frequently become the battlefield in their struggles to live comfortably in a sexual world fashioned largely by men. If they come to perceive specific parts of their bodies (e.g., breasts, buttocks, thighs) to be inadequate based on unrealistic cultural standards of thinness, they may be unwilling to expose these parts to the scrutiny of others or attempt to change them through dieting, exercise, or surgery. The emaciated body of the anorexic is an extreme example of how popular cultural messages can play themselves out in the lives of women, sometimes to the point of self-destruction. In intimate relationships, women may experience guilt and shame related to sexual expression or the focus of their erotic desires. They may lose touch with their "erotic life force"—their creative energy, which is an important source of power and pleasure in women's sexual lives and self-constructions (Lorde, 1984, p. 55).

CONCLUSION

It is the contention of this book that many of the problems experienced by women related to their sexuality occur in attempting to accommodate and make sense of the physical, personal, and interpersonal changes in their lives. These accommodations may be facilitated or impaired based on the meanings that are available to women to make sense of their experiences. In the following section of the book, I explore from a developmental perspective how women's sexualities are shaped, changed, and expressed throughout life based on unique biological, psychological, and social realities. In this exploration, it becomes apparent why the development of a sense of sexual agency can be problematic for women, under what circumstances, and within which particular contexts. Recommendations are provided to assist mental health professionals and educators who work with girls and women to help them live more comfortably in their bodies and to guide them in the development of more personally empowering sexual meanings and self-constructions.

II

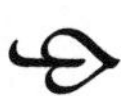

CHILDHOOD AND ADOLESCENCE

2

TEACHING THE CHILDREN

> Marcelle Drouffe was a dreamy, precocious little girl: as early as the age of ten months she gave signs of being extraordinarily sensitive. "When you hurt yourself, it wasn't the pain that made you cry," her mother told her later. "It was because you felt the world had betrayed you."
>
> —SIMONE DE BEAUVOIR,
> *When Things of the Spirit Come First*

The definitions that women come to hold about what body parts and activities they consider "sexual," and how they understand themselves as sexual people have their origins in childhood. Children's conceptions of their sexuality and the meanings they hold begin to be formed in infancy and continue to evolve throughout life. According to Martinson (1991), "Organic capacities, cognitive development and integration, and intrapsychic influences . . . determine the rate and extent of development of the sexual capacity" and understanding of children. "Each child's development will [also] be markedly influenced by the cultural norms and expectations, familial interactions and values, and the interpersonal experiences" (p. 58) she encounters. Sexual meanings are learned in childhood from caretakers, the media and wider culture, as well as from "the child's own slowly unfolding biography with its own set of earlier acquired meanings." The child turns to these sources in an attempt to interpret her "bodily sensations, name the parts and the acts, identify sets of feelings, [and] make sense of emerging relationships" (Plummer, 1991, p. 238).

To understand the development of sexuality for the young girl, and the ways in which sexuality may become problematic to the child, we begin with what the child brings to this interaction in terms of her bodily capabilities and sensations. The kind of physical exploration and behaviors that children typically engage in prior to their teens are also addressed. Next, the psychological development of the child is examined in terms of her evolving sexual self-constructions. Finally, our attention is turned to the social context within which the child learns to make sense of her bodily experiences and sensations and negotiates her sense of herself as a sexual person. It is in this interaction between the physical and psychological realities of the child and the messages she takes in from the her family and from society that problematic meanings are generated and the seeds of sexual discontent are often sowed.

"SUGAR AND SPICE AND EVERYTHING NICE": BIOLOGICAL DEVELOPMENT

Many of us have been taught this popular nursery rhyme. From the standpoint of sexuality, however, what do we really know about what little girls are made of? We know that the developing child has unique biological properties and physical characteristics. These include fetal development and chromosomal composition, neurological and hormonal structures, sexual morphology, and specific physical capacities and anomalies (Friedrich, Grambsch, Broughton, Kuiper, & Beilke, 1991; Martinson, 1991). Chromosomal composition determines the physical attributes and organs that we are born with, and hormones play a critical role in genital maturation and arousal, and in reproduction. There is also some evidence to suggest that individuals have different thresholds of sensory responsiveness (Martinson, 1991). Biology, then, provides the blueprint for determining what the child is capable of physically feeling and experiencing. Cognitive development is also important in setting parameters around children's abilities to understand and make sense of their physical and social environments (Piaget, 1950).

In terms of sexual development, it would appear that children's first sensory experience that might be defined as "sexual" may be the pleasure derived from nursing at their mother's breast (Gil & Johnson, 1993). From birth, girl children have vaginal secretions (Martinson, 1991). Considerable anecdotal evidence suggests that infants and children are capable of experiencing pleasure from sensory and tactile stimulation of their genitals very early in life (Gil & Johnson, 1993; Goldman & Goldman, 1988; Reinisch, Rosenblum, & Sanders, 1987). Not all cultures, however, appear to define this behavior as sexual. In fact, in some cultures in southern Asia, equatorial Africa and the South Pacific, the genitals of infants are intentionally stimulated by adults to calm and soothe their restlessness (Yates, 1987).

So what is considered "normal" sexual behavior and development, then, by North American standards? According to Gil and Johnson (1993) and Goldman and Goldman (1988), children engage in a wide range of behaviors that are culturally defined as sexual.

> Children become interested in, ask about, and obtain sexual information progressively over a period. They appear to become interested in their bodies first, and later develop an interest in experimentation with others. Sexual interests therefore range from self-stimulation, to exhibitionism, to periods of inhibition, to touching others, and finally, to experimenting with kissing, fondling, oral sex, and penetration. (Gil & Johnson, 1993, p. 32)

More specifically, preschool children (ages birth to 4 years) like to be nude and are fascinated by the nude bodies of other children and adults. Not surprisingly, they are also very interested in bathroom functions. They show considerable interest in the genitals of others and, in particular, are curious about differences in the genital configurations of older children, adults, and people of the opposite sex.

Young children also like to touch and rub their own genitals. "It is common for children in this age group to 'discover' that when certain parts of the body are touched, poked, rubbed, or otherwise stimulated, pleasant sensations occur. When something pleasurable occurs, children may seek to repeat the event" (Gil & Johnson, 1993, p. 21). Although this behavior is much more common for boys than girls, children of both sexes appear to be "fascinated by themselves and the fact of their own existence" (McDermott, 1970, p. 13) and by the characteristics and functioning of their bodies. At this stage in their development, their genital exploration is usually limited to self-exploration and self-stimulation. Peer contact, when it occurs, most often involves children visually examining the bodies and organs of other children in an attempt to appease their natural curiosity. Young children also experiment with using "dirty" words to see what effect these words have on others, but they frequently have little understanding of their meaning. They also like to play house and act out the roles of Mommy and Daddy, "impersonating the mannerisms of parents, siblings, or television actors" (Gil & Johnson, 1993, p. 23).

Behavior considered "normal" for young school-age children (ages 5–7) includes genital self-exploration and touching, acute interest in the bodies and actions of others (particularly the "sexual" behavior between men and women), telling "dirty" jokes, playing house and taking on parental roles, kissing, holding hands, and some mimicking of observed "sexual" behaviors. There is increased peer contact and experimentation in this age group. This is fairly limited due to the fact that children at this age vacillate between being drawn to and repulsed by overt sexual activities such as kissing and hugging. They are also quite shy and inhibited about their own bodies and exhibit a desire for privacy around dressing and toilet activities (Gil & Johnson, 1993; Goldman & Goldman, 1988; Martinson, 1991).

During what is referred to in the literature as the latency/preadolescent stage of development (ages 8–12 years) common behaviors include genital self-stimulation, exhibitionistic displays such as mooning, kissing and sometimes even dating, light petting, observing and sometimes touching the genitals of others, and dry humping. Interestingly, the peak period for "playing doctor" is around 9 or 10 years of age. Kissing and fantasy sexual play in which children practice the adult roles of partner, lover, prostitute, and so on (Lamb & Coakley, 1993) are also common among children of this age. This stage of development is marked by increased peer contact, experimental interactions, and disinhibition. Some children experiment with oral sex, but "only 2 to 3 percent of children twelve and younger engage in intercourse" (Gil & Johnson, 1993, p. 42).

Sometime between the ages of 5 and 12 years, children begin to use slang words such as "fuck, faggot, cunt, queer, bitch" (Gil & Johnson, 1993, p. 11). These words are often considered by adults to be sexual in nature. Ironically, children's understanding of these terms and their meaning often lags behind their language acquisition. "Not infrequently, children attach a meaning to words not only from the context, but also from the affect associated with the word when they heard it" (Gil & Johnson, 1993, p. 11). The words appear to gain power because of their connection to something that is taboo, and because of their ability to elicit a response from the listener.

Normal sexual development for children, then, appears to include "autostimulation and self-exploration, kissing, hugging, peeking, touching and/or exposing of genitals to other children, and perhaps simulating intercourse" (Gil & Johnson, 1993, p. 42). Age-appropriate sexual play or exploration is usually accompanied by hushed excitement and silly or giggly reactions. Although children engaged in such exploration "may feel confused and guilty, they do not experience feelings of deep shame, fear, or anxiety" (p. 42). Masturbatory behavior, the use of sexual language, nudity, and sexual play with peers, although more common for boys (Goldman & Goldman, 1988), is developmentally appropriate and normal behavior for all children. These behaviors are generally transitory. Professionals become concerned only if they appear to occur in a vacuum, become "excessive, compulsive, unresponsive to appropriate limits, or escalate in frequency and intensity [and thus] distract the child from other age-appropriate activities" (Gil & Johnson, 1993, p. 97).

We do not yet know how much biology contributes to the developing child's sexuality in terms of her visceral, cognitive, and affective experiencing. It would appear, however, that unless children are born with particular chromosomal and hormonal abnormalities, they are not generally limited by their biology in terms of how they may express and enjoy their sexuality. Assuming that their endocrine functioning is adequate, girls' potential for enjoying their bodies in all their unique capacities appears to be great indeed (Gil & Johnson, 1993; Goldman & Goldman, 1988; Martinson, 1991; Plummer, 1991).

GIRLS' PSYCHOLOGICAL DEVELOPMENT

In terms of psychological development, there is very little literature specifically addressing the sexual development or expression of children, or the problems characteristically experienced by children as they attempt to understand and make sense of their feelings and experiences. The exception is when a child has been sexually victimized by an older person (e.g., Sweet, 1981), is born with specific genital and anatomical abnormalities (e.g., Money & Ehrhardt, 1972; Reinisch et al., 1987), or is exhibiting behavior that may suggest gender dysphoria. We know very little about children's psychological experiencing of themselves as sexual people in general and even less about the sexual self-constructions of children from different ethnic, racial, economic, or religious groups (Gil & Johnson, 1993; Goldman & Goldman, 1988).

Freud's (1948) theory of psychosexual development is the only theory that attends explicitly to the developing sexual self-structure of the child. Freud has been soundly criticized for his heterosexist bias and androcentric assumptions. In recent years, however, psychodynamic theory has witnessed a resurgence among some traditional and feminist theorists. They underscore the importance of early childhood socialization in the psychological development of the child (e.g., Benjamin, 1988; Eichenbaum & Orbach, 1983; Goldenberg, 1990). As such, psychodynamic theory warrants a brief review at this time.

The primary contention of psychodynamic theory is that sexual instincts, in terms of the pleasure principle, are the driving life force motivating all human behavior from birth until death. Freud linked the sexual development of the child with her psychosocial development. He posited that the first 5 years of life are a time of considerable sexual upheaval. Freud believed that during this period, children form attitudes about physical pleasure and about what constitutes appropriate masculinity and femininity. The young girl child learns to differentiate between "right" and "wrong." If she resolves the Electra complex, she comes to terms with her envy over the fact that she does not have male genitals or male power. In identifying with the feminine gender role, her desire to possess her father (the power of the male) is sublimated, to resurface later in adolescence in the form of sexually seductive behaviors.

Freud (1948) conceptualized a period of sexual latency following resolution of the girl's Electra complex from about 6 years old until puberty. During this time he proposed that the child's tumultuous struggles and preoccupation with sexual pleasure and possession are replaced by an increasing interest in the development of interpersonal relationships and the mastery of practical life skills. For girls, this means the acceptance of biological inferiority and the mastery of caretaking skills and nurturing abilities (Walton, Fineman, & Walton, 1996). This is contrary to the literature reviewed earlier in this chapter, which suggests that far from slowing down or terminating, children's sexual explorations and interactions continue with increasing complexity throughout childhood (Goldman & Goldman, 1988; Friedrich et al., 1991; Martinson, 1991).

When the development of the sexual self is understood from an interactionist perspective, the early years are indeed important in the child's developing self-constructions and meanings. Motivated by natural curiosity and sensory pleasure, the child explores her physical and social world. Based on the reactions of others to her body and explorations, she begins very early on to develop some understanding of the meaning of particular body parts and to define particular activities and behaviors as acceptable or off limits. This is not because the child perceives her behavior as "sexual" per se. Rather, based on her limited cognitive capacity, the child will *interpret* the messages communicated implicitly and explicitly by the significant adults in her life and conclude that certain thoughts, feelings, and behaviors are "right" or "wrong." In this way, her bodily sensations and experiences will be imbued with adult meanings (Plummer, 1991). The physical experiences and sensations that for the adult are understood to characterize sexual pleasure and excitement in all probability will be lived, felt, and understood quite differently by the child who has not been fully socialized to the motives and feelings that adults routinely associate with sexuality. These adult meanings, however, will be integrated with the child's own visceral and sensory experiences when engaging in this type of activity. From the often discrepant messages of her caretakers and her body, the child will construct an understanding of her body, behavior, and her "self" as good or bad, clean or dirty, fun or shameful. She will begin to develop a tentative hypothesis about herself as a sexual person. This hypothesis will continue to be shaped and changed throughout childhood, based on her unique personal and interpersonal experiences, and on her interpretation of the values, attitudes, and beliefs of those to whom she turns to help understand herself and her experiences.

It is important to note that based on gender-role socialization, girls and women may be particularly sensitive to the attitudes of others in the development of sexual meanings and self-constructions (e.g., Belenky, Clinchy, Goldberger, & Tarule, 1986; Chodorow, 1978, 1994; Flax, 1990, 1994; Hare-Mustin & Marecek, 1990; Jordan, Kaplan, Baker-Miller, Stiver, & Surrey, 1991; Kaschak, 1992). Of particular interest to this discussion is the contention by several theorists that young girl-children develop greater relational acuity and heightened sensitivity to the opinions and feelings of others. This happens because of their relationships with their primary caregivers. It is also related to the feminine gender-role proscriptions imposed on girls by society. This sensitivity may play itself out in the way desires, needs, and preferences are experienced and acted upon throughout life. It will also influence the development of girls' sexual selves and their emerging sexual meanings. We turn now to an examination of the social world of the child.

MESSAGES AND MEANINGS

Clearly, children vary in their ability to process information and understand their worlds. They may also have different levels of sensitivity to sensory stimulation. It appears to be when biological characteristics interact with context that problems may arise in terms of the developing child's experience and understanding of herself as a sexual person. From this perspective, there is no discrete limit to the number or range of possible meanings and interpretations that might be applied to the child's pleasurable experiences, but the meanings strongly supported by those who influence the child most significantly in her life have the greatest probability of being accepted by the child as she comes to understand herself as a sexual being and certain parts of her body as the source or site of sexual pleasure (Plummer, 1991).

In childhood, caretakers and family members are particularly significant in shaping girls' sexual meanings and self-conceptions. Within North America, the written and visual media are also increasingly becoming a salient source of influence in the sexual development of children (Gagnon & Simon, 1982; Gil & Johnson, 1993; Laws, 1980; McDermott, 1970). The degree of influence of each of these factors on the developing sexuality and sexual self-esteem of the child differs based on the source of the information, the way it is communicated, and the degree of consensual validation. The child's physical development, emotional maturity, and cognitive sophistication are also important.

Don't Touch, Don't Feel: Caretaker Messages

Caretakers are especially powerful sources of influence in a child's developing hypothesis about herself as a sexual person (Chodorow, 1978, 1994; Gagnon & Simon, 1982; Gil & Johnson, 1993; Laws, 1980; Wyatt & Riederle, 1994). It is uncertain exactly how family messages are transmitted and taken in by the child, or why some messages are accepted and others are not. However, it is clear that what produces sexual anxiety for the child depends to a great extent on what produces anxiety for the child's caretakers. "Adult caretakers greatly influence children's perceptions . . . conveying their approval or disapproval" of particular actions and behaviors (Gil & Johnson, p. 93).

> Parents play an important part in instilling values about sexuality in their children. When parents view sex as dirty, inappropriate, or secretive they

> may set rigid and restrictive limits on self-exploration, language, questions, or curiosity considered healthy in children. When children are punished, chastised, or humiliated for their sexuality, they may associate sex with shame and guilt. (p. 26)

To appreciate the development of children's sexual self-conceptions and how meanings may become problematic, it is important to differentiate between the adult's understanding of the child's behavior and the child's understanding of her experiences. The genital touching and exploration typically engaged in by most children may provide a useful example of the relationship between parental imperatives and the needs and understanding of the child. Most parents can recall with some degree of shamed amusement and discomfort their children's curiosity and perhaps occasional obsession with their genitals during various periods of their development. As indicated earlier in the chapter, this type of bodily self-exploration is quite natural and may initially represent nothing more than curiosity and self-discovery—it may or may not even be experienced as pleasurable. However, based on their own childhood socialization, many parents experience considerable discomfort in dealing with this aspect of their daughter's development because they perceive this behavior to be sexual (Goldman & Goldman, 1988). This perception is communicated to the child. If parents prohibit this type of self-exploration, which many do, the message that is communicated is that this aspect of the child's body is "off limits" (Gil & Johnson, 1993; Goldman & Goldman, 1988). Parents may also implicitly or explicitly communicate that the girl's genitals are bad or dirty. It is the imposition of adult sexual meanings attributed to such common childhood experiences as genital exploration and play that results in distress and confusion for the child. This is especially true when these parental sanctions are contrary to the body's messages of pleasure. These pleasurable physical sensations may well motivate the child to continue to secretly pursue self-stimulation, but this may well occur at the cost of sometimes overwhelming feelings of shame and guilt (Goldman & Goldman, 1988).

Similarly, how parents react to catching their child in the act of "playing doctor" or examining the bodies of other children can be quite formative in terms of the child's developing sexual self-constructions. Parents may react with anger and disgust, thereby communicating to their child that her behavior is shameful and wrong. Or they may use this as an opportunity to teach their daughter about her own body and to help her begin to set appropriate boundaries around this type of exploration. In this way, they can underscore the naturalness of the child's curiosity and communicate bodily acceptance. They can also "foster empathic thought and consideration of others" (Gil & Johnson, 1993, p. 94).

In all likelihood, the significance of sexuality to any child will be in direct proportion to its perceived significance (Gagnon & Simon, 1973). The excessive presence or absence of focus on the developing sexuality and embodied sexual feelings of the young child by her caretakers will be reflected in the significance accorded to sexuality in the life of the child. For example, Gil and Johnson (1993) identify the consequences for the child of growing up in a "repressed" family where sex is a taboo subject, something sinful and shameful. This perspective is often supported by religious admonitions against sexual thoughts, much less sexual behavior. In such families, children have little freedom to ask about or explore their own bodies. Some are severely punished for any behavior that may be interpreted by their parents as sexual in nature. One woman I worked with recalled being told by her parents that she was "oversexed" and "promiscuous," when at the age of 4, she was "caught" examining the genitals (or lack thereof) of her girl and boy dolls. This form of sexual repression may result in a "pseudo maturity deplete of spontaneity and playfulness one would expect from a child." Or, paradoxically, like the forbidden fruit "when the subject of sexuality is forbidden and even thoughts are sinful it [may] take on a greater appeal and mystery" (pp. 114–115). These experiences of avoidance or punishment may be interpreted by the child to mean that this aspect of her body is "taboo." They can result in the development of a sexual self-construction based on shame and guilt.

Parents also influence their daughters' sexual meanings and self-conceptions by their apparent comfort with their own bodies, and with the bodies of their children. Because parental communications are subject to interpretation, shame and guilt may inadvertently be communicated through such parental behaviors as the "the hurried changing of the subject, and the frantic covering of bodies when daughters inadvertently [catch] their parents in a state of undress" (Gil & Johnson, 1993, p. 13). The unspoken messages of parents regarding their children's sexuality are often more potent than their spoken messages in shaping children's perceptions of themselves and their bodies. Locks on bedroom doors and directions to knock before entering serve as a sign that sex is something that happens behind closed doors, at night, and in the dark, within the confines of a socially sanctioned relationship (Tiefer, 1995). Being highly sensitive to implications and innuendo (Goldman & Goldman, 1988), "the nonverbal method of warning children off the subject of sex is as strong as if the parent were to tell the child that sex is evil" (McDermott, 1970, p. 13).

The story of one woman whose mother's discomfort with her own genitalia and sexuality represents a particularly poignant example of the consequences of this type of nonverbal parental message. Herself a victim of childhood sexual abuse, the messages of shame passed on by this mother to her children regarding their sexuality were profoundly damaging.

> "I lived in a really schizophrenic world of sex as dirty and not talked about. . . . In all the baby pictures we have my mom has cut all the crotches out. . . . To this day she feels dirty and diseased in her sexual genitalia."

In her symbolic dismemberment of the organs that socially defined her children's sex and sexuality, this mother provided a tremendously negative and debilitating set of sexual meanings for her daughter. As a young woman, her daughter grew up estranged and alienated from this part of her body and from her sensory experiences. Sexual alienation became a persistent theme in her experience of herself as a sexual person throughout her life.

> "My brother and I totally cut ourselves off at the waist. . . . It's like we had dead sexual parts. . . . I still have this kind of image of smelly, dirty, yucky female parts, and that goes so deep."

As well, the language parents use in reference to the body parts most associated with sexuality in our culture—the genitals—is formative in girls' knowledge of, and comfort with their bodies. Depending on their own level of comfort, parents may refer to their daughters' genitals using clinical language or euphemisms. In some cases, there may be no words they are comfortable using. In a study of 115 girls and women, Gartrell and Mosbacher (1984) noted the large percentage of girls who reported learning no names at all for their own genitalia as children (suggesting that this part of their body was metaphorically invisible). Many of the women recalled using pejorative and euphemistic words when making reference to their genitals such as "down there," "privates," "muffin," "shame," "nasty," or "no, no special place." These words connote mystery and disconnection from the part of the young girl's body that is most closely associated with her sexuality in our culture. Faced with an absence of powerful and affirming language, it is not uncommon for parents to use clinical words such as "clitoris," "labia," "vulva," and "vagina" (words that many young girls can barely pronounce, much less understand) in naming their daughters' genitals. Neither option suggests that the young girl's genitals are a source of pride or pleasure—something she has a right to be curious about (unlike the attention paid to the young boy's penis).

Parents may also fail to educate their daughters about the functioning of their genitals. In this way, young girls may grow up quite disconnected from, and unaware of, their own bodies and how they work. Indeed, Tiefer (1996) underscores how the "ubiquitous parental mislabeling of female genitals as 'vagina' (and little else) can lead to lifelong confusion and inhibition for many women." She suggests that women's uncertainty about their genitals and the workings of their own bodies "seems to create an inhibiting insecurity" (p. 57).

> With few messages or even "emptiness" coming from adult worlds, many children are left to sort out their [experiences] with peers, media or alone in secretive and dark corners. It is not that childhood sexuality is being repressed; it is rather that a pattern of communication is being set up which starts to put "sex" into a separate compartment cut off from the

rest of experience—a compartment which may grow tighter and become even more closed in adult life. (Plummer, 1991, p. 239)

Cinderella, Snow White, and Other Myths of Childhood: Media Messages

We turn now to another powerful source of influence on the developing child's sense of herself as a sexual being—the popular media (Gil & Johnson, 1993; Unger & Crawford, 1992). Media images can be very influential in informing the developing girl child about gender-role appropriate behavior and expectations (Gil & Johnson, 1993). These images help to provide meaning to the girl's experiences of herself. The relative presence or absence of particular images serves as a template through which the child makes sense of her sensations, feelings, and thoughts. Clearly, they also inform her understanding of her developing sexuality.

Accounts of sexual agency for girls in childhood are relatively absent in the written and visual popular media. A review of some of the most popular children's movies, fairy tales, and toys indicates few images of childhood sexual pleasure or agency (although metaphorically these stories are filled with images that an adult might construe as sexual). The depictions of most female characters in the popular children's media generally fall into one of two categories, the princess or the witch. Each may be seen to represent the epitome of the stereotypical cultural notions regarding women's sexuality: the pure, chaste virgin or the seductive, dangerous whore (e.g., Madonna's stage image comes to mind here). The messages are pervasive; they begin very early in children's lives and are formative in the developing child's sexual meanings and self-constructions.

As young girls, many of us remember growing up with Barbie as the image of hyperfemininity that we longed to emulate and against which we assessed our own developing bodies. Having recently celebrated her 40th (or was it 50th?) anniversary, it is a testament to the veracity of popular cultural notions regarding the appropriate roles of women that Barbie still endures in popularity.

More current creations are similar in their messages to the young girl regarding her sexuality. The enormously popular recent Disney movie *The Little Mermaid* serves as an excellent example of the media messages that help construct the sexual reality and understanding of young girls in our culture. The heroine of the movie, Ariel, possesses many of Barbie's physical attributes in terms of her flawless complexion and skin color (white), her long hair and eyelashes, large round eyes, small waist, ample bosom, and compact buttocks. Ariel, the youngest and most willful of three daughters, and daddy's favorite, I might add, is all that personifies the virgin side of the sexual equation: good, sweet, kind, gentle, curious, and anxious to please. She also has enough spunk and sense of adventure to be somewhat interesting. To pursue the love of her prince (to awaken her sexuality), however, she must give up her voice (an interesting metaphor in itself), abandon her family, and reject the freedom of movement that comes from her life underwater. The person to whom she abandons these aspects of her "self," the witch, is the antithesis of the Ariel figure, the other side of the sexuality equation. She is large, powerful, all encompassing, mean, and manipulative. When Ariel appears to be winning the heart of the boyish prince, the witch transforms herself in the appearance of the seductress, a sultry, emasculating temptress that is clearly the epitome of sexual evil. Mesmerized by the witch's apparent charms (and his own all encompassing sexual needs), the boyish prince almost succumbs to the feminine wiles of the witch. In the final moment, he is forced to come to his senses, and the witch is revealed for the ugly monster she really is. Good, in this case personified as "slim, young, and beautiful," triumphs over evil, which is characterized as "fat, old, and ugly."

The messages regarding women's sexuality are clear in this Disney tale. These reflect dominant dichotomous good–bad notions regarding women's sexuality and sexual expression. They leave the young girl with only two options in making sense of her sexuality and sexual choices. She can become the sexual temptress, a powerful, evil creature whose behavior eventually is punished through rejection and isolation, or she can be the virgin, the sweet, good creature who needs to be rescued by the prince. He will guard her sexuality and provide for her bodily comforts at the price of her own voice and efficacy. This theme can be seen to run through a host of popular children's fairy tales (e.g., *Sleeping Beauty, Snow White, Little Red Riding Hood*) and movies (e.g., *Aladdin, 101 Dalmatians, Jungle Book, Dirty Dancing*). The messages they communicate to young girls and *boys* about their sexual needs, rights, and responsibilities are disturbing indeed.

It is little wonder, then, that many girls grow up to believe that men should be in charge in sexual interactions, and that to act on their own needs or impulses is undesirable and even dangerous. In this way, the seeds are sewn for the "pleasure and danger" dichotomy that is reflected in many of the media images and messages related to the sexuality and sexual expression of older women, which will be discussed later in this book (Vance, 1992).

Sexual Violence

The incidence of sexual abuse of female children is alarmingly high (Butler, 1978; Courtois, 1988; Finkelhor, Hotaling, Lewis, & Smith, 1990). As such, a discussion of the influences on the developing sexuality of young girls would be incomplete without some attention to the issue of sexual violence. Of all the messages that the young girl-child takes in from her caretakers regarding her sexual self, the one that may present the greatest threat to the child's developing sexuality and self-conception is the imposition of the sexual needs, desires, and will of an adult in the form of sexual abuse. Such an imposition may indeed be physically damaging to the young child in terms of vaginal or rectal tearing (Courtois, 1988). However, the long-term psychological damage to the child may be considerably greater in terms of the young girl's understanding and experience of herself as a female, as a sexual person, and as an active agent in her own life (Butler, 1978; Courtois, 1988; Friedrich, 1990; Herman, 1992; Kaufman & Wohl, 1992; Russell, 1986; Wohl & Kaufman, 1985).

Even young girls who are not directly subjected to sexual violence receive a multitude of messages from their culture and from their parents, who fear for their safety, that they are at risk of sexual violation. Girl-children learn very young that they must be wary of strangers who might "hurt them" or "touch them in bad places," forcing a level of hypervigilance that sends a clear message about their inherent vulnerability as females. These are often paired with messages of passivity and compliance. The young girl comes to understand early in life that she is powerless to protect herself against the threat of sexual violence. She learns that she is, in a sense, potential prey to the desires of more powerful boys and men. The victimized child must contend with many paradoxes in her young life, not the least of which includes the realization that for protection she must rely on the strength and power of men, and yet men are also those she must fear. It is therefore left up to the resources of the developing child to learn to differentiate between the men whom she can trust and the men whom she cannot. She then may feel accountable/responsible when her trust is violated, perceiving this as an error in her own judgment and therefore her own "fault" (having taken in another strong cultural message that violence that is done to a woman, particularly sexual violence, must in some way be the woman's fault).

The enormous damage wrought by sexual abuse may be understood in terms of the child's limited cognitive capacity to accommodate and understand the meanings implicit in this type of interaction. The difficulty arises for the child in attempting to make sense of an experience that takes place in secret, that may involve severe threats of reprisal, that is laced with mixed messages regarding caring and pain, and that is presented *to the child* as consensual behavior. In attempting to interpret the meaning of the abuse, the child is faced with extremely discrepant messages. Her body may at times experience moments of pleasure, but this pleasure will also be accompanied by fear and pain. Her abuser will tell her that his motivations are based on love and caring, and yet the child or her mother will be threatened with punishment if this secret behavior is revealed. The child then must interpret the adult's behavior and her own reactions, based on these highly discrepant messages, and make some meaning of the situation at the time, and retrospectively, that allows her to keep from being psychologically fragmented or shattered.

In any interaction, "participants may fit their acts to one another . . .

on the basis of compromise, out of duress, because they may use one another in achieving their respective ends, because it is the sensible thing to do, or out of sheer necessity" (Blumer, 1969, p. 76). In the case of the sexually abused child, the child may well attempt to deal with these discrepant messages and meanings by complying with the abuse and maintaining the secrecy that is demanded of her. To do so, however, and still maintain some sense of a unitary self-structure, in the face of the shame, secrecy, and trauma associated with the violation of the child's personal boundaries, the child may need to psychologically dissociate from the experience (Miller, 1990).

According to Mead (1934), "the phenomenon of dissociation of personality is caused by a breaking up of the complete, unitary self into the component selves of which it is composed, and which respectively correspond to different aspects of the social process in which the person is involved, and within which [her] unitary self has arisen" (p. 144). When the child's physical and psychological boundaries have been violated, the process of dissociation may require "getting rid of certain bodily memories which would identify the individual to herself" (p. 143). From a psychodynamic perspective, dissociation or splitting "means any breakdown of the whole, in which parts of the self or other are split off and projected elsewhere" (Benjamin, 1988, p. 63). Given the child's limited cognitive abilities to negotiate discrepant messages, dissociation allows the child to reconcile the reality of the violation with the cultural messages she receives, suggesting that adults, and particularly parents, are trustworthy individuals whose job it is to protect children from harm.

However successful she may be at dissociating from the memories of the abuse, the child can never fully separate herself from the trauma. According to Miller (1990),

> The truth about our childhood is stored up in our body, and although we can to repress it, we can never alter it. Our intellect can be deceived, our feelings manipulated, our perceptions confused, and our body tricked with medication. But someday the body will present its bill, for it is as incorruptible as a child who, still whole in spirit, will accept no compromises or excuses, and it will not stop tormenting us until we stop evading the truth. (p. 316)

The consequences of sexual victimization then, pervade all aspects of the developing child's world and frequently accompany the woman into adulthood, distorting her self-perceptions and shaping her interpersonal and intrapersonal world (Butler, 1978; Courtois, 1988; Maltz, 1991; Russell, 1986; Westerlund, 1992). In the case of one infertile client, for example, excessive weight seemed to be impeding her ovulatory cycle, inhibiting her from achieving a desired pregnancy. Exploration of the woman's history revealed sexual molestation and an attempted rape by a stranger at a candy store when the woman was 9 years old. In the words of the client:

> "I guess you could say, actually he was attempting to rape me. He didn't succeed but it scared the hell out of me. I managed to take charge of the situation and get him the hell away from me, but not before I was hurt. . . . I had to tell the police where he touched me, and I couldn't because it was private, because you don't talk about things like that. It's made for a lot of fear in me, and mistrust, figuring I'm safer if I just build a wall of fat between me and the world. If I make myself unattractive, nobody can hurt me, but I'm hurting myself."

Clearly, the imposition of adult sexual needs and desires on the child has profoundly negative and far-reaching consequences. Such violation continues to affect many aspects of the developing child's sexual self-esteem and interpersonal functioning throughout life.

It is beyond the scope of this book to provide specific recommendations for mental health professionals whose work involves helping children heal from the trauma of sexual victimization. However, resources are listed in Appendix A for counselors who work with sexually abused children and adolescents, and for parents who are trying to help their children deal with the aftermath of sexual violation.

SUMMARY AND RECOMMENDATIONS

Wyatt and Riederle (1994) note how "very few American parents provide their children with sufficient, accurate, and meaningful information about sex. Rather, parents and schools often teach only gender specific, basic facts of anatomy and reproduction and ignore other vital aspects of sex education" (p. 613). Certainly, most parents do not intentionally set out to make their daughters feel shame or discomfort related to their bodies, or guilt about their developing sexuality. However, parents are a product of their social worlds and are also limited by the inadequacy of language, repressive cultural norms, and the paradoxical messages that characterize much of the social communication related to the sexuality and sexual expression of girls and women. Despite parents' best efforts, young girls may well become alienated from the parts of their bodies which, in our culture, are most associated with their sexuality. The seeds may be sewn early in life for the development of sexual self-conceptions based on shame and guilt rather than agency and entitlement. These childhood experiences can form the basis for a sense of disconnection from the power and pleasure of the body—from girls' embodied sexuality. Without the benefit of alternate, more affirming messages and meanings, these seeds run the risk of becoming well rooted in the child's developing sexual hypothesis, making the challenges of adolescence considerably more difficult to successfully negotiate.

Parents may feel like they are in a no-win situation when it comes to helping their daughters develop a sense of sexual agency and comfort in their bodies. And yet it would appear that not all young girls experience feelings of shame and inadequacy about their bodies and their developing sexuality. References are made in the literature to the freedom, pleasure, and spontaneity that characterize the embodied experiences of young girls who have yet to take in and accept the rigid restrictions of prescribed femininity and repressive female sexuality. In the words of one mother:

> I watch my daughter. From morning to night her body is her home. She lives in it and with it. When she runs around the kitchen she uses all of herself. Every muscle in her body moves when she laughs, when she cries. When she rubs her vulva, there is no awkwardness, no feeling that what she is doing is wrong. She feels pleasure and expresses it without hesitation. She knows when she wants to be touched and when she wants to be left alone. It's so hard to get back that sense of body as home. (Boston Women's Health Book Collective, 1992, p. 205)

Much of the inner-child work that is used in counseling women (Laidlaw & Malmo, 1990) is aimed at helping adult women recapture the sense of bodily connection and delight that was a part of their experience as children.

Given the significance of familial influences in girls' developing sexual self-conceptions, parents can play an important role helping their daughters learn about their bodies and their developing sexuality (Gil & Johnson, 1993; Goldman & Goldman, 1992). They can play a role in ensuring that girls retain a sense of their bodies as "home." To do so, however, it is important that they are provided with the requisite tools and information. Parents need to know what constitutes "normal" sexual behavior and exploration, and may benefit from some guidance on how to respond openly to their children's questions and concerns. They need to know how to set appropriate boundaries around such issues as nudity, self-stimulation, and reciprocal physical exploration, without reinforcing a sense of shame. A list of resources are provided in Appendix A related to the sexual development and education of children that parents and educators may find useful. In particular, the book *Show Me Yours: Understanding Children's Sexuality* by Goldman and Goldman (1988) provides an excellent overview of the types of behaviors and experiences commonly engaged in by children, as well as providing many specific suggestions on how parents can teach their children about "public" versus "private" activities. It is important that parents are helped to understand that the behaviors that we, as adults, perceive as being "sexual" in nature, do not hold the same meanings for children (Plummer, 1991). This awareness can help to lessen their discomfort with their children's natural exploration and curiosity.

Parents can also be encouraged to help expand the range of messages available to their children through exposure to alternative fairy tales such as *The Paper Bag Princess* by Robert Munsch (1982) or *The Princess Who Stood on Her Own Two Feet* by Jeanne Desey (1986). These, as well as other books and movies (see Hancock, 1989, for a discussion of some of these), depict girls and women as competent individuals engaged in and enjoying a diverse range of roles and activities at all stages of their lives. Although their numbers pale in comparison to the *Snow White-* and *Cinderella*-type genre, such movies and children's books can be a powerful tool in affirming the young girl's self-esteem and sense of agency (e.g., Zipes, 1986). There is also some excellent literature available to help children of all ages learn to set physical and psychological boundaries in their relationships with others and to reinforce a sense of ownership of, and pleasure in, their own bodies (e.g., Dayee, 1982; Freeman, 1982; Girard, 1984). Parents should take care to select material that emphasizes *children's* rights to and ownership of their bodies but does not increase their sense of physical risk or responsibility for unwanted advances.

It is also important for parents to help their daughters find words that they can comfortably and affirmingly use to refer to the parts of their bodies that are most strongly associated in our culture with their sexuality. In naming comes ownership and acceptance, both of which are a necessary prerequisite for young girls to be able to feel comfortable with all parts of their bodies. In an attempt to counter the disconnection and dissociation young girls often come to experience in relation to "down there," it is necessary for parents to acknowledge that "down there" exists. These parts of their daughters' bodies, while considered private in our culture, need not be a source or site of shame. The use of clinically accurate language to describe children's genitals is an approach commonly taken in many family life education programs and in most educational resources and books (e.g., Gatrell & Mosbacher, 1984; Mayle, 1975; Mayle & Robins, 1978). This is certainly preferable to using vague and euphemistic language that reinforces a sense of mystery and stigmatization. However, as stated earlier in this chapter, children may not be comfortable with or able to relate to such clinically accurate terms as "vagina," "labia," and "clitoris." Together with their children, parents can help to create a new, more affirming vocabulary to refer to genitals and to the pleasurable sensations and feelings they sometimes experience in this part of their bodies.

As indicated in Chapter 1, children's sexual self-perceptions influence and in turn are influenced by their self-esteem. Given this reciprocal influence, when parents build on their daughters' strengths and competencies in all areas of their lives (i.e., sports, music, scholastic performance, dance), they help to build positive self-valuations. These, in turn, can go a long way in helping to reinforce self-acceptance and more affirming sexual self-constructions.

3

ADOLESCENCE

Biological and Psychological Development

Chapter 1 discussed how sexual definitions and meanings begin with the physical potentialities of the body and evolve in interaction with the changing contextual realities of each person's life. This chapter looks at the internal reality of adolescent girls in terms of the biological and physical changes girls undergo during this tumultuous stage in their development. It also examines the psychological tasks that ensue as girls respond to the physical and social changes that characterize this period of life. Particular attention is paid to changes in body image, the consolidation of gender identity, and sexual identity formation. These issues are critical to the sexual meanings and evolving sexual self-conceptions of adolescent girls.

BIOLOGICAL DEVELOPMENT

From Girl to Woman: Bodily Changes

A number of biological and physical changes occur during puberty that mark girls' physical and sexual maturation. They may begin as early as 9 years old and are generally complete for most girls by the age of 16. Breast development is frequently the first sign of these changes, occurring on average around 12 years of age (Brooks-Gunn, 1988). Breast buds begin to form, marked by a slight enlargement of the areola and the formation of the breast tissue into small mounds. This is precipitated by increases in the production and secretion of estrogen from the ovaries and prolactin from the anterior pituitary gland (Golub, 1992). At this time, there is a corresponding increase in the amount of body hair, first under the arms and later in the pubic region. Breast development and pubic hair growth are two of the most obvious manifestations of maturity (Brooks-Gunn & Warren, 1988). Sweat glands also become more productive during puberty, and body odor is enhanced due to increased hormone production. These hormonal changes may also contribute to skin problems in the form of acne (Katchadourian, 1977).

The onset of puberty is generally marked by a growth spurt, which involves relatively rapid gains in height and changes in body proportions. These changes result in the bodies of pubescent girls becoming increasingly sexually dimorphic (Unger & Crawford, 1992). Height may increase as much as 4 inches prior to the onset of menstruation (Golub, 1992). Hormonal changes also precipitate a noticeable accumulation of fatty tissue (Brooks-Gunn, 1988). During this time, girls experience an average weight gain of 24 pounds, deposited primarily in the breasts, hips, and buttocks (Golub, 1992; Unger & Crawford, 1992). To put this change into perspective it is interesting to note that prior to the onset of puberty, girls have an average of 10–15% more body fat than boys. At puberty, however, this distribution shifts considerably. Pubertal girls have an average of 24–30% body fat, almost double the average for boys of the same age.

Genetics appear to play an important role in the rate of physical maturation and in each girl's size and shape (Katchadourian, 1977). How quickly each girl matures, where her weight is distributed, the size of her breasts, and the amount of body hair, are affected by diet and nutrition but are to a large degree predetermined by genetics. The physical changes of puberty generally take an average of 4 years. However, each girl develops at her own pace based on her genetic predisposition. For some girls, development is quite rapid and may be completed in only 36 months. For others, development may take as long as 5 or 6 years.

Genetics are also implicated in body type. Some girls tend to have rounder body types with more body fat and softer curves (endomorphs). Some girls are slim, less curvy, and more angular (ectomorphs). Others are more naturally muscular, with wide shoulders and slim hips (mesomorphs) (Friedman, 1993). This fact is rarely reflected in the increasingly homogeneous thin images of the ideal female body. It is noteworthy that only the ectomorphic body type is reflected in the ideal images currently being promoted for women in North American culture (Seid, 1989, 1994).

The precise role played by the sex hormones in regulating weight is still not fully understood. It would appear that an increase in progesterone may be implicated in fat production. This may enhance the perceived palatability of sweet foods for girls of this age (Rodin, Silberstein, & Striegel-Moore, 1984). According to Rodin and colleagues, "Regardless of cultural, ethnic, or social factors, women are fatter than men. Assuming that body size and weight are normally distributed, only a minority of women can be expected to 'naturally' match the extremely thin ideal; the great majority will have varyingly heavier bodies" (p. 285). They note the painful irony of this fact for adolescent girls. At "precisely the time when she is becoming most concerned with her appearance . . . [the pubertal girl] develops the biological machinery that increases her fat-making capacity" (p. 285).

When Hormones Start "Raging": Menarche

Increases in hormone production and the physical changes of puberty signal another significant biological transition in the lives of adolescent girls. Menarche, the onset of menstruation, is derived from the Greek words *men,* meaning month, and *arche,* meaning beginning. It marks a mature stage in the development of the uterus and endocrine system, although it takes an average of 2 more years before eggs are released from the ovaries on a regular basis. In North America, the average age of menarche is 12.8 years (Golub, 1992). Genetic factors appear to play an important role in determining the age at which menarche begins.

The onset of menstruation signals internal changes. The uterus and vagina undergo changes in size and shape in response to the increase in the output of pituitary and gonadatropin-releasing hormone (GnRH), and the increased production of estrogen and androgens. The ovaries, which have been relatively dormant up to this point in development, become responsive to higher levels of two pituitary gonadotropins, FSH (follicle-stimulating hormone) and LH (luteinizing hormone). These hormones trigger the growth of ovarian follicles. Estrogen secreted by the follicles causes the uterine lining to thicken and endometrial tissue to expand in preparation for a possible pregnancy. If, upon release of the mature ovum, fertilization does not occur, the levels of estrogen and progesterone drop, and the endometrium is sloughed off through the process of menstruation. This cycle repeats itself on average every 28 days, although many girls experience highly irregular menstrual cycles for at least 2 years following the onset of menarche (Golub, 1992). Hormonal production can be affected by nutrition, exercise, proportion of body fat, stress, illness, and the use of certain medications, which in turn can affect a girl's menstrual cycles (Brooks-Gunn, 1988; Daniluk & Fluker, 1995; Golub, 1992; Unger & Crawford, 1992).

These hormonal changes associated with women's menstrual cycles have long been the focus of considerable attention in cultures throughout the world (Delaney et al., 1988). Myths and misinformation about women's "raging hormones" led to the systematic excision of literally thousands of healthy ovaries and the bleeding of cervixes with leeches at the turn of the century (Ehrenreich & English, 1978). Similarly, present-day menstrual cycle research is confounded by some of the myths and mysteries that have always surrounded women's reproductive biology (Hubbard, 1990). According to Sommer (1983), "Because the menstrual cycle is such a clear biologically distinguishing feature between the sexes, its correlates, concomitants, accompaniments, ramifications, and implications have become intrinsically bound up with issues of gender" (p. 53).

In assuming a perspective that views mind and body as an integrated whole, it seems foolhardy to discount the importance of hormonal fluctuations and cyclical influences in adolescent girls' experiences of menstruation

(Parlee, 1987). Research tends to confirm that hormonal changes may be associated with changes in sensation and perception, mood and personality, and cognitive and work performance (Choi, 1994; Golub, 1992). For example, it is not uncommon for girls to have particular food cravings during the luteal phase of the menstrual cycle, or to experience heightened sensitivity to high-frequency sounds in the days that precede menstruation (Golub, 1992; Hubbard, 1990). Some women report greater receptivity to genital stimulation during their menstrual flow. Much of the research substantiating a causal relationship between premenstrual symptomatology and psychopathology, however, has been shown to be methodologically flawed and unsound (Choi, 1994; Clare, 1983; Koeske, 1983; Ussher, 1992a, 1992b).

Sexual Awakenings

The role played by these hormones in increasing sexual interest or receptivity is still uncertain; however, there appears to be a clear relationship between the onset of menarche and the initiation of sexual behavior (Udry, Talbert, & Morris, 1986). Udry and Cliquet (1982) report a relationship between ages at menarche, marriage, and first birth among women in the United States, Malay, Belgium, and Pakistan. It would be erroneous, however, to assume these trends can be fully attributed to biological factors in terms of increased sexual desire. These authors underscore the cultural and social significance of menarche as a marker of maturity, which initiates a sequence of events that begin with dating and the increased probability of early intercourse and childbearing.

In terms of sexual responsiveness, our knowledge is relatively limited to genital functioning. As indicated earlier, this is based on the strong adherence in our culture to the notion of genital sexuality and the achievement of orgasm as the sine qua non of sexual behavior and satisfaction (Masters & Johnson, 1966). Readers will likely be familiar with the research of Masters and Johnson (1966, 1970) on the "human sexual response cycle." These researchers propose a four-stage model that begins with *excitement* (vasocongestion in the breasts and genitals) and progresses through a state of high arousal referred to as *plateau* (engorgement of the vagina, decreases in the size of the vaginal opening, vaginal lubrication), culminating in the intensity of *orgasm* (rhythmic contractions of the pelvic muscles), and ending in *resolution* (return of the genitals to their preexcitement state). They suggest that women and men are relatively similar in terms of the way their bodies respond to sexual stimulation. They do acknowledge, however, that women have the physical capacity for a number of orgasms in quick succession in contrast to men, who require a recovery period after each orgasm (Masters & Johnson, 1966).

The work of Masters and Johnson has come under considerable criticism over the past few decades based on their underlying assumption that one four-stage model can account for the range of physical and psychological stimuli that may be experienced as sexual by any person, their emphasis on the importance of intercourse and orgasm in defining sexual "functioning," and their omission of any attention in their theorizing to the notion of sexual drive or desire (Tiefer, 1988, 1991, 1995, 1996). Based on these criticisms, it would appear that our knowledge of what constitutes sexual desire and stimulation for girls and women is, at best, quite limited.

Research does indicate that in terms of physiology, most girls are capable of achieving orgasm from a very early age (Goldman & Goldman, 1988; Martinson, 1991). There are few physiological barriers to the achievement of orgasm. Sexuality and sexual pleasure for girls and women, however, do not appear to be limited to genital development. There are many areas of girls' bodies that are sensitive to touch and stimulation. As discussed in Chapter 1, depending on the context and meaning ascribed to any particular event or encounter, the ensuing sensations may or may not result in orgasm but may be imbued with eroticism and be highly pleasurable. In terms of cognitive development, adolescents generally operate at the level of formal operations (Piaget, 1950). They are therefore capable of elaborate and detailed fantasies and images, some of which may be extremely arousing. It is significant to note that physical stimulation is not essential to vaginal lubrication. Psychological titillation (e.g., fantasies, novels, daydreams) can also elicit this characteristic sign of sexual arousal (Tiefer, 1996).

Because the work of Masters and Johnson has been central to defining what is sexual, and because most research in the area of "human sexuality" and "sexual functioning" has been based on their work, it is safe to say that as yet we know relatively little about "women's sexual response" or responsiveness. There appears to be enormous variation between women in terms of the contextual, situational, and relational variables that are deemed to be erotic, that are sexually titillating, and that elicit sexual pleasure. Sexual desire appears to involve a host of complex biopsychosocial factors, with physical stimulation being only one avenue to the achievement of sexual pleasure for girls and women. It remains to be determined what other aspects of girls' or women's minds, souls, or bodies are implicated in a "sexual" experience.

In concluding this discussion of biological development, it seems that puberty is a time of tremendous physical transition, involving changes over which adolescent girls have relatively little control. Whether or not they are emotionally ready to cope with these changes, based on their genetic predispositions and unique life circumstances (health, nutrition, etc.) at puberty, adolescent girls are faced with adapting to bodies that are significantly altered from their child-like amorphous states. The implications of these changes in terms of girls' developing psychological self-structures are the focus of the next section of this chapter.

PSYCHOLOGICAL DEVELOPMENT

Adolescence as Developmental Crisis/Opportunity: Body Image Changes

In 1923, Freud stated that "the ego is first and foremost a bodily ego" (cited in Plaut & Hutchinson, 1986, p. 418). He underscored the importance of the body as the source and site of the initial and most tangible sense of self. According to Freud, the body ego is central to the development of the self throughout life. Specific life-cycle changes are the stimulus for ego reorganization and development. They may also be the source of considerable anxiety.

From a psychoanalytic perspective, the physical changes that occur for the young girl during puberty in terms of breast development, the accumulation and redistribution of body fat to the stomach and hips, and the growth of pubic and axillary hair constitutes a "dramatic change in the body ego of the pubescent girl" (Plaut & Hutchinson, 1986, p. 418). Signaling an abrupt end of quiescence of sexuality in latency, the onset of menstruation and the corresponding physical changes of puberty inevitably produce a sense of discontinuity in the girl's psychological self-structure. This requires reorganization and reintegration of these changes in terms of her gender-role identity and body image. According to some psychodynamic theorists (e.g., Deutsch, 1945; Plaut & Hutchinson, 1986), puberty and its associated psychological and physical changes represent *the* major developmental transition in the female life cycle.

Many aspects of Freud's theorizing have been soundly criticized. However, most developmental theorists agree that puberty is a critical time period for girls in terms of their increasing physical and psychological maturity and the evolution of a stable and cohesive self-structure (Strober & Yager, 1985). Gender-role identity intensification appears to occur for girls between the ages of 12 and 15 years (Simmons & Blyth, 1987). At this time, girls attempt to integrate the physical changes of puberty with societal definitions and expectations of gender-appropriate behavior and appearance (Crockett & Petersen, 1987; Hill & Lynch, 1983; Petersen, 1988; Rierdan & Koff, 1980, 1985). Negotiating the developmental challenges of puberty is a process "of integrating changes in physical appearance and bodily feelings [that] requires a reorganization of the adolescent's body image and other self-representations" (Attie & Brooks-Gunn, 1989, p. 71). According to Attie and Brooks-Gunn, the formation of identity at adolescence includes the important task of integrating the physical changes of puberty with the girl's old self-image, and with societal definitions and expectations for young women during this transition from childhood to womanhood.

For girls, the onset of menstruation, with its accompanying social significance in marking the transition of the adolescent from girl to woman, appears to be a particularly potent stimuli for maturation. Menarche introduces a new set of changes and challenges to the physical and psychological integrity of the girl. Current theorists view the onset of menstruation and the accompanying physical changes of puberty to be a time of gender identity consolidation and increasing self-definition (Jordan et al., 1991; Kashak, 1992; La Sorsa & Fodor, 1990). Menarche appears to be a pivotal event around which the adolescent girl's body image and sexual identification come to be reorganized (Rierdan & Koff, 1980, 1985). With the onset of menstruation young girls turn their attention to their developing bodies as the distinction between maleness and femaleness becomes more apparent (Rierdan & Koff, 1980; Rierdan, Koff, & Stubbs, 1989; Unger & Crawford, 1992). At this stage, girls begin to reorganize their body images in the direction of greater feminine differentiation and sexual maturity (Golub, 1992; Koff, Rierdan, & Strubbs, 1990). Gender roles are intensified (Hill & Lynch, 1983), characterized by increased attempts for girls to differentiate themselves from boys in appearance and behavior (Simmons & Blyth, 1987).

Body image is generally considered to be a significant component in this process of gender-identity development during adolescence (Blyth, Simmons, & Zakin, 1985; Golombeck, Marton, Stein, & Korenblum, 1987; Jackson, Sullivan, & Rostker, 1988; Petersen, 1988). Emphasizing this connection between the body and the psyche, Hutchinson (1994) refers to body image as "the psychological space where body, mind, and culture come together—the space that encompasses our thoughts, feelings, perceptions, attitudes, values, and judgments about the bodies we have" (p. 153). Body image is "entrenched in the identity" (p. 157) and is both a product of, and contributor to, girls' psychological experience of "self."

The concept of body image is complex and multidimensional. It is composed of an affective response to a visual perception of one's body in relationship to an ideal cultural standard (Fisher, 1986). Body image is not a purely objective phenomenon. Rather, an individual's subjective experience of her body, as well as her observable physical characteristics, are vital to an understanding of body image (Blyth et al., 1985). Hutchinson (1982) suggests that "body image is not the same as body, but is rather what the mind does to the body in translating the experience of embodiment into its mental representation. This translation from body to body image and from there to body-cathexis is a complex and emotionally charged process" (p. 59).

Many theorists believe that body image develops and changes from birth. Like the development of the sexual self discussed in Chapter 1, body image evolves over time and is affected by a complex and interrelated set of sociocultural, interpersonal, and intrapsychic factors (Fisher, 1986; Jaggar & Bordo, 1989). Initially, body image, or bodily ego, as Freud called it, may be based on sensorimotor experiences as young children live in their bodies and experience the world. As girls grow older, cognitive and interpersonal factors appear to become more salient in mediating their body image. As they physically mature during adolescence, girls take in and process feedback from their environments that helps shape their physical self-perceptions.

There appear to be two aspects to body image. One involves the day-to-day experience of living in one's body. This image is rarely static. These more fluid bodily perceptions differ in response to changes in girls' menstrual cycles, shifting affect, mood, life circumstances, and so on (Bartky, 1990; Martin, 1987). The other aspect of body image is commonly referred to as *core* body image (Fisher, 1986). Core body image, the image the girl has incorporated into her self-structure from childhood, is more consistent over time and resistant to change (Fisher, 1986). This helps explain why girls who lose a considerable amount of weight, and who by external standards appear to be quite thin, may still perceive themselves as fat.

Body image also appears to be related to gender-role identity and self-esteem. Femininity and lower self-esteem are correlated with body image dissatisfaction (Jackson, Sullivan, & Hymes, 1987; Jackson et al., 1988; Kimlicka, Cross, & Tarhai, 1983; Unger & Crawford, 1992). Poor body image is related to lower self-esteem and negative feelings of self-worth. More satisfactory body image is correlated with positive self-esteem and self-worth (Jaggar & Bordo, 1989).

Sexual Identity Development

Another important aspect of identity formation in adolescence is sexual identity formation. The physical changes of puberty and the social significance of these changes force girls to begin to integrate a sense of themselves as sexually mature into their broader psychosocial identities (Rierdan & Koff, 1980). In a culture that lacks formal rituals to signify girls' transition into the world of women, menarche and physical maturation serve to mark their identification of themselves as women and as sexual persons (Gagnon & Simon, 1982). It is during this period of development that the issue of sexual attraction becomes salient. During adolescence, girls begin to identify themselves as heterosexual, bisexual, or lesbian. Although this process begins with the sexual experimentation of adolescence, for many, it continues into adulthood. For example, an estimated 24% of lesbians have been previously involved in heterosexual partnerships (Ettorre, 1980). Some bisexual women go through periods of their lives when they are more committed to relationships with women than men, and vice versa (Firestein, 1996). In fact, bisexual women "first self-identify as bisexual in their early to middle 20's . . . somewhat later than the ages of first homosexual self-identification of . . . lesbians" (Fox, 1996, p. 25). Irrespective of when the process of sexual identity formation is complete, the negotiation of attraction and sexual expression within intimate relationships is an important part of the experiences of most girls during adolescence.

The young girl during puberty is faced with the task of attempting to incorporate an understanding of her sexual desires into her self-structure in terms of the development of her sexual identity. This task will inevitably be more difficult if the focus of her desire falls outside of the social norms in her attraction to women, or to women and men. It is difficult to accurately determine the percentage of adolescent girls who will be faced with attempting to negotiate the consolidation of a lesbian or bisexual identity versus a heterosexual identity. Based on behavioral indices alone, the data of Kinsey et al. (1953) indicate that 28% of women reported engaging in a sexual activity with another woman at some time in their lives (13% reported a same-gender sexual experience during adolescence). Three percent reported exclusive sexual involvement with women. In a review of the more current sexual behavior surveys, Fox (1996) reports figures ranging from 64% to 94% for women who had consensual homosexual and heterosexual experiences at some point in their lives. Surveys based on subjective assessment of sexual orientation rather than strict behavioral indices indicate that 9–11% of women self-identify as lesbian (e.g., Golden, 1987; Hite, 1981). An estimated 0.5–3% of women self-identify as bisexual (Fox, 1996). Fox concludes his review of the literature with the following observation: "The large-scale general sexuality surveys . . . clearly indicate that, although some individuals have exclusively same-gender sexual experiences, a substantial proportion of individuals have both homosexual and heterosexual experiences and relationships. . . . Sexual orientation is not dichotomous for everyone" (p. 16).

There is also considerable confusion and disagreement as to what constitutes heterosexuality, lesbianism, and bisexuality. Behavioral indices and identity self perceptions may not be the same. For example, although a large number of women may have erotic encounters with both women and men at some point in their lives, they may not self-identify as bisexual. Rather, their identities may be based on the sex of the people they experience their primary sexual attraction toward, or that represent the majority of their sexual encounters. Alternately, individuals may self-identify as heterosexual, lesbian, or bisexual based on the focus of their erotic desire, but not be actively involved in activities that would be characteristically defined as sexual. Women may self-identify as heterosexual but be celibate (Cline, 1993), or they may be involved in relationships with women that are asexual but include the choice of women as intimate life companions (e.g., Rich, 1980; Rothblum & Brehony, 1993). Also, Firestein (1996) notes how individuals who experience "erotic, emotional, and sexual attraction to persons of more than one gender . . . may identify as bisexual, homosexual, lesbian, gay, heterosexual, transgendered, or transsexual or may choose not to label at all" (p. xix).

Sexual "Identity" and Sexual "Orientation"

So how does sexual identity develop? Some theorists see sexual orientation and identity formation as components of the larger process of gender identity development. The assumption is that in early childhood, girls begin to develop a sense of themselves as separate and distinct from others. A significant part of this awareness centers around their femaleness—the fact that they are physically different from boys. The dramatic physical changes experienced during puberty purportedly initiate a further reorganization of the self during adolescence (Kegan, 1982). More than a process of individuation, this reorganization involves development of a view of the sexual aspects of the self, including the focus of the young woman's erotic desires. (The reader is referred to the discussion of the sexual self in Chapter 1).

Freudian and neo-Freudian conceptualizations regarding gender identity and early love object orientation, and Erikson's (1968) attention to girls' "genital inner space" are two examples of this perspective. Freud (1969) proposed that successful resolution of the Electra complex for girls during childhood required relinquishing the mother as primary love object in exchange for the father (for heterosexuality). He suggested that during puberty, girls' ego consolidation requires a further shift from parental objects to heterosexual peer relationships. Freud placed heterosexuality and vaginal orgasm at the center of mature psychological development for women (Lewis, 1980). According to Plummer (1992), this assumption still forms the basis for much of the current theorizing about normal and healthy sexual development and functioning.

Others link the early programming of sexual orientation with the formation of gender identity. According to Money and Tucker (1975):

> Each person's turn-on has rather fixed boundaries which are set before puberty. . . . They were established in childhood as part of the differentiation of gender identity, by the coding of schemas, and by any quirks or oddities that were incorporated into the schemas. Boundaries may first show themselves at puberty, but they are not set in puberty, and they don't change much, at puberty or later. (p. 164)

From a constructionist perspective, gender identity acquisition and the development of sexual orientation are viewed as quite different processes. These theorists (e.g., Gagnon & Simon, 1973; Parker & Gagnon, 1995; Plummer, 1975, 1992; Weeks, 1981, 1985, 1987, 1995) propose that gender identity is a more stable and enduring aspect of the self. Sexual orientation is more fluid and open to change, based on a multitude of social and contextual influences (e.g., Blumstein & Schwartz, 1976; Rich, 1980). Plummer (1982) suggests that sexual orientation is best understood as a dependent rather than independent variable. It is shaped through the interaction between the drives of the individual and the socially constructed meanings, motives, and norms regulating sexual expression. From this perspective, sexual orientation is about the negotiation and construction of sexual meanings. In this sense, the messages of the body (including a woman's desires, wants, preferences) are interpreted through the set of norms and beliefs that she has come to hold (e.g., heterosexuality, sexual exclusivity, fidelity) based on her membership in, and identification with, certain social groups (families, religious groups, community groups, etc.).

As with other aspects of human functioning, in all likelihood, the determination of sexual orientation probably involves both nature and nurture (Loewenstein, 1985). The body may well be technically responsive to a wide range of physical stimulation, but the impulses of the body are mediated through the mind, and the content of the mind, to a degree, is the product of socialization. And from the standpoint of social and cultural expectations, heterosexuality has been, and continues to be, considered the norm. Until the 1970s, all other forms of sexual identification and attraction were considered aberrant—the sign of psychological maladjustment. The attitudes of mental health professionals may slowly be changing. According to Rothblum (1989), "The prevailing view on lesbianism by mainstream mental health professionals today is one of cautious acceptance" (p. 5). However, the attitudes in mainstream culture still reflect a belief on the part of 75% of American men and women that sexual relations between two same-sex adults is wrong (Hyde, 1990).

Ponse (1980) identifies three types of lesbian identity resolutions that may prove useful in differentiating between lesbians: primary, elective, and women-related lesbians. The primary type sees lesbianism as an orientation that informs and is consistent with her whole character. Unlike elective lesbians, primary lesbians do not see lesbianism as a choice, but rather experience heterosexual involvement as inconsistent with or contrary to their fundamental sense of self. Elective lesbians, on the other hand, see lesbianism as a voluntary choice, a preference with respect to their sexual–emotional behavior. Over time, they may come to view a lesbian sexual orientation as a condition of the self, but this is not necessarily the case. The third group, women-related lesbians, "may hold that lesbianism is the essential, pivotal feature of the identities of other women" but believe that "lesbian describes only an *aspect* of themselves or refers to situated and circumstantial behavior that does not have identity implications." For these women, their "own involvement in lesbian relationships is accounted for more in terms of attraction to a particular personality, though [they] may well express deep commitment to relationship[s] with women" (pp. 196–197). Adoption of a lesbian identity and life structure may be based on a rejection of male dominance, erotic desire, and/or intimacy and attachment to women.

For adolescent girls, the development of a lesbian identity may involve a difficult "coming out" process of awareness and consolidation of a socially stigmatized sexual identity. Sophie (1985/1986) proposes that the formation of a lesbian identity involves the stages of awareness, testing and exploration, identity acceptance, and identity integration. Both Rothblum (1994) and Golden (1987) suggest a multidimensional model of lesbian sexual orientation based on sexual behavior, sexual identity, and participation/membership in the lesbian community. McCarn and Fassinger (1996) extend this theorizing even further in proposing a four-stage model of lesbian identity development that "posits a dual nature of lesbian identity" (p. 509). They focus on the development of both individual sexual identity and the parallel development of an identity based on membership in an oppressed minority group. They propose that this is critical in supporting the development of identity for lesbian women. A more thorough discussion of the process of lesbian identity development is beyond the scope of this book. For information and critiques on some of the more prominent models of lesbian identity formation, I recommend the authors listed above, as well as Coleman (1981/1982), Herdt and Boxer (1993), Kitzinger (1987), Savin-Williams (1990), and Sophie (1985/1986).

Even less information is available regarding the sexual identity formation of bisexual women. Weasel (1996) notes the relative invisibility of bisexuality in most sexual theorizing regarding normal *or* deviant sexual expression. In her book, *Bisexuality,* Firestein (1996) refers to bisexuals as "an invisible minority." These and other authors (e.g., Fox, 1996; George, 1993; Hutchins & Ka'ahumanu, 1991; Weise, 1992) note the greater difficulty that may be experienced by bisexual women in attempting to negotiate a viable and integrated sense of their sexual identities. This is due to their relative exclusion from the heterosexual models of identity development (with the defining criterion for inclusion in this group being not having sexual relations with *women*) and from the homosexual models of identity development (with the defining criterion for inclusion being not having sexual relations with *men*). Weasel underscores how the difficulties of bisexual women may be further compounded by their potential lack of community identification.

> Bisexual women, on the basis of their sexual identification with men as well as women, are often excluded from lesbian communities. This can leave them feeling without a community to belong to, and can often lead to feelings of invisibility . . . abnormality . . . and isolation . . . [making] the coming out process . . . particularly difficult. (Weasel, p. 6)

Research suggests that heterosexuals also carry negative perceptions of bisexuals (Spalding & Peplau, 1994). For more information on the debates and theorizing regarding bisexuality and bisexual identity formation, I recommend Firestein's (1996) book, as well as the works of Hutchins and Ka'ahumanu (1991) and Klein (1993).

CONCLUSION

Adolescence is clearly a time of considerable physical and psychological growth and development for girls. It is also a time of corresponding social changes, as the onset of menstruation and the signs of physical maturation mark girls' social transition into the world of women. This change in status is accompanied by changes in roles and expectations. In the following three chapters, we turn our attention to the social worlds in which adolescents live out these changes, and in particular, to the messages of significant others and the cultural at large about the meanings of these changes. We turn to the interaction between adolescent girls and their worlds to understand how problematic meanings evolve, and to explore how girls might develop more affirming sexual meanings and self-constructions.

4

MENSTRUATION

Initiation into Womanhood

> What would happen if suddenly, magically, men could menstruate and women could not? Clearly, menstruation would become an enviable, boast-worthy, masculine event: Men would brag about how long and how much. Young boys would talk about it as the envied beginning of manhood. Gifts, religious ceremonies, family dinners, and stag parties would mark the day. To prevent monthly work loss among the powerful, Congress would fund a National Institute of Dysmenorrhea.
>
> —GLORIA STEINEM,
> *Outrageous Acts and Everyday Rebellions*

Of all the physical changes experienced by young girls, the one more closely associated with their "budding" sexuality and emerging womanhood is the onset of menstruation. In most cultures of the world, the first sign of menstrual blood heralds a change in the sexual and social status of the girl, from girl to young woman, from child to potential mother (Golub, 1992; Martin, 1987). Menstrual blood is the symbol of this change (Weideger, 1978).

As discussed in Chapter 3, puberty is a time of considerable physical development and psychological change for girls. The physical changes that accompany the onset of menstruation, however, are only one component of a dynamic process rife with psychological significance and social meanings. It is a personal event, but it is also highly social. The physical experience is shaped by the context in which it occurs. How girls come to understand and make sense of the biological realities of menstruation, and incorporate these changes into their sense of themselves as young women and as sexual persons, has a great deal to do with how others in their worlds respond to these changes. Girls' perceptions of menstruation are inevitably shaped by their interactions with others. The personal meanings girls hold about this experience and about themselves are based on the messages and meanings available to them in their cultures. The reactions of parents and peers are particularly important in shaping their experiences. Research confirms that most women, despite their age and life stage, remember with remarkable clarity and detail where they were when menstruation began, how they felt about the experience, and how friends and family members responded to their entrance into womanhood (Delaney, Lupton, & Tóth, 1988; Golub, 1992; Koff et al., 1990; Martin, 1987; Rierdan et al., 1989; Taylor & Woods, 1991; Weideger, 1978). For many, these memories are bittersweet: Feelings of excitement and anticipation were mixed with ignorance, fear, and humiliation. Other representatives of the larger social culture that influence girls' experiences of menstruation and how they feel about this aspect of their femaleness include the popular media, religion, and medicine. To varying degrees, all of these sources shape the personal meanings girls come to hold about this process that is unique to women (Amann-Gainotti, 1986; Brooks-Gunn, 1988; Gagnon & Simon, 1982; Laws, 1980; Unger & Crawford, 1992). We turn now to a examination of some of the more common messages communicated to girls about menstruation and discuss how these messages can become problematic in girls' comfort in their bodies and in their emerging sexual self-constructions.

THE THINGS WE NEEDED MOTHER "AND DAD" TO TELL US: PARENTAL MESSAGES

The onset of menstruation and the physical changes of puberty precipitate changes in parent–child relationships and interactions. Both parents and their children are forced to confront girls' budding sexuality and changing status from child to woman (Leaper et al., 1989; Hill & Holmbeck, 1987). Girls begin to differentiate themselves from their parents and turn to the outside world for direction in making sense of their lives and experiences as young women. Menarche marks a turning point not only in the lives of girls but also in the lives of their parents. With society's emphasis on menarche as *the* marker of sexual maturity for girls, parents are faced with trying to accommodate the physical and psychological changes this transition heralds for their daughter. They must also deal with the change in social status that menstruation represents in our culture with the change from girl to woman, and with the reality that their child now has the biological potential to become a mother.

Research confirms that the onset of menstruation is indeed a social stimulus to which parents inevitably respond. Parents typically become more controlling of their daughters for the first 6 months following the onset of menstruation. There is greater parent–daughter conflict, more emotional and physical distancing, and an increase in struggles over authority (Brooks-Gunn, 1988). This may reflect parental uncertainty about knowing how best to respond to the physical changes of menstruation and to the change in their daughters' social–sexual status as well (Unger & Crawford, 1992). La Sorsa and Fodor (1990) note how parents are often struggling with their own midlife developmental issues at the same time that their daughters are coping with menarche. It may, therefore, be even more challenging for them to respond effectively to their daughters' transition.

Adequate preparation has been found to be an important component in helping girls cope more positively with the initial experience of menstruation (Amann-Gainotti, 1986; Goldman & Goldman, 1988; Golub, 1992; Rierdan, 1983). In terms of information about menarche and the changes a girl can expect during puberty, research indicates that American parents play a relatively small role in the transmission of concrete information to their daughters about menstruation and sexuality. Fathers, in particular, are noticeably absent in this process. They appear to perceive it as the mother's role to discuss issues related to bodily changes and menstruation with their daughters, and implicitly communicate this to their daughters. Not surprisingly, the majority of girls select to tell their mothers when they begin to menstruate. Few tell their fathers due to the "embarrassment" this may cause for both father and daughter (Brooks-Gunn & Ruble, 1983; Golub, 1992; Yalom, Estler, & Brewster, 1982).

Physical development and the onset of menstruation also precipitates other changes in father–daughter relationships. Fathers become more assertive and tend to distance themselves from their postmenarcheal daughters. This may be in response to their own discomfort in knowing how to adequately respond to the change in their daughters' social status from girl to young woman (Amann-Gainotti, 1986). Parental withdrawal may also reflect the fact that men in general appear to have even more negative views of menstruation than women do. Based partially on ignorance about a process unique to women, such attitudes make it even more difficult for men to broach the subject of menstruation with their daughters in an informed and accepting way (Delaney et al., 1988; Hubbard, 1990). These interactions with their fathers reinforce for girls the message that menstruation and reproduction are "women's issues." Fathers' silence is interpreted to signify men's discomfort with this process. From the outset, then, girls come to believe that all signs of menstruation must be kept hidden from view, especially in relation to men.

What girls do learn about sexuality and menstruation within their families, they tend to learn from their mothers. In North American society, it is mothers who are charged with the primary responsibility of finding ways to help their daughters cope with and adapt to these "womanly" changes. This is clearly not an easy task. Adolescence is a time when communication is characteristically becoming strained between girls and their parents. Daughters are experiencing painfully heightened self-consciousness regarding their changing bodies. Also, menstruation is about a physical process involving girls' genitals—a part of the body that many girls have learned in childhood is "off limits." It is a process that is associated with sexuality—a topic that also elicits considerable discomfort in most families. As such, the issue of menstruation is often imbued with embarrassment and shame for daughters, and sometimes for their mothers as well, making open and direct communication more difficult.

These problems are exacerbated by the lack of preparation most mothers received within their own families of origin regarding menstruation and sexuality. While mothers may want to help ease their daughters' entrance into womanhood, they also are products of their own histories and cultures. As such, they may be ill-prepared to take on this task in a way that does not serve to alienate or embarrass their daughters. The difficulty of adequate preparation may be further compounded by ethnic and cultural differences, particularly in cultures where ensuring virginity is critical to facilitating an appropriate marital arrangement. With menstruation marking girls' sexual maturity, the communications between mothers and daughters in these cultures may be colored by their fears of an unwanted pregnancy. In fact, in some cultures, clitoridectomies and vaginal infibulation are still performed at menarche to ensure girls' virginity (Kitzinger, 1985; Omer-Hashi & Entwistle, 1995).

Unfortunately, the information provided by mothers about menstruation is often perceived by daughters to be inadequate (Amann-Gainotti, 1986; Golub, 1992; Madaras & Madaras, 1983). One woman recalled the inadequacy of her mother's attempts to inform her about the facts of life:

> "Actually I remember the day she told us the facts of life, my younger sister and I. I was lying on the floor with my hands under my chin, elbows on the floor, Dad sitting in the chair reading the newspaper, pretending not to listen, and my younger sister was beside me. . . . She read to us from a book. That's all she did. She didn't know how to handle it herself. . . . I remember she was telling us that when you get to a certain age that you are going to bleed, and I said, 'Well, does dad bleed?' 'No.' 'Well how come?' 'Just the girls do.' 'OK, where do you bleed from?' 'Down there.' 'Down there?' 'Down there,' just indicating with her finger, pointing. I was lying on the floor, so I thought I was going to bleed from my breasts, and it sounds so foolish but I never told her up until 2 years ago that I thought for years I was going to bleed from my breasts."

Another woman reflected on the painful and frightening beginning of her period and her mother's apparent casual reaction:

> "One day I was going to the bathroom and wiping myself up, and my legs were full of blood and I thought I was dying. I thought I cut myself and I was bleeding to death. . . . I thought I was dying. I didn't know what was wrong with me. So I screamed for my mother, and she came

> upstairs and didn't say much. She gave me this huge blue Kotex box, and there were instructions in the box, and she said, 'There you go,' and left the room. I had absolutely no idea what to do with the pads and the belt. . . . It took me hours in the bathroom to figure it out . . . and then, of course, my young friends, my girlfriends, all told me about what it was."

Sadly, these recollections of fear, shame, and misinformation are not unusual. Many women remember the onset of their period and their parents' reactions as being "horrible," "awful," "disgusting," and "embarrassing" (Delaney et al., 1988; Leroy, 1993).

Fortunately, times are changing, and in sharp contrast to their predecessors, most pubescent girls of the present cohort are better prepared for the physical changes that they experience. Between parents and sex education classes, most girls are exposed to information about the physiological functioning of the uterus and ovaries, and have seen detailed illustrations of female genitals and reproductive organs. With the educational resources available now (e.g., Bell, 1987; Gravelle & Gravelle, 1996; Madaras & Madaras, 1983), the job of preparing daughters for the physical realities of menarche is certainly easier than in the past. *The Period Book* by Gravelle and Gravelle (1996) is a particularly noteworthy example of a resource that not only explains how to use pads and tampons, but also provides useful tips on how to deal with irregular schedules and breakthrough bleeding. It would appear we have come a long way from the little books put out by pharmaceutical companies in the 1950s and '60s with titles such as *How Can I Tell My Daughter?* Or have we really? Havens and Swenson (1988) note how, even now, many of the educational booklets and tools distributed to prepubescent girls are still developed by manufacturers of sanitary products. These manufacturers emphasize menarche as "a hygienic rather than developmental milestone" (p. 90). This emphasis reinforces a sense of secrecy and shame toward menstruation, rather than feelings of pride and acceptance.

Even girls who feel that they have been given enough information about menstruation and puberty report a lack of attention on the part of parents and educators to menstruation as a "personal" event (Rierdan, 1983). Menstrual preparation rarely includes attention to the social and emotional needs of the girl at this point in her development. There is little recognition of what it feels like to menstruate, whether it is uncomfortable or painful, whether others will know, and how (Rierdan, Koff, & Flaherty, 1985).

In recent years, some parents have attempted to overcome some of the negative connotations associated with menarche by revisiting the old tradition of marking their daughter's first menstruation with a ritual or party. They have attempted to celebrate her initiation into the world of women. Certainly, rituals celebrating the onset of menstruation are evident throughout recorded history. From earliest times, the menstrual cycle was viewed as a life-affirming source of creativity. In ancient Greece, women participated in a ritual known as the Thesmophoria, a ceremony during which the women entered "wholly into the femaleness of themselves" and reaffirmed their connection to the earth through the ceremonial joining of their menstrual blood with the earth (Meador, 1986). According to Meador, rituals "similar to those in the Thesmophoria, have been found in all parts of Old Europe dating from 6000 B.C." (pp. 36–37). These "rites of passage" usually involve older women ritually welcoming the menstruating girl into the circle of womanhood.

Even now, some cultures retain a commitment to celebratory rituals when a girl begins to menstruate. They see the girl's crossing through the threshold into womanhood as a highly spiritual event (Golub, 1983). A woman of East Indian decent recently reflected on her very positive memories of menarche. Echoing a wedding ceremony, her parents adorned her bed with beautiful flower garlands, and family members brought gifts of gold and silk to mark the celebration of her entrance into womanhood. Her parents' continued validation of, and comfort with, her reproductive functioning was evident when they accompanied her to the reproductive health clinic where she and I first met.

While it certainly seems more affirming to have parents approach menstruation as a time of celebration, not all girls will react positively to these attempts to provide validation and support, irrespective of the positive and affirming attitudes of parents (Stoltzman, 1986). Not surprisingly, without a corresponding commitment on the part of the culture to view menstruation as a celebration, familial attempts to honor their daughters' transition into womanhood may heighten girls' discomfort with menstruation and increase their self-consciousness about their changing bodies (Delaney et al., 1988; Golub, 1992; Martin, 1987). One young woman reported being "absolutely mortified" when her mother proudly announced to the entire family at the dinner table that she had now "become a woman." This declaration was followed by a toast from both parents and embarrassed snickers from the girl's younger siblings. Logan (cited in Golub, 1992) investigated the ritual preferences of pubertal girls and their parents regarding the public acknowledgment of menstruation. She found that girls appear to be very sensitive to maintaining boundaries of privacy around this event. Certainly, they preferred some sign of positive acknowledgment of menarche to parental silence. However, most indicated that they would prefer to be given a display of affection or a material token such as flowers or a gift by their parents to mark their transition into womanhood, rather than having to endure any type of public display or declaration.

In light of the prevailing cultural climate and menstrual taboos, it may be difficult for parents to help their daughters through this important transition in a way that is informative and supportive. It it hard for parents to be validating while also being respectful of their daughters' privacy and sensitive to their individual needs. This difficulty may be further compounded by young women's identity struggles. Kitzinger (1985) suggests:

> The way in which a mother decides to react to the advent of her daughters' menstruation has to be wrong, in a way, because a major task for a girl in adolescence is to differentiate herself from her mother. The scenario in which the first menstruation takes place is just one part of that process of differentiation . . . a highly significant one. And to differentiate she has to make boundaries, to draw back from her mother, to define herself as distinct from her with different ideas and feelings. (p. 179)

Despite parent's best efforts to inform their daughters about menstruation and their developing sexuality, many young girls report feeling quite unprepared for the personal and physical changes that are associated with menarche. In particular, many girls feel ill-prepared to deal with an event that has such significant social implications (Golub, 1992; Rierdan, 1983; Unger & Crawford, 1992).

A FRIEND IN NEED: MESSAGES OF PEERS

Menarche seems to mark a shift in the greater influence of peers. Based on their shared reality, the beliefs and opinions of friends often are given more credence and validity at this life stage than those of parents. Research by Stoltzman (1986) suggests that even when parents are perceived as having very open and positive attitudes, daughters are more likely to seek information about menstruation and puberty from their friends. Dynamics in relationships with opposite-sex peers also increase in complexity as girls (and boys) attempt to deal with the physical and social demands of their new status as young "women" (Unger & Crawford, 1992). The acute interpersonal sensitivity that characterizes this stage of development and girls' receptivity to the messages of others have considerable implications for the meanings they come to hold about menstruation and their changing bodies, about their developing sexuality, and about the way they express their sexuality within intimate relationship.

Most girls turn to their same-sex friends for information, support, and guidance about dealing with menstruation. It is with a few close confidantes that they share their curiosity, fears, and apprehensions about menstruation (Rierdan & Koff, 1985). So what do girls learn from their peers regarding menstruation? On the one hand, discussions with friends can serve to normalize the process of menstruation and help girls feel less isolated and unusual. Well-informed friends can be a valuable source of information and validation in preparing for the *social* as well as *physical* changes that characterize menarche. They can help fill in some of the gaps in girls' information about the pragmatics of dealing with periods, as well as helping to demystify the experience. One woman reflected on the important role played by her friends in her menstrual and sexual preparation and education:

> "I honestly don't know what I would have done without my friends. . . . I was so naive, and felt so stupid. I didn't have a clue about anything. My friends told me about periods and tampons and how to use them. I didn't even know where to put them. Can you believe it? I didn't know I had a vagina, and I use to listen to friends talk about sex and 'doing it' and I was petrified 'cause I couldn't imagine anyone sticking their whatever in my bum. . . . God, I was naive."

These sentiments underscore the way in which shared experience may well serve as a buffer against adolescent girls' insecurities, apprehensions, and fears. On the other hand, exchanges between less-informed, albeit well-meaning friends can result in erroneous and inaccurate information being passed on about menstruation. In their hushed whispers and veiled communications, girls can also pass on their sense of embarrassment and shame about this aspect of being female.

Beliefs and values regarding menstruation are also reflected in the language used by family members and both female and male peers to describe and define this experience. Language, in turn, shapes a girl's experience and understanding of menarche. Unfortunately, the words used to describe the "womanly" process of monthly bleeding are at best inadequate and at worst derogatory. Reflecting an early Christian theme of menstruation as "pollution" and menstruating women as "unclean" (Letson, 1987), words commonly associated with menstruation include "the curse," "the plague," being "on the rag," and being "under the weather" (Delaney et al., 1988). More neutral but still inadequate terms include "your period," and "that time of the month." Unger and Crawford (1992) list a host of menstrual expressions that have been historically used by American women, including terms like "a weeping womb" and "bride's barf." According to Golub (1992), a file in the Folklore Archives at the University of California, Berkeley, on American menstruation folkspeech cites 128 euphemistic expressions used to describe this physiological event. Unfortunately, the majority are negative and are intended to maintain secrecy or avoid embarrassment. These words reflect a sense of shame and degradation related to the process that marks girls' entrance into womanhood.

In examining the language used by 133 women in reference to menstruation Hays (1987) reports an absence of the use of more clinical terms such as "menstruation" or "menses." Rather, the words most frequently used by the women were more indirect and inferential. Sometimes they were in reference to the cyclicity of the menstrual cycle (e.g., "monthlies," "in my cycle," "that time of the month"), sometimes they involved menstrual products (e.g., "on the rag," "using the paper dick"), and sometimes they were related to illness or the inconvenience associated with menstruation ("the plague," "the curse," "under the weather," "woman trouble").

Even now, when browsing through books on sex education, problems with language persist. Girls are faced with an either–or choice of using words to describe their menstrual experience that are highly medical, or using slang terms that emphasize the secrecy and shame associated with a process that has for centuries been viewed as disease (Delaney et al., 1988; Weideger, 1978). With such problematic language, how are adolescent girls to find appropriate words to express the changes they experience at puberty, much less celebrate the event that marks their entrance into womanhood?

OF CLEANLINESS AND WOMANLINESS: MEDIA MESSAGES

Another very formative influence in the construction of menstrual meanings in North America is the media. At a time in their lives when they are looking to the outside world for cues by which to identify themselves, the media serve as a significant source of information. Research indicates that girls get more information about menstruation from the media than from their parents (Stoltzman, 1986).

What is most noticeable about media representations of menstruation are their relative absence. Apart from premenstrual syndrome (PMS) jokes made, usually by men, in reference to their wives', girlfriends', employees' or bosses' "raging hormones" in some popular sitcoms, we never see the activities or sex lives of female stars or heroines being in any way affected by the fact that they are "on their period." There is no evidence of the bloating, cramping, pimples, or fatigue that sometimes accompany menstruation. There is no sign of their appearance or behavior being in any way circumscribed by menstruation. It is as if menstruation does not exist.

A notable exception to this is in advertising. Most magazines directed at a female audience contain several ads aimed at informing the reader about menstrual pain relief and "sanitary protection." In attending again to language, even the choice of words is telling. The implicit message is that girls and women need to be "protected" against the byproduct of menstruation and that our bodies need to be made more "sanitary." In turning to my dictionary, I note that the definition of "sanitize" is "to make more acceptable by removing unpleasant features." These ads have recently even made it to prime-time television. It is no longer unusual to see images of tampons soaking up "blue" (not red) fluid from a container, with corresponding commentary about the comfort and safety of products "designed by a woman gynecologist."

Havens and Swenson (1988) analyzed the imagery associated with menstruation in the advertisements for sanitary products in a popular teen magazine over a 10-year period. They reported two primary approaches in these ads to dealing with sanitary "protection": the scientific and the athletic approaches. The scientific approach emphasizes the dimensions, schematics, material, absorbency, and design of the products. The athletic approach emphasizes the freedom of movement, comfort, confidence, and "safety" associated with menstrual amenities (no unsightly or unexpected leaking). Many of the ads are aimed at assuring the consumer that menstruation will remain unnoticeable, thereby giving her added "security" and "peace of mind." These researchers also analyzed ads for medications directed at the relief of menstrual "cramps, headache, backache, swelling, bloating, breast discomfort caused by swelling, and leg aches" (p. 94). The focus of these ads is on the need to overcome menstrual limitations if girls are to look their best (no bloating) and not let their physiology get in the way of having a good time. The implicit message communicated to young women is that menstruation is an inconvenience that can successfully be made invisible with the right products. Rather than supporting menstruation as a natural and healthy human process, it is presented as a "feminine hygiene crisis" that requires cleansing, fixing, and deodorizing (Delaney et al., 1988; Rothbaum & Jackson, 1990).

It is not surprising, then, that a primary concern for women in general and for adolescent girls in particular is to "make sure" that they completely cover up any evidence of menstruation (Patterson & Hale, 1995). They may well see menstruation as a sign of their advancing maturity. However, premenarcheal girls report that the feeling most associated with beginning their period is fear (Delaney et al., 1988; Golub, 1992). Many are "petrified" that when their period begins, the bleeding might break through their clothing, and then others will know. They might boast with close friends about having "gotten theirs." Certainly, the experience of beginning menstruation is accorded some status among adolescent girls. They may secretly gloat about the change in role status that their menstruation signifies, but they also experience shame. The messages are paradoxical. On the one hand, through the process of menstruation, they have now attained the status accorded adult women in our culture. The marker of that status, however, must be sanitized and hidden.

RELIGIOUS AND MEDICAL MESSAGES

Religious and medical messages also shape girls' experience and understanding of menstruation. Being linked to fertility, menstruation has been a central focus in defining and circumscribing the purpose and roles of women in the teachings and beliefs of most religions throughout time. Widely held Judeo-Christian beliefs regard this monthly bleeding as a symbol of women's inherent inferiority and associate menstruation with impurity and uncleanliness (Rothbaum & Jackson, 1990; Sevely, 1987). To cite an often-quoted example in Leviticus 15:19, it is written that "when a woman has a discharge, *if* her discharge in her body is blood, she shall continue in her menstrual impurity for seven days." Leviticus goes on to indicate that anything or anyone who comes in contact with a menstruating woman is, by association, also unclean. This perspective is echoed in the teachings of other religions as well. For example, most Orthodox and some Conservative Jews still practice *mikvah*. This involves a ritual bathing at the end of the woman's menstrual cycle plus 7 days, to make the woman pure after being *niddah,* or spiritually unclean (Siegel, 1986).

The view of menstruation as "pollution," and menstruating women as unclean, is still reflected in the period of seclusion required of menstruating girls and women in some religions (Delaney et al., 1988; Kitzinger, 1985). These religious beliefs and teachings reflect a common theme of the menstruating woman as pariah. Ironically, the physiological process that allows women to give life and continue to propagate the species is the very capacity that is viewed as embodying women's inferiority. Girls who are raised in families that adhere to these anti-woman religious beliefs will, to varying degrees, incorporate them into their developing self-structures. They may well come to believe in their inherent inferiority as women and perceive themselves as unclean and defective because they menstruate.

The medical profession also has a long history of interest in women's reproductive biology and functioning. Echoing Judeo-Christian religious beliefs, 16th-century physicians came to view the uterus as the primary "controlling" organ for women. This "highly unpredictable" part of the female anatomy was considered responsible for emotional volatility and erratic shifts in temperament and behavior (i.e., "raging hormones"). The brain was viewed as the controlling organ for men (Ehrenreich & English, 1978). Women's uterus and ovaries have been, and continue to be, a primary site of medical intervention. By the turn of the century, the removal of the ovaries, or female castration, was *the* most commonly performed surgical intervention in the United States (Ehrenreich & English, 1978). Today, hysterectomies have replaced the ovariotomy as the most performed "elective" surgery in North America (Pokras & Hufnagel, 1988). The development and perfection of "advanced" reproductive technologies and the study and control of menstrual cycle fluctuations (PMS) is now a multibillion dollar industry (Arditti, Klein, & Minden, 1984; Corea, 1985).

These medical perceptions are significant in shaping girls' understanding of their bodies at menarche. For most girls, the onset of menstruation marks the beginning of a long-standing relationship with the medical profession. As children, girls may have visited the family doctor for yearly physical checkups and routine inoculations. Once there is evidence of reproductive maturity, however, many girls are required to undergo regular gynecological exams and yearly Pap smears. With the onset of menstruation, the part of their bodies that they have been encouraged to keep private and covered becomes subjected to medical examination and scrutiny. They are faced with having to expose their genitals to the view and touch of a physician, which in itself can be a very difficult and even traumatic experience. The implicit connection between menstruation and disease is obvious. Girls also learn that the management of their reproductive functioning (dealing with menstrual irregularities or discomfort, birth control, etc.) is not under their own control but, rather, requires medical intervention.

SUMMARY: PROBLEMATIC MEANINGS

The process of responding to the biopsychosocial changes that accompany menstruation is a complex one. It involves a host of intrapersonal, interpersonal, and social variables. Menstruation is a monthly reminder of the girl's deficiency—a "curse." With its connection to fertility, it is, paradoxically, also a symbol of her value.

In light of these conflictual messages, it should come as no surprise that most girls experience the onset of menstruation as confusing and equivocal at best. The literature on adolescent development suggests that few experiences in a young girl's life are as conflictual as menstruation. Research indicates a doubling in the likelihood of severe depression for girls in the year after the onset of menstruation (Golub, 1992). Early maturers are particularly vulnerable to psychosocial difficulties (Attie & Brooks-Gunn, 1989; Petersen, 1983; Rierdan & Koff, 1985). Even adolescents with accepting parents and a supportive and accepting peer group must still find ways to cope with and make sense of contradictory messages. These suggest that menstruation is a distasteful and embarrassing aspect of being a woman—and yet the hallmark of womanhood.

In the next section, a number of exercises are provided that can be used to help girls critically examine the explicit and implicit messages that have been communicated to them about menstruation. Suggestions are made to begin the process of creating more positive, woman-affirming meanings and self-constructions related to menstruation and to women's menstrual cyclicity.

CHALLENGE AND CHANGE: CREATING NEW MEANINGS

How can counselors help girls more positively respond to the changes that accompany menstruation? Clearly, the task is not an easy one. In working with pre- and postmenarcheal girls, the goals of counseling should be the promotion of menarche as a normal, developmental event, one that may, at times, be physically challenging but also affords opportunities for creativity and enhanced energy (Golub, 1992; Kitzinger, 1985; Martin, 1987; Meador, 1986). In offering the possibility of alternative meanings, it is necessary for counselors to abandon the disease-oriented language that is so prevalent in referring to menstruation. It is important to normalize the hormonal and physical changes that characterize this process as a healthy and positive component of female development and experience (Delaney et al., 1988; Kitzinger, 1985; Martin, 1987).

When working on these issues, it is first necessary to assess girls experiences, feelings, and attitudes toward menstruation. To what degree have girls internalized the messages of others and of the larger culture about the meaning and significance of this process? Any number of activities may help gather this information. For example, questionnaires can be used to assess attitudes toward menstruation (e.g., Oyefeso & Osinowo, 1990; Petersen, 1983). Or girls can be asked to respond to a list of statements regarding menstruation. Individually, or in a group, girls can be asked to indicate "true or false" to the following types of statements:

Menstruation is a painful process.
Menstruation makes you feel fat, and makes your hands and feet swell.
Some women have more energy at particular times in their menstrual cycle.
Menstrual blood has an unpleasant odor.
Periods usually last 5–7 days.
Girls have their periods once every 28 days.
Girls cannot get pregnant when they are on their period.
Girls need more rest when they are menstruating.

The types of statements can be easily geared to the age and developmental level of the girls involved and should be aimed at identifying many of the erroneous myths and assumption commonly associated with the menstrual cycle (see Bell, 1987, and Madaras & Madaras, 1983, for examples of myths and misconceptions commonly held by adolescent girls regarding menstruation). When working with a group of girls, a useful adaptation to this exercise is to have the girls themselves generate the statements of things they have heard about menstruation, both positive and negative. Group leaders can also engage girls in a discussion of the *source* of these statements, providing important information about who the most significant socializing agents in the girls' lives appear to be. Activities such as those identified below can then be undertaken to help counter the negative attitudes that have been taken in by the girls, and to correct false perceptions and misinformation.

It is also important to assess girls' feelings regarding menstruation. What is the meaning and significance of menarche in terms of their self-perceptions? Given the prevalent cultural ethos regarding menstruation, it is important to determine the extent to which young women have accepted the notions of menstruation as "disease" or "pollution." Feelings of shame and fear are often experienced by girls prior to the onset of menarche. Because of this, an activity may be useful that provides some emotional distance for the young adolescent, while still accessing important information regarding her own affective responses to this transition. Story completion may serve as a useful activity in this regard. For example, Petersen (1983) used an incomplete story about menarche adapted from Blume's book, *Are You There, God? It's Me, Margaret,* to explore girls' feelings about menarche. After being presented with the story excerpt, girls were asked to indicate what happened and how the character felt about beginning her period? Another variation of this activity is to have the girl write her own story about a character who has reached this crossroad in her development, placing emphasis on how the character feels about this experience and what it means to her in terms of her sense of herself. In reviewing the story together, the counselor can ask questions that help move the story from the fictitious character's frame of reference to that of the adolescent girl, in terms of exploring *her* feelings regarding the impact and significance of this event in her life.

Finally, with postmenarcheal girls, it is important to assess how they have experienced the onset of menarche. What are their feelings associated with this "transition to womanhood"? What have been their experiences so far with their menstrual process and cyclicity. It is especially important to attempt to identify negative and shame inducing interactions or circumstances experienced by young women in relation to menstruation (e.g., breakthrough bleeding, being caught without adequate menstrual protection, comments from or withdrawal by significant others, embarrassing lack of knowledge or information). Counselors can help girls work through these experiences using some of the activities identified below. A particularly negative experience around menstruation can be quite devastating for the young girl (Bell, 1987), resulting in debilitating feelings of shame and inadequacy related to this aspect of her feminine identity. Not surprisingly, a high degree of safety and rapport is usually required before most young women can feel comfortable sharing with others those experiences that are often a source of tremendous shame.

When counselors have had an opportunity to assess the attitudes, feelings, and meanings associated with menstruation, it is possible to select activities and strategies that build on the more affirming aspects of this experience. These help to counter more popular notions of menstruation as debilitation or as a "hygienic crisis." For premenstrual girls, it is important to validate their fears and apprehensions and to help them adequately prepare for integrating this new experience into their lives. Postmenarcheal girls may also need assistance in comfortably living with both the physical and psychosocial changes they have experienced as a result of menstruation.

Girls can begin to examine the attitudes of others that have shaped their perceptions and feelings about menstruation, and can start to get in touch with their in-the-moment experiences of living with the reproductive rhythms of their bodies. With enhanced self-awareness and exposure to more affirming menstrual images and meanings, they can begin to reject messages that produce feelings of shame and inadequacy and start to appreciate what menstrual cyclicity *adds* to their experience of being women.

The exercises presented below are examples of how counselors might begin to achieve these goals when working with young adolescent girls. In selecting interventions, counselors must be sensitive to the developmental differences in the needs and maturity of pre- and postmenarcheal girls.

Information Is Power

Whether pre- or postmenarcheal, research indicates that adequate information is valuable in helping girls develop a more positive experience of menstruation. This is information that many adult women retrospectively perceive as largely missing from their own menstrual preparation (Golub & Catalano, 1983; Rierdan, 1983). Adequate menstrual education can be undertaken on an individual basis or in mixed or same-sex groups (although same-sex groups are often helpful at the outset in overcoming feelings of shame and discomfort), or on an individual basis. Adequate information means coverage of both the physiological process, and the personal experience. In the area of physiological process it should involve a detailed but accessible review of girls' reproductive anatomy and information on the specific physiological, hormonal, and affective changes that are commonly experienced during the various stages of the menstrual cycle, as well as ways to cope with these changes. Characteristic alterations in body weight and shape should also be addressed. Attention needs to be paid to differences in body types and sizes, so that girls might understand the importance of genetics in the determination of their own morphology and menstrual process (Rierdan & Koff, 1985). Information on menstrual hygiene is important, but care should be taken to emphasize each girl's comfort with her bodily experiences rather than ensuring the comfort of others by covering up any signs or traces of menstruation (Patterson & Hale, 1985).

There are a number of excellent resources (films and books) available that can be used to help educate girls about their changing bodies and about the hormonal changes that characterize particular points in the menstrual cycle (e.g., Gardner-Loulan, 1991; Madaras, 1993; Madaras & Madaras, 1983). In particular, Bell's (1987) revised edition of *Changing Bodies, Changing Lives* provides excellent, detailed, and accessible information about the physical changes that are commonly experienced during puberty. It also addresses the range of feelings and attitudes that are often experienced by girls in response to these changes. I also made reference earlier in the chapter to a self-help book for teens by Karen Gravelle and her daughter Jennifer (1996), called *The Period Book: Everything You Don't Want to*

Ask (but Need to Know). This book is filled with useful information, including suggestions for dealing with breakthrough bleeding. Within a relaxed and comfortable environment characterized by safety and trust, girls should be encouraged to ask any questions they may have about puberty and menstruation, although given the shame that often accompanies such a discussion, anonymous written questions may prove more useful in generating questions. Questions commonly include what it feels like to menstruate and to wear tampons, whether menstruation is painful, whether one can have intercourse or get pregnant while menstruating, and so on (Bell, 1987; Madaras, 1993). It is also useful to have girls who are comfortable talking to their mothers about these issues ask their mothers about their own menstrual cycle experience. Research evidence confirms some similarity in menstrual process and cyclicity between mothers and their daughters (Golub, 1992).

Girls also require information about the phenomenological experience of menstruation, about menstruation as a *personal* as well as physiological event (Rierdan, 1983; Rierdan et al., 1985). Same-sex groups of 8 to 10 girls who are at a similar stage of development can provide an excellent forum for such exploration, a forum in which feelings, fears, and myths regarding puberty and menstruation can be shared and explored. In dyads, premenarcheal girls can share with each other their "worst fears" about menstruation, and group leaders can help counter these fears by dispelling common myths and normalizing girls' apprehensions about menstruation. Using guided imagery, girls can be encouraged to live out their worst fears and find creative ways of coping with and working through these fears should they ever be realized. For example, a girl whose worst fear is that she may begin menstruating while in school, resulting in bloodstained clothing and feelings of shame and mortification, can be assisted in living through this scenario in a guided fantasy. Group members can serve as resources to each other and can brainstorm ideas and suggestions as to how they and their peers might best respond if their "worst fears" should actually happen. In a later session, the inclusion of older peers who have been living with the changes of puberty and menstruation for a few years can also prove to be very validating for the premenarcheal girl, providing her with role models of girls who have found positive ways to deal with the changes and challenges of puberty and to more comfortably incorporate menstruation into their lives and sexual identities.

For postmenarcheal girls who have experienced situations that resulted in feelings of humiliation or shame around their menstrual process, a guided imagery exercise or rewriting the script of their experience(s) can prove to be powerful tools in providing a corrective experience, helping the adolescent move past her feelings of embarrassment, shame, or humiliation, and assisting her in the re-creation of a more positive and affirming experience. Ambrogne-O'Toole (1988) emphasizes the value of having girls share their personal stories about menarche as a way of breaking down the secrecy that is characteristically associated with menstruation and normalizing the menstrual process. Encouraging the exploration of meanings and feelings about menstruation, with an emphasis on *both* the positive as well as the negative meanings associated with menarche, can help girls expand their frame of reference and begin to generate feelings of pride in, and respect for, this aspect of their womanhood. Having girls maintain a daily journal of the physical and emotional changes and sensations they experience throughout the menstrual cycle can be a useful tool in helping them become more attuned to their bodies and to the cyclical nature of their experience. Also, painting, drawing, and other forms of art can be creative ways to help girls explore the meanings that menstruation holds for them and may help expand their conceptions of the meaning of menstruation through the symbolic or metaphorical representation of this process in their artwork.

Another powerful tool that serves to counteract media messages about menstruation *and* to help generate the creation of more positive meanings involves having girls construct a collage of the messages portrayed in the media (particularly teen magazines) about menstruation. When constructing their collages and discussing these in a group, adolescent girls come face-to-face with the stark visual representation of popular media messages that characterize menstruation as a "hygienic crisis." After processing the impact that these messages have on the menarcheal girl and discussing the degree to which each girl takes in these messages, group members can be asked to create new collages that more accurately reflect their menstrual experiences. Participants can also be encouraged to select small ways in which they might reject the hygienic crisis hypothesis in their everyday lives, as a concrete way of rejecting the assumption that menstruation and its accompanying odors and sensations must be covered up. For example, an adult woman in a group that I led on women's sexuality selected to reject the "unnaturalness" of menstrual blood by refusing to hide her bloody tampons and pads in wads of tissue or innocuous brown paper bags. Her lack of willingness to "cover up" the signs of her menstrual process served as a powerful representation of her rejection of the messages she received from her culture. For the adolescent girl, symbolic rejection of these messages might involve refusing to hide her menstrual products in the back of the bathroom cupboard or insisting on using unscented pads or tampons, rather than accepting the contention that menstrual odors are distasteful. Depending on the individual girl's comfort level, even a small step toward rejecting these messages can be experienced as highly validating.

Bridging the Gap

There are few experiences in a girl's life subjected to as much secrecy and privacy as menstruation. Shaming can be a powerful tool of control (Ussher, 1989). The silence, secrecy, and innuendo that characterize our communications about menstruation are powerful in shaping adolescent girls' sense of feminine self-worth and value. As such, it is important for counselors to help take menstruation "out of the closet," to challenge this secrecy, and to help facilitate communication between adolescent girls and the significant people in their lives. Certainly, one of the most difficult areas of communication occurs for girls in attempting to talk with their parents about menstruation and the psychosocial changes that are associated with this event (Golub, 1992; Rierdan, 1993). Role plays and two-chair techniques are particularly effective activities to help girls begin a dialogue with their parents about their experiences and feelings regarding menstruation and the role changes and shifting expectations that accompany the onset of menstruation within their families and within our culture. This technique, or its empty-chair equivalent, is also quite useful in reworking painful interactions that have already occurred between adolescent girls and their parents. Counselors can role-model by assuming the role of the daughter and/or of the parent(s). In so doing, the client is provided with an opportunity to assume the perspective of her parent(s) and to get in touch with and practice what she would like to communicate to them. Letter writing is also a useful vehicle in opening up the process of communication between adolescents and their parents, a tool that can be particularly beneficial in maintaining the boundaries of comfort and security on the part of parents and their children, while also providing *both* parents *and* their daughters with a relatively safe avenue of communication about this often difficult topic. A poignant example of the power of this type of communication is the following excerpt from a letter an adult client received from her father when she began to menstruate:

> I know I'm not very good with words and I'm not sure how to talk to you about these things. But I wanted you to know how proud I am of you. I've watched with wonder over these past 13 years as you grew up and turned into the beautiful, sensitive young woman you have become. . . . I feel so fortunate having you for a daughter and love you very much.

Whenever possible, counselors can also work with parents, providing them with resources and material to help prepare their daughters for menarche, and helping them understand and cope with the psychosocial changes that typically accompanying this stage in an adolescent's development.

In attending to the issue of communication, it is also important for counselors to address the language of menstruation. As stated earlier, the majority of words used to describe menstruation are negative and derogatory (Golub, 1992; Unger & Crawford, 1992). Within a group setting or individually, girls can be asked to free-associate in response to words such as "menstruation," "periods," "menstrual blood," and so on, generating a list of euphemisms that are commonly associated with menstruation. Participants can then assign each word to a positive, negative, or neutral category, depending on its implicit tone and meaning. In increasing girls' awareness of the negative language associated with menstruation, a discussion can ensue about how this language makes girls feel about their bodies and about having their periods.

Participants can then be assisted in generating more positive menstrual words and metaphors that serve to reinforce the naturalness and acceptability of menstruation. For example, following completion of this exercise, one group of girls chose to call themselves "Sisters of the Moon" in honor of their shared womanhood and the significance to them of the connection between the 28 days of the menstrual cycle and the 28-day lunar cycle. Regarding this popular theme with strong historical roots (Eisler, 1988), other girls that I have worked with have chosen to refer to their period as being "in their moon." Still others have selected metaphors (e.g., "high tide") that have symbolic as well as personal significance. Although words such as "menstruation" or "menses" generally are placed in the neutral category by most adolescent girls, the use of medical language may well reinforce a medical model and hence disease-oriented perspective on the menstrual cycle. Girls should be encouraged to become creative in expanding their menstrual vocabulary.

Celebrating Womanhood

Contrary to popular notions of menstruation as a hygienic crisis or disease, it is important for counselors working with adolescent girls to acknowledge the more creative and affirming aspects of this uniquely female process. Certainly, many adult women will attest to experiencing enhanced energy and creativity at certain times in their menstrual cycles (Golub, 1992). In reference to the Yurok view of menstruation, Skultans (1988) reports on the belief that

> a menstruating woman should isolate herself because this is the time when she is at the height of her powers. Thus the time should not be wasted in mundane tasks and social distractions, nor should one's concentration be broken by concerns with the opposite sex. Rather, all of one's energies should be applied in concentrated meditation on the nature of one's life, "to find out the purpose of your life," and toward the accumulation of spiritual energy.

A much more powerful and affirming perspective on menstrual cyclicity, this view is one that is absent from the experience of most girls and women in our culture. As aptly stated by Skultans, "What in the right context might be released as powerful creativity or deep self-knowledge becomes, in the context of women's everyday lives in our societies, maladaptive discontent" (p. 172).

How can counselors help to create more affirming experiences to mark this "rite of passage" in the life of the adolescent girl? One way is to help premenarcheal girls design a ritual to mark the onset of menstruation and their corresponding entry into young womanhood, a ritual that is personally meaningful and that affirms their connection to the world of women (and perhaps to nature). It may be a ritual that includes significant others, such as friends and parents, or it may be one that the adolescent shares only with herself. It may involve something as simple as writing a poem or capturing the experience in a piece of artwork or music, or it may include a type of ceremony. For example, shortly after she began menstruating, one young client and her mother went on a women's retreat weekend together to celebrate their shared experience and signify the daughter's transition into the world of women. Another daughter I worked with recalled receiving a special piece of her grandmother's jewelry to mark her transition into womanhood, something she still cherishes today as a symbol of their shared experience and connection. Counselors can also encourage parents to be respectful of their daughter's needs and boundaries at this sensitive juncture in her development, staying open to her wishes, and taking care not to impose their own agenda in their enthusiasm to make her transition a positive one (Golub, 1992). Rituals may also be helpful for postmenarcheal girls, particularly when the onset of their menarche was met with little or no parental acknowledgment. Even those who can never realistically expect parental participation or acceptance of their new status can be encouraged to create rituals that include another significant, older woman (e.g., an aunt or a friend's mother), who by her age and status can serve the function of welcoming the girl into this new stage in her life.

Another powerful way in which counselors can help reaffirm the positive, life-affirming aspects of the menstrual process is by exposing young girls to some of the wonderful stories and literature about cultures and times in history when women's cyclicity was praised rather than feared. Some of the stories in Estes's (1992) book, *Women Who Run with the Wolves,* provide beautiful examples of this type of affirming imagery. Some anthropological literature and tapes, such as *The Goddess Remembered* (1990), can also help powerfully to underscore the importance of culture in shaping current attitudes about menstruation.They can expose the young girl to the ways in which her cyclicity and womanhood have been worshiped and valued for their connection to the central, life-giving forces of the earth (Mother Nature) and for their creativity—messages that are largely absent in our present-day communications about this basic aspect of female experiencing. Clients can be referred to Dena Taylor's (1988) book *Red Flower: Rethinking Menstruation,* in which she presents a positive and affirming view of menstruation as "a time for sleeping and dreaming, meditation, yoga, and dancing. A time for healing, being creative, figuring things out. A dark and inward time, a sexual time, a powerful time" (p. 109).

CONCLUSION

Both for women and men, menstruation serves as a cyclical reminder of our difference from men. It is a symbol of women's ability to give life—not of biological destiny but of biological possibility. While it is not without its requisite hassles, it is a truly remarkable aspect of human experience. Counselors can serve an important role in helping girls prepare for and appreciate this important aspect of their development and in presenting more positive, woman-affirming messages that reinforce the significance and value of this uniquely female process. As Weideger (1978) so accurately points out, "In order to change the social evaluation of women it is necessary to change our attitudes about the biological and emotional foundations of female existence, as well as our attitudes toward cyclicity and modes of hormone variation" (p. 233).

5

"BAWDY" IMAGE

From Subject to Object

> But, above all, the life to which the adolescent girl is condemned is that she must pretend to be an object, and a fascinating one, when she senses herself as an uncertain, dissociated being, well aware of her blemishes. Make up, false hair, girdles, and "reinforced" brassieres are all lies. The very face itself becomes a mask: spontaneous expressions are artfully induced. . . . The eyes no longer penetrate, they reflect; the body is no longer alive, it waits; every gesture and smile becomes an appeal. Disarmed, disposable, the young girl is now only an offered flower, a fruit to be picked.
>
> —SIMONE DE BEAUVOIR, *The Second Sex*

Based on their experiences in childhood, as discussed in Chapter 3, girls enter puberty with a preconceived set of perceptions about their bodies—a core body image. The physical changes experienced during puberty must be incorporated into each girl's evolving sense of herself as a person, as a woman, and as a sexual being. Girls' perceptions of the bodily changes they experience at this time are based on this core body image, on their current experiences of their body, and on the messages they receive about their developing bodies from significant people in their worlds. These external messages in turn reflect cultural expectations and attitudes toward the bodily development that characterizes mature womanhood. The often-dramatic physical changes of puberty invariably heighten girls' self-consciousness. This helps to explain why, particularly during adolescence, the reflected appraisals of others can profoundly alter or shape girls' perceptions of, and relationships with, their bodies—their core body image (Fisher, 1986; Pike & Rodin, 1991).

There can be little question that sociocultural influences are critical in contributing to the development of body image, particularly during adolescence (Hutchinson, 1985, 1994; Pike & Rodin, 1991). Adolescent girls are faced with attempting to accommodate the physical changes they experience during puberty with the reflected appraisals of others in their worlds. The sources that are discussed below are those that appear to be most significant in influencing how young women appraise their developing bodies. These include the expectations, reactions, and beliefs of family members and peers, and the images of feminine beauty portrayed in popular media.

CHANGING ROLES AND EXPECTATIONS: MESSAGES OF SIGNIFICANT OTHERS

Family members and peers provide an important set of external criteria against which girls evaluate themselves (Golombeck et al., 1987; Holmbeck & Bale, 1988; Isberg et al., 1989; Kamptner, 1988; LeCroy, 1988). This evaluation includes an assessment of their physical adequacy (Fisher, 1986). Mothers and fathers are especially influential in girls' body image development. As noted in the previous chapter, the relationships between adolescent girls and their parents often become quite strained during puberty. In particular, the period just after menarche is one of heightened stress between parents and their daughters (Hill, Holmbeck, Marlow, Green, & Lynch, 1985; Unger & Crawford, 1992). This has implications in terms of parents' effectiveness in communicating their expectations and perceptions to their daughters. Also, as daughters attempt to differentiate themselves from their parents during adolescence, this relationship strain may make it more difficult for them to accurately interpret the explicit and implicit meanings of parental communications.

Considerable attention is paid in the developmental literature to the importance of the mother–daughter relationship during puberty (Eichenbaum & Orbach, 1983; Holombeck & Hill, 1986; La Sorsa & Fodor, 1990; Pike & Rodin, 1991; Usmiani & Daniluk, 1997). However, adolescent girls' relationships with their fathers are also important in shaping their evolving self-conceptions. As their children's bodies start to take on a more womanly appearance, research suggests that fathers characteristically begin to distance themselves from their daughters (Unger & Crawford, 1992). Many fathers become increasingly uncomfortable with physical contact. They begin to redefine the physical and emotional boundaries between themselves and their child/woman daughters. Fathers appear to struggle with how to set appropriate boundaries around such things as nudity and physical contact with their maturing daughters (Unger & Crawford, 1992). They characteristically become more assertive and controlling of their daughters. Perhaps this is in response to their own concerns and uncertainty about the meaning and significance of the changes their daughters are experiencing (Hill, 1988). Whatever their motivation, girls are left to make sense of these changes in their relationships with their fathers. They may well interpret this distancing to be a consequence of their changing bodies.

Fathers also communicate their own values and perceptions regarding feminine attractiveness in their actions and in their reinforcement or admonishment of their daughters' physical appearance. Within girls' lives, fathers often serve as the representatives of the adult male world. Fathers who continue to reinforce the adequacy and acceptability of their daughters' appearance throughout the changes of puberty will help to strengthen positive physical self-perceptions. On the other hand, even subtle comments made by fathers about their daughters' increasing weight, size, or eating habits may be interpreted by girls as critical reflections of how their bodies are perceived by members of the opposite sex. Because of girls' heightened self-consciousness, they may interpret these messages to mean that their developing bodies are inadequate. This may serve to weaken their positive childhood body image, or may further reinforce their already negative self-perceptions.

Adolescent girls' relationships with their mothers are significant in the development of gender-role identity (Miller, 1983; Moen, Erickson, & Dempster-McClain, 1997; Rubin, 1984), body image, and self-esteem (Holmbeck & Hill, 1986; Isberg et al., 1989; LeCroy, 1988; Striegel-Moore, Silberstein, & Rodin, 1986; Usmiani & Daniluk, 1997). In response to their daughters' physical development, and in conjunction with their own midlife changes and accommodations, mothers are faced with negotiating new roles with their daughters who are no longer children but are not yet mature adults (La Sorsa & Fodor, 1990; Usmiani & Daniluk, 1997). Mothers are charged with the responsibility of preparing their daughters for entrance into womanhood. This entrance includes awareness of their changing bodies and what these changes mean in terms of their developing self-conceptions and their position in the world (Usmiani & Daniluk, 1997).

When girls are making the transition from girl to woman, mothers serve as role models and important sources of information. From mothers, girls learn about how their bodies measure up in the world of women. There is a close link between self-esteem, gender-role identity, and body image of mothers and their adolescent daughters (Isberg et al., 1989; La Sorsa & Fodor, 1990; Striegel-Moore et al., 1986; Usmiani & Daniluk, 1997). Daughters' observations and interpretations of their mothers' relationship with their bodies appear to shape girls' relationships with their own bodies. From mothers who are comfortable with and accepting of their own bodies, daughters learn to develop relationships with their changing bodies that are based on self-respect and acceptance. If, on the other hand, mothers are distressed by their own failure to meet impossible cultural standards, their distress may be transmitted to their daughters (Wooley & Wooley, 1980, 1985). Daughters may well become harshly critical and rejecting of their own bodies. If mothers experience shame about their bodies and are disconnected from this embodied aspect of their experience, they may inadvertently pass their shame on to their daughters (Usmiani & Daniluk, 1997). Mothers who themselves are products of a restrictive and oppressive socialization may inadvertently reinforce unrealistic cultural standards of beauty or attractiveness in their implicit or explicit communications with their daughters. In underscoring the importance of girls' relationships with their mothers Chernin (1986) suggests: "The problem with female identity that most troubles us, and this is most disguised by our preoccupation with eating and body size and clothes, has a great deal to do with being a daughter and knowing that one's life as a women must inevitably reflect upon the life of one's mother" (p. 37). Bonita Brigman (1994) discusses the legacy of embodiment that is passed on through generations of women in families, including mothers, grandmothers, sisters, and so on.

However, this is by no means a one-way street. Daughters also bring their own developing self-constructions and beliefs to these interactions. Depending on their assessment of the adequacy of their mothers' bodies, girls will evaluate their own bodies as adequate or inadequate. This does not mean they necessarily want to mirror their mothers' images. Quite the contrary for some daughters, it may be in their physical difference from their mothers that they evaluate their bodies as adequate. They may be very accepting of the traditional values related to the standards of physical appearance for women that were reinforced in their families, or they may rail against these proscriptions in their attempts to define themselves as different from their mothers.

The responses of both mothers and fathers to their daughters' developing bodies will also be influenced by parents' fears for their children's safety. While the risk of physical and sexual violence is ever present in the minds of parents from the time their children are young, that risk increases as girls begin to exhibit the physical characteristics of mature womanhood. As girls venture into the adult world in adolescence, parents are confronted with the harsh reality that their daughters' changing status as young women and changing bodies puts them at greater risk of being considered sexual prey. Changes in body shape and size, combined with social pressures to adorn the symbols of sexual maturity in terms of makeup, clothing, mannerisms, and so on, place the adolescent girl at greater risk of being assaulted. Research evidence confirms that postmenarcheal girls are more likely to wear makeup and bras, to shave their legs, and to act and be treated as older than they are (Golub, 1992). Although emotionally they may still be children, in their attempts to "try on" the accoutrements of adulthood, they may appear to be much older and more sexually mature than they actually are. It can be difficult, then, for parents to find a balance between validating the changes in their daughters' bodies that herald their entrance into the adult world, while at the same time preparing them to deal with the increased vulnerability that accompanies physical and social development during adolescence.

Parents may be very accepting of the developing bodies of their daughters. They may be quite constructive in helping their daughters cope with the psychosocial and physical implications of pubertal changes. This still may not be enough to circumvent the powerful impact of other influences outside of the family that result in many girls appraising their bodies in a harsh and critical manner. In the words of one woman,

> "No matter how accepting my family is, I still live with those outside messages. I still conduct myself in a world that has a particular ideal. It's really hard to walk away from that and say no matter what you think I should be, I know who I am. . . . It's great to have those people in my life initially who tell me that I'm OK. That's a real good start, but it's not enough."

As noted in Chapter 4, peers in particular are a tremendously important source of influence in girls' developing physical self-conceptions during puberty. At this stage in their development, teenage girls are often acutely receptive/sensitive to the opinions of others. Adolescent girls draw their cues for appearance and behavior primarily from their peers (Laws, 1980). Their sense of identity and self-esteem is very closely tied to peer-group acceptance. This approval is contingent upon similarity of experience and viewpoint.

During puberty, girls turn to their peers as a basis for assessing the timing and adequacy of their own appearance and physical development (Golub, 1992; Rierdan & Koff, 1985). The style and color (or colors, as the case may be) of their hair, their manner of dress, if and where they pierce their bodies, and whether they sport tattoos are all signatures of their group membership. This need for identification helps to explain some of the difficulty experienced by the early maturer, and by girls who physically mature quite late relative to their peers (Attie & Brooks-Gunn, 1989; Petersen, 1983; Rierdan & Koff, 1985; Rodin et al., 1984). Being developmentally out of sync with their peers makes it more difficult for these girls to "fit in."

Peer-group membership can also serve as a buffer against the assessments and criticisms of others during this critical period of identity development and self-definition. In this way, negative comments about their developing bodies from friends and acquaintances outside of their peer group may be taken in, but generally have less impact in girls' self-assessments. Comments from friends within their peer group, however, are very influential in adolescent girls' assessments of the adequacy of their bodies and appearance. The opinions of peers are central in girls' developing self-constructions. For example, many parents of teenage girls can probably recall how a particular piece of their daughters' valued clothing was permanently retired after only one wearing, because of an offhanded comment by a valued peer that their daughter interpreted as being critical of the item in question. The same is true for comments about weight, size, and physical appearance. Based on the direct or indirect comments of friends, many girls restrict their eating or take up smoking in an attempt to conform to the values and standards of their peers. In her personal and collective accounts of adolescent sexual experience and bodily development, Wolf (1997) notes the power of peers in shaping girls' experiences of their developing bodies, particularly during early adolescence, before the gaze of sexual intimates becomes more critical. Wolf quotes a woman she interviewed: "No one has shamed my body like women have. The shaming experiences I have had, when I was just beginning to develop, were from other girls first" (p. 45). The power of peer communications and values cannot be underestimated in the development of body image and esteem during adolescence (Isberg et al., 1989; Laws, 1980; Pike & Rodin, 1991).

Research suggests that girls who show the characteristic physical changes of weight gain and breast development before the other members of their peer group, and who begin to menstruate early, find this transition particularly problematic (Attie & Brooks-Gunn, 1989; Golub, 1992). During adolescence, girls feel a tremendous amount of pressure to "fit in." To do so requires physical and behavioral conformity. Such conformity is more difficult for the girl whose early physical development triggers a host of psychosocial changes. Early developers can be propelled into womanhood without the requisite social and emotional maturity and peer support necessary to cope with these changes. Not surprisingly, girls who mature early have lower self-esteem, poorer self-image, higher self-consciousness, and a more negative menarche than those whose maturation is more consistent with the members of their peer group (Attie & Brooks-Gunn, 1989; Rierdan & Koff, 1985). According to Unger and Crawford (1992), "The early-development girl faces a double handicap. She is in a minority vis-à-vis her peers, and her physical changes have socially ambiguous implications. Her difficulties in comparison with comparably aged boys and later-maturing girls illustrate the contradictions implicit in being a mature woman in our society" (p. 287). Girls who experience late maturation, unlike their early-onset counterparts, appear to fare much better socially. They have a greater level of emotional and psychological readiness in dealing with these changes. They also have the added advantage of watching their peers negotiate this transition first (Golub, 1992).

Other factors that reportedly mediate girls' reactions to the changes of puberty include class and race. White, adolescent girls experience greater psychological disruption in response to early development and menstrual onset than black, adolescent girls of the same age and class (Simons & Rosenberg, cited in Unger & Crawford, 1992). However, white, adolescent, middle-class girls appear to adapt more comfortably to early maturation than their working-class counterparts (Golub, 1992). This may be due to the differing social expectations and responsibilities that accompany physical maturation for girls in the working classes.

This discussion of family and peer influences in the developing self-constructions of adolescent girls during puberty would not be complete without attention to the importance of language. The words most often used to describe young women who meet the current cultural standards of thinness and acceptability include "slim," "slender," "petite," "slight," "attractive," and "svelte," to name just a few. A girl who does not meet these cultural standards of slenderness, or who is experiencing the increase in body fat that is characteristic of pubertal development, may be referred to by significant others as "chubby," "hefty," "chunky," "stocky," "large," "big-boned," "stout," "husky," "pudgy," "plump," "heavy," "cuddly," or "voluptuous." If her body size is particularly disparate to the cultural standards, she may be called "rotund," "immense," "overweight," "fat," or "obese." Those who use words as weapons may refer to the pubertal girl as a "pig," "cow," "porker," "pork chop," or "oinker," all references to meat-producing animals that are bred for their large size. In a society that perpetuates a cult(ure) of thinness, these words are often more powerful mechanisms to hurt and control than being called stupid. When girls are admonished for their weight or appearance by parents, family members, or peers, even in jest, feelings of shame and inadequacy are often the consequence.

OBJECTS OF DESIRE: MEDIA MESSAGES

During puberty, when girls begin to look to sources outside of the family for information and guidance about what it means to be beautiful and desirable, they need not look far to find one of the most pervasive and significant sources of indoctrination into prevalent sociocultural attitudes toward female appearance—the media (Kilbourne, 1994; Rodin et al., 1984). Bartky (1990) and others (e.g., Faludi, 1991; Wolf, 1991) underscore the "growing power of the image in a society increasingly oriented toward the visual media" (Bartky, 1990, p. 80). Media messages are virtually everywhere. They are on billboards and television, in movies and rock videos, and in grocery stores and shopping malls. The $1.3 billion advertising industry tutors young women in the nuances of obtaining the "right look." As one woman said in reference to her teenage daughter,

> "My 14-year-old brings home one of those teen magazines. She picked up another one today, *Vanity Fair.* You know, I mean big glossy magazines. She goes into the bathroom for a long time, and when she comes out, she has transformed her look—and I'm not just talking makeup. It's her essence, to come out with the same nuance as the magazine cover."

This woman also commented on the connection between her own insecurity about her midlife body and her daughter's desire to redefine her image based on external standards.

> "And I do the same thing. I still put on my nuance, or my mask, or my presentation. . . . I don't sit in front of the mirror without any makeup or without anything done, and just look at myself and say I love you and I accept you just the way you are. Maybe I can't. . . . Maybe my daughter and I are really doing the same thing."

What is particularly striking about the current female images being promoted in the media is the increasing emphasis on excessive thinness. Today's popular models are waif-like creatures whose body size and shape represents only 5% of women in the normal weight distribution (Kilbourne, 1994). The current reality of at least 95% of American women is not represented in the media. When they measure themselves against these ideal images, many girls and women feel woefully inadequate (Grogan, Williams, & Conner, 1996). So demanding is our present cultural ethos of thinness and restraint that it requires a $20 billion cosmetics industry and an $8 billion diet industry to maintain (Wolf, 1991). According to Kitzinger (1985), the message to women is clear: "You are deceiving yourself if you think that what you are is good enough. You are more inadequate than you realize" (p. 184).

Adolescent girls who are faced with matching their development against these largely unattainable standards of physical beauty and appearance that are promoted within our culture are clearly at risk of developing distorted and negative perceptions of their bodies. Many develop relationships with food and with their bodies that are ambivalent at best and highly destructive at worst. In a study of 203 adolescent girls between the ages of 14 and 18 years, Storz and Greene (1983) found that 83% desired to lose weight, even though 62% fell well within the normal weight range for their height and sex. In light of the messages young women receive from their culture "extoling the virtues of slenderness while promoting a fear of fat" (Dionne, Davis, Fox, & Gurevich, 1995), it should come as no surprise that a drop in self-worth, negative body image, and serious preoccupation with food and weight are significant problems for many adolescent girls (e.g. Brown & Jasper, 1993; Gilligan, 1991; Steiner-Adair, 1986). From the portrayal of girls and women in the popular media, girls learn that they are literally and figuratively to take up as little space as possible, and that their bodies are their tickets to a successful life (Currie, 1997). Their success, however, is contingent upon their ability to control nature through personal denial and restraint.

Adolescence is a time when body image dissatisfaction and eating disorders have their genesis for many young girls (Attie & Brooks-Gunn, 1989; Fabian & Thompson, 1989; Mendelsen & White, 1985). The indoctrination into restraint that generally begins in childhood is reinforced by the media, particularly during adolescence, in terms of what and how much girls eat. When the only available images they see are of tall, thin young women with perfect, air-brushed complexions, they cannot help but feel insufficient. Unaware of the increased fat production during puberty, many girls feel they are personally responsible for the changes in the size and shape of their bodies based on their lack of restraint and control. They believe that the pimples on their skin or the condition of their hair is a result of their inadequate diet. They come to believe that the inability of their bodies to replicate the cultural ideal reflects their own personal inadequacy. For many girls, this results in a type of hypervigilance about what they put in their mouths. Many learn early to count calories and to monitor their "appetites." Intense and sometimes debilitating feelings of guilt and shame are often the price of "failure."

There is growing evidence that increasing numbers of adolescent girls express dissatisfaction or discomfort with their bodies. Research confirms that the unrealistic images portrayed by photographic models in the popular media are a primary factor in contributing to decreases in body-esteem and satisfaction for young women (Grogan et al., 1996). Negative body image is one of the greatest risk factors in the development of eating disorders (Boskind-White & White, 1983; McKinley & Hyde, 1996). Estimates indicate that 10–15% of adolescent girls develop a full-blown eating disorder (Fabian & Thompson, 1989; Striegel-Moore et al., 1986). The onset of eating disorders is most significant for women during their adolescent struggle for identity, when their bodies undergo considerable change.

White women in particular appear to exhibit more body image dissatisfaction and weight preoccupation than black or Native American women (Unger & Crawford, 1992). Eating disorders such as anorexia have been primarily identified in the white female population (Dolan, 1991). This may be related to the preponderance of images in the popular media of women who are "white, Western, and wealthy" (Chapkis, cited in Wooley, 1994, p. 37; Plous & Neptune, 1997). Bodily dissatisfaction appears to be greatest among the women who are the targets of fashion ads, "white women who are old enough to have some money to spend, and still young, powerless, and insecure enough to be manipulated by the criticisms implicit in fashion adds" (p. 19).

The incidence of eating disorders appears to be spreading, however, across class and ethnic boundaries (Steiner-Adair, 1986). McKinley and Hyde (1996) underscore the importance of not concluding that body dissatisfaction is limited only to "young, middle-class, European-American women." They note how "researchers have only begun to explore the relationship of cultural body standards to body esteem in other groups of women . . . from diverse ethnic groups as well as other groups not usually thought of at high risk of body image disturbance, such as lesbians" (p.

211). Research by Thompson (1992) suggests that while the invisibility of certain groups of women (e.g., women of color, lesbian women, disabled women) in popular media images may appear to protect marginalized groups from developing a negative body image, these girls and women may actually be multiply oppressed. They are confronted with the reality that they do not meet the cultural standards of beauty, not only in terms of their size, but also based on their race, color, sexual orientation, or disability (Jaggar & Bordo, 1989).

Sexual objectification in the media is also instrumental in the body image dissatisfaction of many young women (Wooley, 1994). The naked bodies of women appear in whole or part in media images and ads everywhere. Parts of women's bodies are used to sell everything from cars to beer. The prominent message is that breasts, buttocks, and legs are women's most valuable assets. Since the so-called "sexual revolution" and perhaps in response to the gains made by women toward economic and reproductive autonomy, women's bodies have been undressed in popular fashion and in the media (Grant, 1994; Plous & Neptune, 1997). The percentage of women's bodies that is now characteristically available for consumption in the popular media has increased quite dramatically over the years, exposing over 90% of the body to public scrutiny. Even the slightest evidence of fat on "women's buttocks, breasts, hips, abdomens, and thighs" (Wooley, 1994, p. 37) are now evident. This leaves little room for visible "imperfections."

Wooley (1994) attributes part of girls' body image dissatisfaction to their culturally constructed embarrassment about their own naked bodies. For adolescent girls who are already painfully self-conscious of their changing bodies, continual exposure to scantily clad (half-naked) female bodies and body parts, and the objectification and commodification that this represents, necessarily heightens their sensitivity to their own bodily development and "inadequacies" (Fredrickson & Roberts, 1997; McKinley & Hyde, 1996). These images also engender feelings of embarrassment and shame. Bartky (1990) refers to women's shame regarding their bodies as "a pervasive sense of personal inadequacy that, like the shame of embodiment, is profoundly disempowering" (p. 85). She goes on to say that "sexual objectification occurs when a woman's sexual parts or sexual functions are separated out from her person, reduced to the status of mere instruments, or else regarded as if they were capable of representing her. To be dealt with in this way is to have one's entire being identified with the body" (p. 35). The "greater cultural scrutiny of the female body-as-object" (Franzoi, 1995, p. 420) may help to explain why young women appear to hold more positive attitudes toward their bodily functions (e.g., health, coordination, agility, etc.) than toward their body parts. This is especially the case for young women who identify more closely with stereotypical feminine attributes.

Media messages are quite paradoxical. On the one hand, they warn the young woman to be "afraid of her body because it can let her down by becoming fat, emitting odors and bleeding. At the same time she receives messages that her body is her passport to happiness" (Ussher, 1989, 1992a). Current media images reinforce the message that a girl's inherent value is in her ability to adequately package and sell herself. They promote a vision of feminine success and acceptability based on sexual objectification and physical desirability rather than female agency (Rodin et al., 1984).

Clearly this is a "no win" situation. The young girl learns that her body is both her asset and her liability. It is the site of her success and the source of her shame. As articulated by Greenspan (1983), "Woman in contemporary patriarchal society is fundamentally identified with her body. Her body is her power." Ironically, however, "if a woman's body is her only real asset, it is thus also her greatest liability" (pp. 164–165). She learns that she must exert control over her body even though she has no ability to control the physiological changes that are happening to her. The price of her success is deprivation and denial. The cost of her inability to do so is humiliation, shame, and a sometimes profound sense of inadequacy (McKinley & Hyde, 1996).

Being in a time of developmental transition, young girls at puberty may be particularly vulnerable to accepting the narrow and restrictive standards of bodily acceptability that are promoted in the popular media (McKinley & Hyde, 1996). "Our culture tells the adolescent girl, almost invariably, that her body is not good enough, that it is too fat, too thin, that her breasts are too small or too large, she is pear-shaped or top-heavy, her bone structure is wrong and so on" (Kitzinger, 1985, p. 184). The underlying theme is one of inadequacy. According to Kilbourne (1994), "An internal voice rages at us: 'You are too fat. You are ugly. Your thighs are like jelly. You have cellulite. You have pimples. You have vaginal odor. Your hair is drab. Your skin is dry.' We are taught to hate our bodies and thus learn to hate our selves" (p. 396).

SUMMARY: PROBLEMATIC MEANINGS

Western culture has for centuries placed the body at the center of women's value and usefulness. During puberty, then, girls come face-to-face with the cultural ethos of "Woman as Body" (Greenspan, 1983, p. 181). With pubertal development, girls are thrust from the world of "self as subject" into the world of "self as object" (McKinley & Hyde, 1996; Fredrickson & Roberts, 1997; Ussher, 1989). This shift results in a sense of opposition being set up between the experiences of embodiment and embodied sexuality that often remain a source of tension throughout the lives of girls and women. It is here that the seeds are sown for what Rodin et al. (1984) refer to as women's "normative discontent" (p. 267) with their bodies, a discontent that for many women persists long after adolescence. In reference to the bodily discontent of adolescent girls, Pipher (1994) notes how young girls are suffering needlessly by putting so much energy into changing their bodies. She argues that we need to revolutionize our values by defining attractiveness within much broader parameters.

The degree to which each young woman incorporates the negative and often paradoxical messages she receives from the significant influences in her life into her self structure and body image will differ based on the timing and pacing of pubertal changes, her self worth, and the extent to which her shape and size conforms to cultural standards. "Unique combinations of ethnicity, class, sexuality, age, and other physical and personal attributes undoubtedly create unique sets of experiences across women, as well as experiences shared by particular subgroups" (p. 174). However, the pervasiveness of the "cult of thinness" within North American culture and the experience of sexual objectification—"of being treated *as a body* (or a collection of body parts) valued predominantly for its use to (or consumption by) others" (Fredrickson & Roberts, p. 174), combined with the heightened self-consciousness of girls at puberty, makes it difficult for most to escape the tendency to turn a critical eye on their own bodies (McKinley & Hyde, 1996; Raudenbush & Zellner, 1997). Whatever their size or shape, or however accepting their parents and peer group are of their developing bodies, when faced with the unrealistic standards of attractiveness that are promoted in our culture, body image dissatisfaction is bound to be fostered for most adolescent girls.

Research confirms that early adolescence is a period of high stress for many young women. The rapid accumulation of fat and changes in physical morphology are often difficult to accommodate with cultural messages that reinforce the importance of thinness in defining female attractiveness (Gilligan & Brown, 1992; Gilligan, Rogers, & Tolman, 1991; Golombeck et al., 1987; Tolman & Debold, 1994; Ussher, 1989). Paradoxically, "On the one hand, adolescence presents girls with the challenge of coming to terms with their adolescent bodies; at the same time, society judges girls according to their looks and the culture encourages girls to change their body to fit a narrowly defined cultural ideal" (Steiner-Adair, 1986, p. 100).

So prevalent and powerful is this discourse around food and weight in women's lives that one writer suggests the language of fat becomes an avenue for the expression of a host of other, less acceptable feelings for girls and women. These include depression, anger, fear, loneliness, inadequacy, powerlessness, and insecurity. According to Friedman (1993), " 'feeling fat' (and its corollary: 'needing to be thin') becomes a way of describing the myriad situations a woman encounters in life in which she feels she has little control" (p. 288). Food intake becomes one of the few areas in life in which the young woman has, and is expected to exhibit, some control. The success of her efforts are gauged by her ability to force her body to conform to the largely unattainable cultural standards of thinness.

Not surprisingly, girls' levels of self-esteem and body image perceptions appear to plummet at adolescence compared to earlier and later stages of development (Davies & Furnham, 1986; Dionne et al., 1995; Rodin et al., 1984; Storz & Greene, 1983; Striegel-Moore et al., 1986). A national survey of adolescents in 1984 (cited in Rodin et al., 1984) indicated that normal development produces dissatisfaction with body weight for most adolescent girls. Increasing numbers of young women (and men) express dissatisfaction or discomfort with their bodies, causing Raudenbush and Zellner (1997) to suggest that "nobody's satisfied" with their bodies. Although black teens appear to be generally more satisfied with their bodies, "many middle-class blacks who are assimilated into the white culture . . . want to be thin, thinner, thinnest" (Chapman, cited in Schneider, 1996). Increasingly, adolescent girls have eating disorders, obtain cosmetic surgery to change their appearance, and attempt to lose weight through dieting, weight-loss programs, rigorous exercise regimens, and smoking (Wooley, 1994).

Unfortunately, it would appear that many young women develop a relationship with their bodies at adolescence that is at best ambivalent and at worst highly conflictual and self-destructive. This is not limited to the North American context. A very recent study of Australian teenage girls "demonstrated once again that young women are overwhelmingly dissatisfied with their current shape and rate their current figures as larger than their ideal and attractive figures" (Dyer & Tiggemann, 1996, p. 135).

In defining negative body image, Rodin (1992) includes behaviors such as avoiding looking in the mirror, distorted perceptions of body size, preoccupation with one's body, and feeling physically flawed and defective. People may portray a negative body image by distorting their internal visual representation of their body, and by harboring negative feelings such as shame and inadequacy associated with their bodies. They may display any number of behaviors that indicate dissatisfaction with their body, such as eating disorders, weight preoccupation, compulsive fitness regimens, cosmetic surgery, and so on.

Hutchinson (1982) refers to negative body image as being on a continuum "from complete dissociation or denial of the body to open warfare with the whole or parts of the body" (p. 59). During adolescence, girls characteristically experience confusion regarding the changes in their bodies and in what is expected of them as adult women (Martin, 1987).

> The transformation of a body during the pubertal changes of adolescence—which conforms to society's present stereotype of feminine beauty—into one which is heavier and rounder, and therefore perceived as less attractive, causes distress for many adolescent women. It is at this stage that a major split can develop between body and self as the young woman develops insecurities about a body which is seemingly out of control. (Orbach, 1985, pp. 38–39)

Ussher (1989) suggests that "it is during adolescence that the young woman first experiences a split between her body and herself: between her own experience and the archetype she is expected to emulate" (p. 18).

Reinforcing the importance of reflected appraisals in the adolescent's self-construction, in 1972, Berger (cited in Wooley, 1994) spoke of this split:

> A woman's self [is] split into two. A woman must continually watch herself. She is almost continually accompanied by her own image of herself. . . . From earliest childhood she has been taught and persuaded to survey herself continually. . . . The surveyor or woman in herself is male: the surveyed female. Thus she turns herself into an object—most particularly an object of vision. (p. 40)

According to Bartky (1990), these messages women receive regarding their bodies produce "a duality in feminine consciousness. . . . What occurs is not just the splitting of a person into mind and body but the splitting of the self into a number of personae, some who witness and some who are witnessed" (p. 42). "The adolescent girl, just beginning to grasp the role she is to assume becomes an object and sees herself as object; she discovers this new aspect of her being with surprise: it seems to her that she has been doubled; instead of coinciding exactly with herself, she now begins to exist outside" (p. 38).

The body becomes numb and begins to feel alien to her. She becomes disconnected from the experience of her somatic self and, in the process, is cut off from the pleasure, excitement, and joy that is a vital part of her experience of her body and of her embodied self. Given that the body is often a primary vehicle for the expression of sexuality, she is at risk of becoming disconnected from her sexuality in its most visceral (embodied) form. Debold (1991) suggests that "girls in adolescence experience deep dis-ease in and with their bodies" (p. 177). Strengthening the "bodily ego" and reinforcing a sense of connection and enjoyment in girls' experience of their bodies is an important component in their embodied sexuality. This is the focus of the next section of this chapter.

CHALLENGE AND CHANGE: CREATING NEW MEANINGS

The following exercises and techniques may be helpful in assessing adolescent girls' body image perceptions and the relationship between their experiences of their bodies and their evolving self-constructions. These exercises can be adapted to the age and level of development of most young women and may be used individually or in groups. Group work on these issues can be especially powerful in dealing with body image issues. Girls are often surprised and comforted to learn that the peers they perceived to be "more beautiful," or "better developed," also suffer the same insecurities and uncertainties regarding the adequacy of their changing bodies. In the words of one woman, "If only there had been some sorts of events for us, where girls were there to support one another about their changing bodies—*something,* saying that we were all of like gender, and this is what to expect and that there's . . . a *goodness* for us in it" (Wolf, 1997, p. 46).

Counselors should be aware, however, that issues related to body image are often quite "loaded" for young women. As indicated in the previous chapter, care must be taken when working in groups to ensure a high level of safety and trust before clients are asked to participate in this type of personal exploration. Also, it is important for counselors to attend to both the implicit and explicit communications of young women regarding their self-perceptions, self-esteem, and their level of satisfaction with their maturing bodies. Finally, counselors should ensure that clients are fully informed of the nature and intent of each of these exercises, that they are aware of the range of feelings that may be elicited as a result of their participation, that they have full control over stopping the activity at any point in the process, and that there is plenty of time following each activity to fully debrief and process the content and affect engendered by the experience.

Given the prevalence of body image dissatisfaction among adolescent girls, an assessment of eating disorders is necessary at the outset. There are a number of standardized instruments available for such an assessment (e.g., Eating Attitudes Test; Garner & Garfinkel, 1985), although a focused counseling interview can also be very effective in identifying serious body image disturbances. The treatment of eating disorders is a highly specialized area of clinical practice and one that is clearly beyond the scope of this book. For further information on the literature in this area, the reader is referred to Appendix B.

Mirror, Mirror

The construction of body image is about reflected appraisals. Although initially these appraisals are external, over time, an inner voice develops. An often harsh and critical internal chorus appraises the body as wanting and deficient. The internal voice monitors what girls eat and how they feel. Acknowledging and learning to silence this critical voice is an important step on the road to bodily acceptance.

Reflections (e.g., mirrors, photographs, symbols) can be powerful tools in assessing girls' perceptions of their bodies (Weiser, 1990). In particular, the ability to stand naked in front of a mirror and to allow the chorus to speak its truths can be very instructive in identifying negative self-perceptions, as well as building on positive self-perceptions. In her book *For Yourself: The Fulfillment of Female Sexuality,* Lonnie Barbach (1975) refers to this as "the body mirror exercise." In the privacy of their own homes, clients are asked to stand naked in front of a full-length mirror and monitor their reactions to their bodies as they slowly and carefully appraise the various parts of their bodies, as well as the whole, looking carefully at all angles. This exercise can be very difficult for clients. To give them some distance and objectivity, Meadow and Weiss (1992) suggest that the exercise be adapted by asking clients to pretend that they are from another planet and that they are looking at their bodies for the first time. Using a guided fantasy and mental imaging, the exercise provides even greater emotional distance. However, counselors should exercise caution, as even this may prove to be too threatening or difficult for some clients in the early stages of counseling.

Assuming that clients are comfortable with proceeding with the exercise, they are instructed to tap into the evaluative voice that they carry within them as they assess each part of their bodies (including their hands, feet, hair, face, eyes, and so on, as well as their breasts, buttocks, stomach, and hips). They are asked to note not only those areas that make them want to avert their eyes, but also those parts of their bodies that they assess to be attractive and appealing. When they have thoroughly appraised their bodies, clients are then asked to systematically review each part of their bodies, from head to toe, and write down their positive or negative evaluations, and, where possible, to try to identify the source of these evaluations. For example, a client may be particularly critical of her hips or stomach, making comments such as "too fat," or "too wide," but she may appraise her hair or her eyes as being "shiny" and "bright."

After the exercise has been completed, it is important in the subsequent individual or group session to process this information with the client, first asking her to share her response to the experience of doing the exercise, and then discussing her reactions to the various parts of her body. Engaging clients in a discussion of the source and strength of their self-evaluations (media, parents, peers, etc.) will provide useful information in working to disempower some of the more negative influences on their self-perceptions and reinforce the strength of the more positive sources of influence, including within the clients themselves. It is often particularly helpful for counselors to disclose some of their own reactions to completing this type of exercise (and their own appraisals of their bodily strengths and deficiencies), helping the client to appreciate that her struggles are not unique to her but, rather, are part of women's shared fate in a society that objectifies the female body.

Counselors can then ask clients, having had an opportunity to assess their physicality, to draw a picture of their bodies as they visualize them, and to color the parts that give them the most pain and discomfort, and the parts that give them the most joy. Both of these exercises are extremely useful in helping to assess body image perceptions and the degree to which the critical voice of others has been internalized. Counselors should also be alert to themes of bodily objectification and disconnection, the experience of being separated from their own experience of their bodies that may be manifested in young women's inability to separate the messages of others and their own internal evaluations of their embodied selves.

Parts Party

This activity is particularly useful for girls between the ages of 10 and 14, who are dealing with the physical changes of puberty. The purpose of this activity is to assess their awareness of their bodies and to identify their comfort and discomfort with particular body parts. In this activity, attention to the body parts girls select to focus on or ignore will provide important information about their beliefs, feelings, and self-perceptions. This will also be useful in assessing areas of potential misinformation and/or difficulty. This activity may be undertaken individually. It is also very powerful in a group, although, as with many of these exercises, group comfort and safety must first be established.

Assuming the activity is conducted in a setting of 8–10 girls of a similar age, the group leader should introduce the activity by indicating that each group member is invited to a "Parts Party." Depending on the objective of the group leader(s), the theme of this party may be on "scary" or "taboo" body parts, on the body part(s) each participant is most (or least) comfortable with, on the parts that are hardest to talk about, on the parts that most define them as girls, and so on. Clearly, the variations are numerous, with each adaptation providing slightly different information regarding girls' perceptions of their own bodies and their relationship to particular parts of their bodies. The group members themselves may participate in setting the agenda, based on their own interests and level of comfort in sharing their feelings about their changing bodies and developing sexuality.

Having identified the theme of the "Parts Party," the facilitator asks the participants to assume that they are invited to a party where they are to come as a particular body part related specifically to the theme (best part, worst part, most shameful part, most interesting/exciting part, etc.). While at the party, the participants are instructed that they must relate to each other, *without words,* "as if" they personify that body part—using body language, motions, and sounds that are specific to the body part in question and to girls' feelings regarding this part of their body. Based on how they present themselves, verbally and nonverbally, it is the responsibility of the other "guests" at the party to identify the body part each girl has brought to the group *and* the predominant feelings of each girl related to this aspect of her body. Participants can carry with them a small placard indicating what body part they are, which can be relinquished to the person who correctly guesses the "part" that they are playing.

In observing the activity, the group leader can learn a great deal about the meaning and feelings associated with particular body parts for the girls in the group. As well, particular issues each girl may have in negotiating her relationship with her body may be identified. One of the primary benefits of this exercise is found in doing the "postmortem" (debriefing) after the party, when the group members have an opportunity to discuss their experiences of having their identities represented by and limited to a particular body part. Group leaders can help identify girls' common areas of discomfort, and emphasis can be placed on the difficulty in accurately communicating about their bodies without the appropriate and accurate language. Also, misconceptions regarding particular body parts and their functioning can be corrected.

Party-Perfect

The following is an adaptation of an exercise, called "The Fat and Thin Fantasy," proposed by Suzie Orbach (1978) in her book *Fat Is a Feminist Issue* (pp. 140–142). The purpose of this exercise is to help explore the meanings and feelings clients hold related to body size, in terms of being perceived as fat or thin. The completion and subsequent processing of this exercise lends itself well to group work, although it can easily be adapted for work with individuals. In the first stage of the activity, clients are put through a basic progressive relaxation exercise to facilitate a level of calm and centeredness. When clients feel ready, they are guided through a fantasy in which they are to imagine themselves at a party filled with people whose opinions are important to them (parents, peers, intimate friends, etc.). They are asked to imagine that as they enter the party, they stop briefly to look into a mirror in the hallway and realize that they are much larger than their normal body size. They are asked to take note of their size and their reactions to looking in the mirror. How are they dressed? Are they comfortable with their size? Do they want to hide or escape? How do they feel about being here? The fantasy continues, and they are asked to join the party, which is now full of laughter and cheer. There is plenty of food and spirits, and they are asked whether they feel comfortable partaking in this cheer. What are they drinking? Do they feel comfortable eating? As they experience being at the party, they are asked to keep track of their interactions with others. Do others initiate contact, or do they? Are they easily invited into the group, or are they left out? Do they feel welcomed, or do they feel like an outsider? They are asked to take note of how others react to them and their body. They are asked to take note of how they feel being in this large body and in this room. Then, they are asked to imagine that all the fat is melting off their bodies, and they are now as thin as they had every hoped to be. They are at the same party and are asked the same questions about what they are wearing, how they are feeling, their comfort level, and their interpersonal interactions with others at the party. When they have had a chance to take note of the differences in their reactions based on their body size and to sit with these differences, they are then asked to come back to their own bodies and return to the present.

When the exercise has been completed, it is important to debrief and process the experience with the other members of the group. Participants should be encouraged to share their fears and expectations of being in a "fat" body and being in a "thin" body. Group leaders should attempt to draw parallels between the beliefs and expectations of the group members while also highlighting the pervasiveness of the myths and stereotypes that are commonly held regarding women's bodies and body size. In debriefing the exercise, it is important to note the size that participants selected to be for the "thin" portion of the exercise, the size they "always hoped to be." It is also important to explore their expectations of what they believe being this thin would actually *mean* to them in terms of their comfort with their bodies and their relationships with significant others. During this processing, group leaders can assess the *meaning* of "fat" for individual members of the group. Subsequently, participants can be asked to go back into the fantasy, with the bodies they presently inhabit. Their experience of living in their current bodies can then be explored. During this exploration, participants can be encouraged to identify a metaphor that represents the relationship that they presently have with their bodies. They can then be asked to identify a metaphor that represents the type of relationship they would ideally *like to have* with their bodies.

Clothing is also an important indication of the way young women experience themselves and their bodies. Clothes make a statement about how girls feel about themselves in their bodies. It is helpful for counselors working with adolescent girls to keep a portfolio of pictures of girls dressed in different types of clothes (e.g., baggy and nondescript, skin-tight, short, long, flamboyant, dull, bright, colorless). As the counselor goes through the pictures one by one, clients can be asked to answer the following question for each: "Given the clothes she is wearing, how do you think this girl is feeling about her body, about herself, and about her life?" Having reviewed the pictures, clients can then be asked to "take a mental walk through their closets at home," asking themselves what their clothing tells them about themselves and about the feelings they have toward their bodies. Counselors can then engage clients in a discussion of the meaning of the clothing they wear, what their clothing communicates to others about how they feel about themselves, and about their relationships with their bodies. In the ensuing discussion, it is important to emphasize how dressing in ways that celebrate their bodies can help to facilitate feelings of pride and pleasure, and serve as an antidote to shame.

Feeling Full-Up

When working with adolescent girls around issues of body image, it is also important to assess their relationship with food. The prevalence of eating disorders is alarmingly high among adolescent girls (Brown & Jasper, 1993; Brumberg, 1989; Dolan, 1991; Fallon, Katzman, & Wooley, 1994; Hirschmann & Munter, 1995; Steiner-Adair, 1986, 1991). Many authors contend that food is actually a metaphor for girls to cope with and express many of their unacceptable feelings such as anger and rage, and their discontent with other aspects of their lives (e.g., Chernin, 1986; Friedman, 1993; Roth, 1982). Consistent with the theoretical model proposed throughout this book, it is important to determine the meaning of food in the lives of girls. The following activity is an adaptation of a "Letters-to-Food Technique" proposed by Mariette Brouwers (1994). It can help counselors to identify the dynamics of girls' relationships with food and to understand the symbolic meaning of food in the lives of young female clients.

Prior to initiating this exercise, it is helpful to first situate clients in terms of the many complex ways food plays a role in their lives. Beginning with a relaxation exercise, clients can then be asked to take a stroll through a typical grocery store. While in the store, they are to slowly walk through the store as they are guided through the various departments (vegetables, meats, dairy, bakery, etc.), observing the range of foods on the shelves and keeping track of their inner/gut reactions to the types of foods in each section of the store. They are asked to take note of the departments in which they feel most comfortable, and the ones in which they feel least comfortable. Having browsed through the entire store, they are then instructed to pick up a shopping cart and, in response to each of the feeling situations identified by the facilitator, select an item from the store that best represents that kind of food and put it in the cart. For example, participants may be asked to select food items that they desire when they are feeling "happy," "sad," "hungry," "angry," "silly," "carefree," "lonely," and so on. When the shopping list is complete, clients are asked to take a last look in their baskets, noting the types of food that they have selected and the purposes these foods serve in their lives.

Having completed this exercise, clients are then asked to write a letter to food, expressing the way they feel about food and the role of food in their lives. When completed, the letters can later be read aloud in the group, or they can be processed individually. In either case, it is the role of the counselor to help identify the salient themes that emerge from the letters. Themes that may be identified include a sense of hatred, feelings of being out of control, feeling trapped, food as comfort, and so on. Identification and discussion of these themes provides valuable information about the meaning and purpose of food in the lives of adolescent girls.

A central task of working with young girls at adolescence, then, is to help these young women cope with, understand, and ultimately become comfortable with the physical and corresponding psychosocial changes that are a part of their development during puberty. It is important to remember that the "cultural meaning of a pubertal event may be more important than whether it is observable to others" (Brooks-Gunn, 1988, pp. 1067–1069). Girls receive paradoxical cultural messages regarding their maturing bodies. Disconnection can result as a consequence of these messages, particularly for girls who mature early. It is necessary, therefore, to address the split in body consciousness that often occurs in adolescence, between girls' phenomenological experience of their bodies and what is culturally expected of them (Fredrickson & Roberts, 1997; Martin, 1987; Ussher, 1989, 1992b). It is also necessary to help girls deal with the sometimes debilitating sense of inadequacy and shame that is engendered by others related to their changing bodies during puberty and throughout their lives. In its most profound sense, shame "contains the derisive accusation . . . that one is at core a deformed being, fundamentally unlovable and unworthy. . . . It is the self regarding the self with the withering and unforgiving eye of contempt . . . a feeling not of having crossed to the wrong side of the boundary but of having been born there" (Karen, 1992, p. 43).

To help heal the split or dissociation between self and body, in which the body becomes an object of criticism and attack, reembodiment work that directly engages the physical body is necessary (Hutchinson, 1994). This work promotes a reconnection with girls' experiences of bodily pleasure and sensation that for most was a part of their childhood. According to Hutchinson, "to be embodied is to experience the body as the center of existence—not as a focus, but as a reference point for being in the world. It is to feel alive, to perceive bodily states as they change from pleasure to pain, from hunger to satiety, from energy to fatigue, from vitality and excitement to calm and tranquility" (p. 155). If girls are to feel centered in their bodies and move through the world with greater ease and self-confidence, it is necessary to help facilitate the "emergence of an authentic delight in the body" (Bartky, 1990, p. 42). If a sense of integration is to be achieved Bartky suggests that

> the personae who affirm the body must be strengthened. Those who are introjected representatives of agencies hostile to the self must be expelled. . . . As part of our practice, we must create a new witness, a collective significant Other, integrated into the self but nourished and strengthened from without. . . . This collective Other, while not requiring body display, will not make it taboo either; it will allow and even encourage fantasy and play in self-ornamentation. Our ideas of the beautiful will have to be expanded and altered. (p. 43)

In working with adolescent girls, then, the goal is to help them reconnect with their bodies, to trust and respect their bodily rhythms and messages, and to come to a place of self-acceptance, where the body and self can coexist in relative harmony. The following exercises are examples of ways to begin to achieve these goals.

I'm OK: Rejecting External Standards

The media are some of the more pervasive and debilitating sources of objectification and disempowerment for young women. As such, they are a necessary target in counselor's attempts to exorcize the demons that reinforce a sense of shame and inadequacy, and keep girls disconnected from an important source of their own power—their bodies. There are many ways to challenge media conceptions of women, but one that I have found quite powerful is to ask clients to bring in any magazines that they can get their hands on, preferably running the gamut from adult-oriented magazines such as *GQ,* to teen magazines, to magazines such as *Good Housekeeping, Life,* and *Time.* This material, particularly effective in a group format, is used by participants in an attempt to make a two-sided collage. On one side, they are to portray their lives as they are led to believe they should be, based on the representation of girls and women in the pages of these magazines. On the other side, they are to portray their lives (and bodies) as they actually are. As participants are completing this activity, it is important to ask them to take note of the types of images of girls and women that are projected in these magazines, and of the explicit and implicit messages that accompany these images.

When the collages are complete, each participant should be provided with an opportunity to share her collage with the others, discussing the process she went through creating her "ideal" life and her attempts to locate images that reflect her real life. In my experience in using this exercise with groups of girls and women, there is usually a paucity of images available in most magazines that reflect the bodies, lives, and experiences of most women. When asked, most participants, in fact, are hard pressed to identify the similarity of these *ideal* images with the lives of anyone they know personally. In particular, women of color and different ethnic backgrounds find that their images and lives are virtually invisible in most of these publications. This exercise is often a stark reality for the group members, one that underscores the artificiality of media portrayals of women's bodies and lives.

Another very useful exercise in reinforcing bodily acceptance, diminishing shame, and rejecting external standards of bodily acceptability involves a follow-up to and extension of the "Mirror, Mirror" exercise discussed earlier. In her book, *Body Love: Learning to Like Our Looks—and Ourselves,* Rita Freedman (1988) proposes an exercise called "Making Mirrors Work for You." Meadow and Weiss (1992) also suggest a similar exercise using mirrors to identify the areas of the body that a girl assesses positively, and building on this with strength affirmations. What these and other leaders of body image workshops suggest is that, as in the earlier exercise, clients be instructed to stand nude in front of a full-length mirror and again slowly scan their bodies from all angles. Clients are asked to choose one part of their body that they like and think is attractive (for some clients, this sometimes proves to be an extremely difficult request, requiring that the instructions be adapted; i.e., select one part of your body that you think is at least acceptable), and to focus on and admire this feature. They are then asked to come up with a word (e.g., silky, smooth, bright, solid, tight) or an affirmative statement ("These are proud shoulders," "These hips are sturdy hips," etc.) that best describes that part of their body about which they feel positive. Next, they are to close their eyes and picture this body part and how it is characterized by the word or statement that they have created for it. They are to repeat the part and the word or phrase until the two merge into each other, and the body part seems to take on the positive characteristic ascribed to it by the client—until the two become one. Having completed this part of the exercise, clients are asked to focus on a part of their body that they find less attractive/acceptable, and to attempt to find a positive word or phrase that they can apply to the part in question. Sometimes, the affirmation is less about attractiveness and more about utility (e.g., "These legs are strong legs—able to walk great distances," "These eyes are compassionate eyes—able to see the pain of others"). This exercise can be repeated several times over a period of many days or weeks, slowly progressing to the body part(s) that causes clients the greatest dis-ease. Clients can be encouraged to keep a list of the affirmations they make about the various parts of their bodies, committing themselves to speaking at least one affirmation each time they look in the mirror, rather than looking at their images with a harsh and critical gaze. In so doing, they can begin to set internalized standards against which to measure their acceptability, rather than relying on the external standards imposed by others.

Finally, an exercise that is particularly useful for helping clients to identify and learn to accept parts of their bodies that they feel are shameful or produce considerable discomfort involves a follow-up to the earlier assessment exercise. This is the activity in which clients are asked to look in the full-length mirror and identify the parts of their bodies that they feel the greatest comfort with, and those that they perceive most critically and harshly. For the purpose of this exercise, it is best to have clients identify a part of their body with which they are uncomfortable. Having identified this body part, clients can be encouraged to engaged in a two-chair activity, metaphorically placing the body part in the opposite chair, thereby distancing themselves from this part of their embodied experience. Clients should then be encouraged to have a conversation with the body part they have negatively targeted. Counselors can gently direct clients to tell this body part how they feel about it, why it causes them such pain, and what they need it to do to make the pain stop (e.g., become larger or smaller, longer or shorter). As the exercise progresses, clients can be encouraged to sit in the place of the body part in question, allowing themselves to feel what it is like for this part of their bodies to live with their accusations and rejection, and with the negative judgments of those in their external worlds (which is often a significant factor in girls' negative self-perceptions). Clients should be directed to begin a dialogue about healing and acceptance, exploring ways that they and these disenfranchised aspects of their bodies are in fact interdependent. They should be encouraged to explore the consequences of being "cut off" from each other. Depending on the specific goals, this very powerful exercise can be adapted to focus on the body part most associated with shame, the part that clients have disowned, and so on.

Remaking the Body Home

Learning to feel comfortable is difficult for any adolescent girl as she attempts to live in a body that is objectified, sized up, and frequently found wanting when compared to the impossibly thin, white, idealized images portrayed in the media (Fredrickson & Roberts, 1997; Wolf, 1997). Bodily disconnection and discontent are "normative" (Rodin et al., 1984) within North American culture. If young, female clients are to live comfortably in their bodies and be more fully in tune with their embodied experiences, it is necessary to help make the body a place of peace and harmony, rather than a site of combat and contest. This requires not only the rejection of the negative and disempowering messages of others, discussed earlier, but also facilitation of girls' experiences of bodily pleasure and connection, and the strengthening of the bodily ego.

According to Hutchinson (1994), to heal the split that occurs between a young woman and her body, reembodiment work that directly engages the physical body is useful. She recommends a psychophysical approach, developed by Feldenkrais, "that uses movement exercises to retrain the nervous system, enhancing body image and promoting embodiment" (p. 165). The emphasis is on facilitating clients' connection or reconnection with their subjective body experience, helping them "to develop respect for the integrity of their bodies" and to "feel more grounded in their bodies" (p. 166). She also emphasizes the utility of imagery as a clinical tool for "accessing primary-process material and affective memories" (p. 157), to explore meanings, to create new patterns and ways of experiencing the self and the world, and as an avenue to facilitate deep emotional healing.

Certainly, there are many ways that counselors may help young women clients become more engaged with and connected to their bodies, some involving relaxation and imagery, and some involving touch, movement, and sensory training (e.g., see Laidlaw & Malmo's [1990] *Healing Voices*). Depending on the comfort level (and physical capacity) of the young women in question, dance and movement can be used to help girls begin to reconnect with the experience of childhood, when they lived more comfortably and freely in their bodies. For some excellent examples of exercises that can be used to heighten body awareness and help clients connect with and learn to feel comfortable in their bodies, the reader is referred to Anne Rush's (1975) book *Getting Clear: Body Work for Women,* and Joan Borysenko's (1988) book *Minding the Body, Mending the Mind.*

In her chapter, "The Body at Play," Debold (1991) talks about "the unconscious, loose-limbed movements" of girls involved in the simple and unconstricted play of childhood, "singing, walking, eating fruit on the street, playing marbles." For many this was a time when the body's messages were "an invitation to play" (p. 173). For most adolescent girls, this was a time before they crossed the threshold into the adult world and lost this connection with the freedom and pleasure of living in their bodies without the heightened self-consciousness related to how their bodies measure up to external standards. To help young women reconnect with the vitality of their bodies, guided imagery, art, and photographs are very useful tools. Readers are referred to the work of Judy Weiser (1990) for examples of the many ways that photographs can be used to facilitate client self-awareness and change. For example, clients can be asked to draw a picture of themselves as children, or to select a photograph from their childhood, depicting a time and place when they recall feeling free and "at home" in their bodies (clients who have suffered considerable deprivation or trauma, or clients who are physically disabled, may find this request particularly difficult to fulfill, requiring the counselor to adapt the activity to the needs of the specific group members). Individually or in a group, clients can be asked to share their drawings or pictures, and to try to get in touch with the tastes, sounds, sensations, smells, and feelings associated with being centered and comfortable in their bodies. They can be asked to think of times in the present when they feel this way, as compared to times when they feel disconnected and alienated from their bodies. Counselors can help clients to explore the differences in these experiences, and to identify the factors that seem to facilitate or impede their sense of bodily comfort.

Simonds (1994) also offers wonderful examples of nonverbal modalities in the treatment of adult survivors of childhood sexual abuse, many of which can easily be adapted for work with girls and women on issues related to body connection, comfort, and ownership. Nonverbal exercise can serve as a powerful stimulus for self-awareness and can help girls identify the sources of dis-ease within their bodies (Debold, 1991). Guided imagery can also be used to help provide clients with the permission, space, and opportunity they need to experiment and play with their bodies as they did in childhood, "in a spirit of lighthearted joy" (Janeway, 1980, p. 18). They can be encouraged to return to these "safe places" during times when they are feeling particularly inadequate, ashamed, or disconnected from their bodies.

Finally, an important factor in girls' experience of discomfort in their bodies is the ever-present threat of sexual violence and the systemic perpetuation of the belief that girls and women are somehow accountable for the violence that is done to them. In reference to an attempted attack by a adult male on her way to summer camp, Wolf (1997) reiterates the painful acknowledgment of this reality:

> "What happened?" they asked. And I told them. But even as I told—using the only language I had—I understood that what had happened to me was not like what happens to children when someone has put a razor into an apple on Halloween. Here there was neither sympathy nor outrage. . . . There was an imperceptible withdrawal from me and my fear. . . . The tears I was not permitted to shed stung. They were a lesson to me: whatever the man had done, no matter how it had harmed me, no matter that no one had said this—it was all, somehow deeper than reason, my own fault. (pp. 32–33)

We live in a world in which men are not considered responsible for their acts of violence against girls and women. For girls to feel "at home" in their bodies, then, it is necessary to help them explore common cultural myths regarding the "type" of girl who gets sexually assaulted or who "deserves" what she gets, and the "type" of guy who is a "danger" to women. It is necessary to help clients find ways to reject the "woman as accountable" ethos that is so pervasive in the socialization of girls and women in North American culture. In a group setting, counselors can help girls identify and confront common rape myths in a number of ways. A method that I have found particularly useful is to create two case scenarios of a sexual assault, one in which many people would hold the victim accountable for the assault (dressed in tight, skimpy clothing; drinks too much at a bar; takes a ride home from a guy she does not know, etc.), and one in which the "woman as accountable" hypothesis is much less apparent (at home behind locked doors, out for a run in broad daylight on a busy street, attacked by a stranger hiding in the bushes, out on a date with a high school "sweetheart," etc.). Depending on the age and maturity level of the group members, they can actually be asked to create two scenarios. In one, the woman "deserved what she got." She "should have been more careful" or "should have known better." In the other, the victim is not viewed as accountable for the violation. Group members are then asked to assess the victims' responsibility for the attacks, rating their opinions on a scale from 1 to 10 (with 10 being very accountable). In the ensuing discussion, counselors can help young women examine the myths and misconceptions inherent in their attributions, and can counter some of these common beliefs with facts (data) about the actual incidence and circumstances of sexual assault. Challenging the accountability hypotheses is critical in this exercise. It is an important step in beginning to free young women from the burden of responsibility for living in a woman's body in a sexist and often violent world. In her book, *Changing Bodies, Changing Lives,* Ruth Bell (1987) also provides a list of common myths about rape (pp. 129–130) that counselors may incorporate into their work with young women.

As a follow-up to this exercise, it is useful to have clients read fiction or view movies for the purpose of identifying scenes describing the "token resistance response" (she says "no," but she really means "yes") and rape scenes in which a woman is portrayed as actually "enjoying" being violated and brutalized (e.g., Anne Rice's [1990] *Witching Hour* comes to mind). Having been sensitized to the prevalence and power of these rape myths, discussion of the pervasiveness of these myths in books and the popular media can prove to be very enlightening and liberating for young female clients.

My Mother, Myself (or In the Company of Women)

As indicated earlier, the literature suggests that there is a relationship between the body image perceptions of mothers and the ways in which daughters assess their developing bodies. The way young girls perceive and experience their relationships with their mothers may be particularly important during adolescence. Exploring the mother–daughter relationship may be a powerful tool in helping girls to understand and appreciate the significance of this relationship and of the relationship between lineage and girls' present embodied experiences (Debold, Wilson, & Malave, 1993; La Sorsa & Fodor, 1990).

The following is an adaptation of an exercise suggested by Judith Ruskay Rabinor (1994, pp. 280–281), which she uses in groups with girls who have eating disorders. The goal of this exercises is to help "honor the positive connection inherent in the mother–daughter relationship" (p. 272) and "deepen participants' awareness of how their body image development is interwoven with their relationship with their mothers" (p. 280). This exercise can be used individually or in groups to promote exploration of the mother–daughter relationship and to deepen daughters' understanding of, and appreciation for, the significance of this relationship in their own understanding of self.

This exercise can be undertaken in a group setting as a homework assignment between group sessions. Group members are instructed to spend some time browsing through family photographs. They are asked to select carefully a photograph of their mothers that "has something important to tell" them (Rabinor, 1994, p. 280), focusing on how their mothers felt about their own bodies and their lives.

During the next group session, there is a relaxation exercise and an opportunity to reflect on the photograph each girl has brought in of her mother. Rabinor (1994, p. 281) suggests that the group leader then announce the following:

"Your mother is the most important woman you will ever know."
"Your mother welcomed you to the world."
"Your mother welcomed you to the world of womanhood."

Participants are instructed to select a title for their photograph of their mother, based on what the title tells about their mothers and how their mothers felt about their bodies and their lives. Each girl is then asked to introduce herself to the group by stating her name, indicating that she is the daughter of (mother's name), and completing the following line with the title she selected for her picture: "I was welcomed to womanhood by (mother's name), (picture title)." Rabinor (1994) gives the following examples:

> "I am JoEllen, daughter of Meg."
> "I was welcomed to womanhood by Meg, Happy and Smiling."
> "I am Marnie, Daughter of Rita."
> "I was welcomed to womanhood by Rita, Angry at the World."

After all group members have completed this introduction, they should be asked to spend some time in the group (in pairs if the group is large) to talk about their experience of browsing through their family photographs and selecting the particular photograph of their mothers. They should be asked to examine their perceptions of their mother's body image and be encouraged to answer the questions: How do you think your mother's body is similar to and different from your own? How do you think your mother's feelings about her body and her life are similar to your own feelings?

While the mother–daughter relationship is considered by many to be important in girls' development, many other factors are also salient in shaping girls' body image perceptions during adolescence (Fisher, 1986; Jaggar & Bordo, 1989; Steiner-Adair, 1986, 1991). Counselors should take care not to ask questions that imply that mothers are accountable for their daughters' feelings about their developing bodies (e.g., Do not ask: How do your mother's feelings about her body *influence* your feelings about your body?). Little is served by blaming mothers for the experiences of bodily dissatisfaction of their daughters. Rather, the purpose of this exercise is to facilitate daughters' understanding of the genetic and psychosocial links between their own lives and embodied experiences, and those of their mothers. The purpose is to build bridges in these relationships, and to celebrate, not denigrate the mother–daughter heritage.

As a follow-up to this exercise, group members can be encouraged to examine the themes related to body and body image in their families, drawing links between their own experience of their bodies and the experiences of their mothers and their grandmothers. Brigman (1994) offers an excellent and compassionate example of this in her chapter entitled "Four Generations of Women: Our Bodies and Lives." The goal of this activity, which can be facilitated by the use of genograms or photographs, is to help young clients see the common threads in their experiences of their bodies and lives, and those of the other generations of women in their families. This review can help to decrease their sense of isolation, and to help them feel more connected to the lives, struggles, and strengths of these women—their ancestors—through their shared stories. Clients can be encouraged to identify one woman in their family who appears or appeared to live and move comfortably in her body, and to explore the ways this family member's experiences, personality, and way of being in the world are similar to her own. Clients who are unable to identify positive and affirming themes in the lives of the women in their families, or those who have little connection to the lives of these women, can be encouraged to look outside their families to other women they know and admire. They can be encouraged to identify the themes of embodiment and centeredness that they would like to emulate, which are apparent in the life of a significant, female role model.

CONCLUSION

The exercises discussed in this chapter are only examples of the many ways that counselors can help adolescent girls challenge the messages of objectification and inadequacy that they are faced with as they attempt to live comfortably in their changing bodies. With their emphasis on strengthening the bodily ego, these and similar exercises can reinforce the experience of bodily pleasure and ownership, and can help to establish a sense of familial inheritance and connection that is often lost in girls' transition to womanhood. When young women can look in the mirror with acceptance and appreciation rather than disdain, when they can honor the vitality, agility, and utility of their bodies, and when they can open themselves to the rhythms and range of sensory experiences that are a part of living in a woman's body, they will have come a long way toward embracing and owning their embodied sexuality.

6

WHO LOVES YA, BABE?

Sexual Intimacies and Expression

> Settle for nothing
> less than the
> object of your desire.
>
> Desire. The weight of. The weight of our
> desire. Then laugh, cry, but laugh
> more than you cry, and when you hold
> the world in your hands, love Her.
>
> —ALMA LUZ VILLANUEVA,
> *The Object*

The onset of menstruation and the physical changes that accompany puberty signify a girl's initiation into womanhood. In our culture, they also represent the attainment of sexual maturity. As long as girls are still child-like in appearance and physiological functioning, they generally escape the demands and expectations of mature womanhood. However, once they exhibit the characteristic signs of physical maturity, they are confronted with sorting out their emerging needs and desires against a social backdrop that presents often paradoxical constructions of female sexuality. In the words of one woman: "People come into their sexuality at different times. And people think that as soon as you get a woman's body, or something remotely resembling one, you're a sexual person" (Wolf, 1997, p. 129).

During adolescence, young women are faced with a challenging task. They must try to make sense of the sensations of their developing bodies in terms of their awakening passions and desires, and to incorporate these into their sexual self constructions. This process of sexual self-definition and understanding is complicated by the often-contradictory messages girls receive from the culture regarding the appropriate expression and nature of their emerging sexuality. According to Palladino and Stephenson (1990),

> Three major changes occur in adolescence which impact on the female's sexual development: she becomes aware of physical sexual impulses, she learns that her sexual feelings are not given validation by males, and she begins to question her right to sexual desire and her need to fulfill those desires. . . . Adolescence is a time when girls not only begin the experience of sexual maturation, but it is also a time when they begin to confront the barriers placed around their sexual selves. . . . (pp. 236–237)

Parents, peers, and the media appear to be particularly influential in shaping girls' understanding of their sexuality at this stage in their development (Gagnon & Simon, 1982; Laws, 1980; Moffat, cited in Unger & Crawford, 1992; Ward & Wyatt, 1994). The language of sex and the threat of sexual violence are also important factors in girls' developing sexual self-constructions and perceptions of choice. Let us look more closely, then, at both the explicit and implicit content of some of the more prevalent messages communicated by these sources regarding the sexuality and sexual expression of adolescent girls.

SEX AS LOVE: PARENTAL MESSAGES

As girls begin to show signs of physical maturity, parents are confronted with the reality that their children are entering a world that holds both promise and danger. They are aware of their decreasing ability to influence and protect their children from the dangers of the adult sexual world. Having been adolescents themselves, parents are very cognizant of the excitements inherent in tasting the "forbidden fruit." Yet they are also painfully aware of the potential landmines that their daughters must negotiate as they traverse this sexual terrain (e.g., unwanted pregnancy, AIDS, sexual violence, lack of emotional readiness, tainted reputations).

So how do parents characteristically handle their daughters' budding sexuality? Research indicates that mothers are the primary purveyors of sexual information in the family, although there are limits as to the aspects of sexuality mothers are comfortable talking about with their daughters. There are also limits to what daughters are comfortable hearing from, and sharing with, their mothers regarding their erotic feelings, desires, and behaviors. For example, in their study of the communications between 184 Stanford sophomores and their mothers, Yalom et al. (1982) report "menstruation, marriage, abortion, pregnancy, and love relationships with a male as the most frequently discussed sexual topics in mother–daughter conversations. . . . Masturbation, orgasm, multiple sexual relations, and love relations with a female ranked as the least frequently discussed subjects for both groups" (pp. 148–149). Reproductive pragmatics, then, and sexual behavior within the context of a socially sanctioned, loving relationship, seem to be easier subjects to broach for mothers and daughters. Topics related to the more "taboo" aspects of sexual and erotic behavior present a greater challenge.

Unlike their predecessors, most young girls today enter adolescence with a fair bit of specific information related to sexual anatomy and physiology (Andre, Dietsch, & Cheng, 1991). They are generally more informed about reproductive health and functioning (e.g., birth control, sexually transmitted diseases). For many reasons, however, not the least of which include implicit negative sanctions against preparing to become "sexually active," this knowledge does not necessarily translate into more responsible sexual behavior (Moore & Rosenthal, 1996). Girls' understanding of their sexuality and sexual relationships is often limited to the pragmatics of physical functioning and what they can glean from the popular media about the dynamics of intimate relationships (this issue will be discussed more fully later in this chapter). Many girls are relatively unprepared for the actual experience of sexual intimacy and for the range of emotions that accompany their sexual explorations and experimentation (Wolf, 1997).

In addition to concrete information, mothers also pass their sexual values and beliefs onto their daughters. In their role of preparing their daughters for the realities of the adult world, their communications frequently reflect the values of the dominant culture. These include beliefs about the appropriate context for sexual behavior, usually a loving relationship, as well as beliefs about girls' safety, responsibility, and accountability. Their freedom and comfort with their own sexuality and sexual expression are also implicitly and explicitly communicated to their daughters. Kitzinger (1985) underscores how the relationship between mother and daughter may be especially important in terms of daughters' embodiment of their mothers' way of sexually being in the world. She notes how mothers "visit on our daughters our unrealized dreams and longings. We burden them with our own unlived lives" (p. 186).

In their legitimate fears for their daughters' physical and emotional safety, mothers may inadvertently reinforce messages of sexual restraint. Mothers are also products of their own sexually repressive socialization. As such, even those who attempt to ensure that their daughters develop a sense of agency and entitlement in their experience of their sexuality often "end up unintentionally repeating both the disconnection and pain of their lives in their children's lives" (Miller, cited in Debold, 1991, p. 177). According to Debold,

> The transformation of the playing girl's body to the restrained woman's body marks a transition from mother's home to the man's world. The mother, friend of childhood and exemplar of womanhood, stands as a guide from the one body to the next. When she protectively warns her daughter of the dangers of desire in a violent androcentric culture—warnings that resonate loudly in countless images and ideas—the mother may unwittingly participate in her daughter's dis-ease with her body. (p. 181)

Alternately, some mothers may feel that their sexual development was prematurely truncated in early marriages, or that their sexual needs and desires remain unfulfilled in their current relationships. They may encourage their daughters to experiment and explore the boundaries of their own sexuality while still walking that fine cultural line between being sexually autonomous and liberated, and being promiscuous (Wolf, 1997). It is a difficult balancing act that few girls are able to master with ease (Fine, 1988).

And what about the role of fathers in girls' sexual education and development? As with menstruation, fathers appear to be conspicuously absent in the direct communication of information to their daughters about female or male desire and sexual experience. Parents, and particularly fathers, are reported to respond to the signs of sexual maturity in their daughters with attempts to "protect" them by restricting their access to sexual situations (Hill & Holmbeck, 1987). As noted in Chapter 5, fathers tend to become quite controlling of their daughters when they begin to display the physical signs of feminine maturity (Hill, 1988). They are often painfully aware of the cultural ethos that permits and encourages adolescent boys to gain sexual experience through the conquest of "certain types" of girls before settling into a long-term, committed relationship. Fathers do not want their daughters to be "used" in this way. Also, within certain cultural and religious groups, the responsibility falls on the shoulders of fathers to ensure that their daughters are not sexually "deflowered" prior to marriage (Omer-Hashi & Entwistle, 1995).

Fathers may also adhere to the long-standing cultural belief that it is their daughters' responsibility to maintain sexual propriety. They may believe that it is up to their daughters to limit the advances and actions of boys who would "have their way" with them. In this way, they may rail against their daughters' attempts to adorn the symbols of female sexuality, in terms of makeup, high heels, short skirts, and so on. Many fathers fear for their daughters' safety, reputations, and marriageability. Implicitly and explicitly they may communicate their fears.

Most parents are aware that "sexuality opens the daughter to the possibility of love as well as the danger of being labelled a 'slut' " (Debold, 1991, p. 173). While they may turn a blind and somewhat amused eye to the sexual experimentation engaged in by their sons ("Boys will be boys"), daughters rarely receive parental sanction for gaining similar sexual experience. Parents generally place more restrictions on their daughters' behaviors and movements than their sons' as they venture into the adult world during adolescence. They are concerned about their safety and their reputations. They also tend to set more rigid limits on the kinds of male and female friends their daughters are allowed to have.

Tolman (1991) notes the importance in many families of daughters being able to "wear white" for their weddings (a cultural symbol of chastity and purity). This reflects the continued cultural significance of "virginity" for girls. In spite of the relaxing of sexual mores over the last 30 years, it would appear that within most families, girls are still not given the same permission as boys to explore their sexuality, nor are they encouraged to experiment sexually. Unlike their male counterparts, girls are encouraged to restrict the exploration and expression of their erotic desires to the context of a committed, socially sanctioned relationship. Within their families, girls learn that it is their responsibility to rebuke the sexual advances of men and to guard their bodies, their virginity, and their reputations with care. They learn that the consequences of making a mistake rest squarely on the their shoulders, in terms of tarnished reputations, unwanted pregnancies, sexually transmitted diseases, and sexual violence.

SEX AS STATUS: THE MESSAGES OF PEERS

Peer influences become very critical in the developing sexual self-structures of girls during adolescence. During their teens, girls spend a great deal of time fantasizing, discussing, and exploring with their same-sex peers their ideas and beliefs about sexuality, sexual intimacy, and relationships. Within their peer groups, they try on different ways of acting and looking sexual, and of being "sexual" in the world. Indeed, the peer groups girls select as their referents reflect specific sexual mores, norms, and behavioral codes that fit their sexual self-conceptions or the sexual conceptions to which they aspire.

It is with their female friends that girls share their sexual fears, uncertainties, and anticipations. It is with their closest friends that they often experience their first real erotic and emotional intimacy outside of their families. In her book on adolescent sexuality, Wolf (1997) reflects on the emotional intensity of these adolescent friendships: "As adult women, those of us who are heterosexual sometimes have a sense of a lost Eden. We are determined to seek out a love as perfect again: a love at once so intimate and so charged; to be once more as teenage girls are when they are in love with each other" (p. 55).

Close girlfriends seem to serve several important roles in the developing sexuality and self-conceptions of adolescent girls. They are purveyors of information and wisdom (including information on contraception and sexually transmitted diseases). They are confidants and coconspirators. They are the confessors to whom girls turn to share their experiences of sexual pain, disappointment, joy, and delight (Andre et al., 1991; Lear, 1997; McKinney & Sprecher, 1989; Sprecher & McKinney, 1993). It is in reference to the sexual behavior and exploits of their friends that girls gauge their own sexual maturity. And it is to these relationships that girls often turn to process their early sexual experiences with boys and, in some cases, with other girls. In the words of one woman after she had "gone all the way" for the first time: "I would have loved to have called up one of my girlfriends to say, 'Something must be wrong with me because this feels *funny*' " (Wolf, 1997, p. 127).

Girls' peers can support or undermine their efforts to negotiate an authentic sexual identity and agentic sexuality. Peer-group pressure can force girls to engage in sexual activities that they are not yet ready for emotionally, most notably intercourse. Or group kinship and solidarity can serve to protect girls from the premature entry into the adult world of sex. Group identification can also be a powerful weapon to shun those who appear to transgress the limits of appropriate female sexuality in terms of their sexual behaviors or the focus of their erotic desires (McCarn & Fassinger, 1996).

> Young women tend, in their peer groups, to act out in the microcosm the splitting off of female sex from "legitimate" identity that the larger culture is intent upon imposing on them. We learn to identify the girl who most embodies that sexuality and do to her, in a form of scapegoating that is a ritual to ward off the fate she represents, what the culture is doing to us. (Wolf, 1997, p. 72)

"INTIMATE" PARTNERS: MIXED MESSAGES

Adolescence is indeed a heady time of life. Just as they are attempting to define themselves as individuals, with identities separate from their families, girls are also attempting to define themselves as sexual persons. In the sexual realm, it is a time filled with the raw heat, lust, passion, intensity, anticipation, excitement, and titillation. It is a time of being on the threshold of something that seems terribly significant. In adulthood, the depth, intensity, and power of erotic passion can reach new levels. However, it is difficult, if not impossible, to recapture the raw excitement and anticipation—the newness—of adolescent sexual awakening. Few adult sexual relationships are characterized by the months and sometimes years of adventure and exploration as girls first investigate the terrain of another's body and of their own erotic potential. And few aspects of adolescent development are more conflictual and paradoxical than sexual relationships.

Sex is the currency of opposite-sex relationships in adolescence (Lear, 1997). It is the socially sanctioned role of boys to encourage girls to let them sample the fruit, and the role of girls to resist the "harvest." If we view sexual behavior on a continuum from kissing and petting to intercourse, the dance between young men and women is often one of seeing how far along the road the two can progress before going too far to turn back. According to Kitzinger (1983), once they begin dating, adolescent girls today experience a tremendous amount of pressure to "go all the way"

(p. 181). It is important that they initially resist the mandate to "put out" or "come across" sexually, so that they do not appear to be too "easy" or "loose." They run the risk of being punished for their "indiscretions" in being labeled "sluts," "tramps," and "whores." It is interesting to note that boys and young men who have multiple partners and "casual" sex are more likely to be praised rather than condemned for their exploits. If adolescent girls act assertively on their own sexual needs and abandon themselves to their desires, however, they run the risk of being labeled "nymphos." On the other hand, too much resistance is also problematic. Girls who do not go all the way may be viewed as "frigid" or as "cock teases."

Eventually, a point is reached where there appears to be no turning back. Sometimes she gives in to "please" her boyfriend. Sometimes she finds herself in a situation where she feels powerless to stop her partner's advances. Sometimes she makes a conscious decision to "get it over with" and planfully initiates intercourse. And sometimes erotic passion and desire allow her to be "swept away" (Cassell, 1984). Unfortunately, for many girls, today, the erotic dance leading up to intercourse appears to be quite brief. While in the 1960s and early '70s petting was the most common adolescent sexual practice, more teenagers today see petting or "foreplay" as: "kid stuff. Believing that intercourse [is] the real thing, they . . . rush into bed with almost no sexual preliminaries. Between the instant ejaculation characteristic of teenage boys' sex and the absence of sexual preparation, many girls say they barely realize what is happening before it is over" (Thompson, 1990, p. 345).

In the absence of other rituals to mark their transition into the adult world, for adolescent girls (and boys), intercourse serves as a major turning point. As noted in Chapter 1, "going all the way" is the hallmark of sexual initiation in our culture. Among their peers, it is a sign of status and prestige. Having entered the realm of the sexual, which means having engaged in heterosexual intercourse, the girl is viewed by her peers as having become an adult. In their eyes, she has gained adult status. Paradoxically, however, in terms of cultural meanings, her male partner is perceived as having gained something in bedding a virgin (i.e., "her cherry" or hymen—like "notches" on the bedpost). She, on the other hand, is viewed as having lost something in terms of her innocence and her virginity.

It is hard to imagine how an experience that is so overpromoted and that is accorded such import can ever live up to the expectations placed upon it. Indeed, it would appear that for many adolescent girls, it clearly does not (Lear, 1997). Thompson (1990) interviewed 400 adolescent girls about their first sexual experiences. She noted the absence of accounts of sexual pleasure and desire in the narratives of the first sexual encounters of three-fourths of these young women. Sadly, the prevalent themes were of coercion, pain, and even boredom. In attempting to legitimize their choice to engage in intercourse, some couched their stories in romantic rhetoric. Others reported feeling let down—physically, emotionally, and romantically—by the experience. "Sex is suppose to be great—a major deal, some of the girls in this narrative group [said] accusingly. By report, it 'makes' love and pleasure, but for them, it made boredom and disappointment" (p. 346).

Prior to acknowledging the legitimacy of their sexual orientation, boredom was the sentiment most commonly expressed by the lesbian girls in Thompson's (1990) study in reference to their experiences of heterosexual coitus. For other adolescent girls, their first sexual encounters were reportedly devoid of intimacy. These sentiments were also expressed by several of the women in my study (Daniluk, 1993). As expressed by one participant: "Sex has always been a very isolating experience for me, especially at the beginning. I always felt very lost and very alone because I always thought it was the biggest irony that this is a sexy experience because I couldn't find anything remotely intimate about." Intimacy, trust, and power take time, self-confidence, and maturity to develop. Without these, a physical act as purportedly intimate as intercourse can be an experience of tremendous emotional detachment and disconnection. In the words of one woman: "We were having sex, but we didn't have much power. So . . . it was not always empowering sex" (Wolf, 1997, p. 129).

The accounts in Wolf's (1997) recent book on adolescent sexuality highlight the qualitative difference in the experiences of *sexual play* versus the actual act of first intercourse. The experience of "going all the way" for this select group of women reflected similar themes of isolation, disconnection, and anti-climax. However, these women underscored the pleasure and eroticism of the physical intimacy and exploration that *preceded* their entry into the adult sexual world (i.e., first intercourse). In the words of one woman: "The intercourse part wasn't much fun but the stuff that led up to it I *loved* . . . I liked the kissing and the touching and the erotic feelings—very sensual and exciting" (p. 128). Others talked about "empowering . . . cuddling" and "empowering companionship" with their boyfriends, and of the absence of "empowering sex." They lacked personal power and did not feel ready to enter this world (p. 129). Some talked about being "too young . . . for the actual act" but not "too young to feel aroused" (p. 126).

Indeed, several factors seem to be implicated in girls' experiences of sexual pleasure. Emotional readiness seems to be important. The specific circumstances of the event are also significant (mutual consent and desire vs. perceived obligation or coercion). Girls also report greater satisfaction with their first sexual encounters when these relationships are characterized by respect, warmth, and caring (Kitzinger, 1985; Thompson, 1990). A women in my research group talked about the importance of mutuality and respect in her first sexual encounter. She credits this experience for her subsequent ability to embrace her own sexuality and sexual desire as a central part of her life:

> "I really feel blessed that I was introduced to sex in such a positive way, in such a loving way, and I still enjoy it, and I have a wonderful relationship with my whole body and with men's bodies that I am involved with, and it feels good."

For some adolescent girls, their experiences of sexual exploration and first intercourse are marked by a sense of pleasure and entitlement. Approximately one-fourth of the girls in Thompson's (1990) study reported such agency-enhancing sexual experiences. Characterized as "pleasure narrators" (p. 350), these lesbian and heterosexual girls perceived their "early sexual experience [to be] a voyage of discovery" and their bodies as "a treasure chest that they take with them." These girls

> believe in pleasure . . . think masturbation and childhood sexuality are good omens, not sins, and that the double standard is a dead issue; . . . encourage the search for the body's wellsprings and for supportive and exciting lovers . . . describe taking sexual initiative, satisfying their own sexual curiosity; instigating petting and coital relations. . . . from earliest childhood, they seem to take sexual subjectivity for granted. (pp. 350–351)

A woman in my research group reflected similar sentiments in her recollection of her early initiation into heterosexual intercourse:

> "I was 14 when I had my first sexual experience. It was very, very positive, and I've always loved sex and sex loved me, and I was always kind of wild, and I've always felt that way about my own sexuality, free and good, and always have had the pleasure of enjoying very positive sexual relationships."

For some young women, it is the experience of heterosexual coitus that proves to be critical in clarifying their lesbian identity (Coleman, 1985; Loewenstein, 1985). In a sample of 197 self-identified lesbian women, Chapman and Brannock (1987) report that 89% had sexual contact with men as they attempted to sort out and clarify their sexual orientation. As discussed throughout this book, heterosexuality is strongly endorsed in most cultures of the world. It is not surprising, then, that many young women attempt to fulfill this social mandate in engaging in sexual relationships with men. Some have their sexual desires for women confirmed through these experiences. In the words of one woman in my research group,

> "I had a very intimate and emotional relationship with a man, and when I slept with him, I knew, and I wanted desperately to just

> continue with him because my life would have been so much easier, . . . but instinctively, I knew. . . . I can still remember being in bed with him just at that point and knowing, that no, there was nothing wrong with this man. He was a wonderful, gentle, loving man, it's just that I mustn't be with a man and I knew that instantly."

For these women, such an acknowledgment has a number of implications. They are faced with having to negotiate a positive lesbian identity in the face of considerable social discrimination (Rothblum, 1994). Their relationships with their same-sex peers may also be threatened. Decisions around disclosure and negotiating issues of attraction can be particularly difficulty for these young women, given the risks of rejection and stigmatization by their family members and friends (Heyward, 1989; Kleinberg, 1986). Many models of lesbian identity development support the need for lesbian women to seek out group membership in the lesbian community as a part of their development of an integrated lesbian identity (see McCarn & Fassinger, 1996, for a current review of these models).

Language also contributes to making sexuality and sexual expression equivocal for adolescent girls. In her book, *Changing Bodies, Changing Lives: A Book for Teens on Sex and Relationships,* Bell (1987) identifies a host of slang words commonly used to describe the "sexual" parts of women's bodies. Such euphemisms as "cunt," "box," "hole," "beaver," "snatch," "twat," "pussy," and "muff" are used to refer to the pubic area, including women's vaginas and vulva. Words used to describe women's breasts include "tits," "knockers," "boobs," "melons," "jugs," "bonkers," "set," "pair," "bedposts," and "knobs," to name just a few. Each of these words represent an animal or an inanimate object, but none reflect any sense of "the woman in the body" (Martin, 1987). Most, in fact, have a derogatory inference to them. They serve to objectify and depersonalize the body part in question. They figuratively sever the part from the person and metaphorically distance girls from their bodies and their sexuality.

These same body parts are also frequently the focus of jokes between boys and men (e.g., breast jokes) as well as verbal jeers. Being very large-breasted as an adolescent girl, I can remember only too well how painful it was to be the focus of endless jeers and jokes, often by total strangers (e.g., "Wouldn't you just love to get your head between those bedposts"). Friends who were less physically endowed were not exempt from this type of harassment either. They were admonished for the smaller size of their breasts (e.g., "Look at those fried eggs"). How can girls feel confident with their embodied sexuality when the representations of this aspect of their experience are the subject of men's admiration and lust on the one hand, and ridicule and scorn on the other?

The words used to describe men's sexual organs are also problematic in girls' constructions of their experience of their sexuality. There are literally dozens of words used to describe what is socially considered to be *the* male sex organ, the penis ("cock", "prick," "dick," "rod," "meat," "gun," etc.). Most of these reinforce the sense of the phallus as being a powerful "tool," "thrusting" its way into the woman in what is purportedly an act of "love." The male language of sex is equally pejorative, including terms like "porking," "fucking," "banging," "humping," and comments such as "I had her," "I layed her," "I screwed her," or "I did her." These words emphasize sex as conquest, as a depersonalized act, as something that is done to a woman's body, with or without her consent.

Young women must also find a way to make sense of the fact that the words commonly used in "lovemaking" are also used as weapons in times of anger and rage. The same language that is used to describe erotic and sexual pleasure takes on entirely different meanings when words such as "fucking bitch," "stupid cunt," or "filthy whore" are hurled in anger. These words are often used as weapons to frighten, abuse, and control.

In her discussion of sexual discourse, Fine (1988) underscores the "missing discourse of desire" that characterizes the education of adolescent girls. Consistent with the sexual scripts of male sexual entitlement and female accountability, popular discourse consistently reinforces the connection between adolescent sexuality and both danger and victimization. This "ideologically separates the female sexual agent, or subject, from her counterpart, the female sexual victim" (p. 30). According to Fine, "The naming of desire, pleasure, or sexual entitlement, particularly for females, barely exists. . . . When spoken, it is tagged with reminders of 'consequences'—emotional, physical, moral, reproductive, and/or financial" (p. 33). In the last 15 years, these consequences have become even more dire. Teenage girls now must negotiate their sexuality under the increasing threat of AIDS. Unfortunately, they appear to know relatively little about this disease (Wyatt & Reiderle, 1994). Research suggests that many girls also lack the confidence to prevent the transmission of AIDS (Lear, 1997; Moore & Rosenthal, 1996). It takes quite an assertive and self-confident young woman to insist that her partner wear a condom.

The consequence of this missing discourse of desire, and of the paradoxical communications about adolescent girls' sexual expression, is to "disable young women in their negotiations as sexual subjects." They are turned "away from positions of sexual self-interest" (Fine, 1988, p. 42). The result is girls' failure to know themselves as the subjects of their own sexuality.

SEX AS SURRENDER: MEDIA MESSAGES

If parents do not easily talk to their adolescents about more than the functional pragmatics of sex, then girls today need not worry about being completely "in the dark" about the dynamics of sexual "relationships." The popular media provide a virtual cornucopia of information on how people behave together sexually. Although years ago, actors doing love scenes in bed each had to keep one foot on the floor (thereby making it almost impossible to actually consummate the act), the rules have been thrown to the wind, and there is little left to the imagination. Far more advanced than a course in Sex 101, not only have the actors in love scenes abandoned their clothing, but also they have apparently abandoned their inhibitions. They grope, grab, lick, suck, poke, and prod each other in a frenzy of erotic delight—usually after the first date (it is little wonder, then, why teenage girls appear to be prematurely rushing into intercourse). The appetite of the voyeuristic audience seems insatiable. More and more frequently, the images of sweating bodies, captured in a heated embrace, grace the television or movie screen. The movie *9½ Weeks* is a good example of this, leaving little to the imagination and promoting sex devoid of intimacy. This arrangement appeared to work just fine for the male figure in the movie (Mickey Rourke), but it took an emotional toll on the female lead (Kim Basinger). The implicit message of the film was that men need sex irrespective of relationship, and that women must have a relationship really to enjoy having sex.

Clearly, from the standpoint of the popular media, sex is "out of the closet," so to speak. At least, heterosexual sex is. The sexual images and stories that appear in most magazines, movies, and television shows are resoundingly heterosexual (other than Ellen having recently disclosed her lesbian identity orientation on prime-time evening television, and Melissa Ethridge and her lesbian partner announcing their pregnancy on the cover of *Time*). Even books that portray lesbian relationships are often rewritten to reflect heterosexual values when they are made into movies (e.g., Flagg's 1997 book, *Fried Green Tomatoes at the Whistle Stop Cafe*).

So how influential are the popular media in shaping adolescent girls' understanding of "adult" sexuality? It is estimated that most North American children have spent an average of 15,000 hours watching television by the time they reach 18 years of age (Orbuch, 1989). The media would appear to be a principal educator of young women and men regarding sexual experience and expression. Numerous studies indicate that magazines, romantic novels, and the mass media are *the primary* sources of information for teens about sexual relationships, sexual behaviors, sexual techniques, and sexual problems (Andre et al., 1991; Bereska, 1994; Evans, Ruthberg, Sather, & Turner, 1991; Lees, 1986).

In a recent study of 251 single female University students (Bielay & Herold, 1995), *Cosmopolitan* was reported to be their leading source of information with regard to most sexual topics. This magazine boasts a mean rating of 4.2 articles dealing with sexuality per issue. The most frequently read topics were those dealing with "sexual skills, techniques and pleasuring." The emphasis was on how a woman can "please" and keep her man (p. 254). In his study of the sexual attitudes of college students at a large U.S. university, anthropologist Michael Moffat (cited in

Unger & Crawford, 1992) confirmed that the major influence reported by respondents on their ideas about sex and love

> was contemporary American popular culture. The direct sources of the students' sexual ideas were located almost entirely in mass consumer culture: the . . . exemplars displayed in movies, popular music, advertising, and on TV; Dr. Ruth and sex manuals; *Playboy, Penthouse, Cosmopolitan, Playgirl,* etc., Harlequins and other pulp romances. . . . (p. 326)

And what are the messages about women's sexuality being promoted by the media? According to Orbuch (1989), "The messages taught to young people . . . are that sex outside of marriage is acceptable, sex is often superficial, power and violence are allowable in the context of sex, and contraception need not be a fundamental element of sexual behavior" (p. 443).

Unfortunately, although the images are far more explicit, the sexual paradigms and scripts have not really changed much over the years. Women's sexuality is still generally portrayed in two ways. It is portrayed as something that lies dormant until awakened by the "right" man—the skilled lover. Or it is depicted as something that is dangerous to the woman who dares to act in her own self-interests based on her own sexual needs and desires. Women's sexual pleasure is juxtaposed with danger. "Good" women are sexually discrete. They eschew the lusty advances of other men until the "right" one comes along. They bless him with the gift of their bodies, and he awakens their sexuality. He keeps the woman safe. On the other hand, the woman who acts on her own sexual needs and desires, or places these above those of her male partner, pays dearly for her selfishness. In the sensual movie *The Piano,* Holly Hunter loses her finger, and almost her life, for daring to fulfill her erotic desires outside of her marital relationship. Glenn Close ends up being bludgeoned to death for her seduction of a nice family man in *Fatal Attraction* (Ellis, 1990). The sexuality of the woman who eschews the norms of monogamy and sexual exclusivity by having multiple sexual partners is inevitably squelched (e.g., Diane Keaton in *Looking for Mr. Goodbar*). Even "good" women must exercise care in their selection of a sexual partner, in case they make the wrong decision. For example, in the enormously popular show *X-Files,* the intelligent, pragmatic heroine Dana Scully's first romantic encounter ends up being with a psychotic serial killer. Women's sexual pleasure is again juxtaposed with danger, a reality even smart women cannot escape.

Advertisers are no better at serving the needs of young women in their tireless commitment to presenting disembodied images of women's sexuality, objectified in the form of breasts, buttocks, and legs. It is becoming common for children of 9 to 13 years to be dressed up in advertisements to look like sensual, adult women (Faludi, 1991; Wolf, 1991). These young girls are prematurely thrust into the role of sexual object long before they are emotionally ready to deal with the consequences of this objectification. Even billboards and placards on buses are filled with images of scantily clad women and men in various erotic poses. As Wolf (1997) notes, children are "exposed, just by walking to our schools and playgrounds, to fantasies that [are] in no way appropriate to [their] psychic ages, that belong to the daily-more-expressive imaginations of adults" (p. 36). In fact, researchers estimate that the average U.S. citizen is exposed daily to over 1,500 advertisements (Kilbourne, 1994).

Rock videos also promote an ethos of goal-oriented sex, the success of which is marked by the achievement of "multiple orgasms." Metts and Cupach (1989) analyzed some popular rock videos. They concluded that "this uniquely adolescent entertainment medium is even 'sexier' than traditional television." The visual presentation of sexual behavior appeared in "more than 75 percent" of these videos. In their content analysis of several rock videos, these authors noted "an average of 4.78 sexual activities being displayed per video" (pp. 141–142). As for the messages in magazines, Kathryn McMahon (1990) notes how even in the acknowledgment of the reader's desire to be an active subject in her own sexual satisfaction, her role, appearance, and behavior are prescribed. In her article, "The *Cosmopolitan* Ideology and the Management of Desire," she identifies the consequences of these messages in terms of the way girls' inherent sense of inadequacy and their tenuous sense of sexual and physical agency are further undermined.

Finally, the romance novel completes the picture. These novels are the source from which many young women draw their understanding of "normal" and "desirable" intimate relationships (Bereska, 1994). These souped-up versions of the fairy tales of childhood (*Snow White, Sleeping Beauty, Little Red Riding Hood,* etc.) are repackaged for an older and, in some ways, even more impressionable audience. This audience is hungry for happily-ever-after versions of relationships based on love and security—relationships filled with all-consuming passion (Bereska, 1994). In none of these standard romance novels does the heroine actively seduce the hero, nor does she reject his sexual advances. Rather, she passively and anxiously awaits his recognition, casting furtive glances and coy looks in his direction. She laps up his meager attention like crumbs being thrown to a bird. Finally, he takes notice of her, whereupon she willingly (hungrily) accepts his animal-like advances as he "ravages" her body and "captures" her sexuality, like a warrior in battle. The stories end with the heroine being "swept away" (Cassell, 1984), literally and figuratively (with no acknowledgment of the work and drudgery that awaits her back at the castle now that she is enslaved to the hero).

The prevalence of this romantic discourse as a way for girls to legitimize their sexual feelings and desires was apparent in the first-sexual-intercourse narratives of Thompson's (1990) participants, discussed earlier in this chapter. Most of these young women couched their personal stories in the "quest for romance" rather than in the context of their own embodied sexual feelings and desires. This can be understood as a consequence of trying to negotiate the impossible cultural paradox of their sexual objectification and corresponding lack of sexual entitlement.

So what does the young girl learn about her sexuality from these sources? What messages does she take in to help her understand her role in the sexual drama? She learns that sex is located in particular body parts (genital focus), and that it is her responsibility to guard and protect these parts from the unwanted advances of men who have insatiable sexual needs. She learns that sex is something played out between a man and a woman (heterosexual), that it involves surrender (consent is relative and assumed), and that once given over, it can never be reclaimed (used goods). She learns that if she is worthy (has the right attitude, body, etc.), she will be chosen, that she must wait for the right man to choose her (she must be in love), and that to act on her own sexual self-interests is a highly risky enterprise. Sexual pleasure necessarily courts danger. In reference to this indoctrination into fear and restraint, Wolf (1997) notes that

> it is no wonder that even today fourteen-year-old girls who notice, let alone act upon, their desire, have the heart-racing sense that they are doing something obscurely, but surely, dangerous. It is also in part because of this inheritance that a modern woman wakes up after a night of being erotically "out of control" feeling sure, on some primal level, that something punitive is bound to happen to her—and that if it doesn't it should. (p. 82)

How can girls develop a sense of sexual agency and entitlement when continually faced with this pleasure/danger paradox? As Fillion (1996) accurately observes,

> What girls desperately need are some positive images of women desiring, women as sexual subjects, women taking charge—taking responsibility. Currently, many don't even have a realistic idea of what female sexual pleasure looks like. Instead, they have some half-baked notions from Hollywood films in which there is zero foreplay and women are portrayed as ecstatic enthusiasts of intercourse. (p. 41)

Unfortunately, however, other than in lesbian literature and erotica, such images are virtually absent in the popular media.

SEX AS WEAPON: SEXUAL VIOLENCE

This chapter would be incomplete without some discussion of the reality of sexual violence. The threat of sexual victimization is a powerful force that inevitably shapes the adolescent girl's experience of her sexuality. As discussed in Chapter 4 in relation to learning to live in a woman's body, as the adolescent girl ventures into the adult world, she runs the increased risk of being the victim of sexual violence. Statistics on sexual assault and sexual harassment suggest that many adolescence girls experience some form of sexual victimization. When the definition of sexual assault is extended to include sexual experiences that involved coercion, force, or threat of force, and are not limited to penile–vaginal penetration, an estimated 54% to 73% of young women report at least one such experience (Koss, Gidycz, & Wisniewski, 1987).

The teen years are a time of particular vulnerability for girls to sexual assault. Many girls begin to date in their early teens, increasing their risk of acquaintance rape (Koss, 1990, 1993; Parrot, 1989). In a survey of 834 students entering college, White and Humphrey (1991) found that 13% of the women reported being raped between the ages of 14 and 18 years. Another 16% experienced at least one attempted rape. Over half (53.7%) of the more than 3,000 college women who participated in a study by Koss et al. (1987) reported some form of sexual victimization during their teens.

It may be bosses and/or co-workers who make lewd and suggestive comments or physical advances. It may be boyfriends who believe it is their right to have their sexual desires met. It may be acquaintances who feel entitled to impose their sexual will (Koss, 1990; Parrot, 1989). Or it may be strangers who lurk in bars and dark alleys, waiting to sexually overpower and terrorize young women. Whatever the scenario, the risk of sexual violation is an ever-present reality in the lives of girls and women. It restricts girls' movements and circumscribes their choices. The reality of sexual violence also carries with it a considerable psychological aftermath (Koss, 1993; Shapiro & Schwartz, 1997; Valentich, 1990). More often than not, it is men who are known to the young women, men who appear typical and "normal," who are the perpetrators of sexual violence. This makes it very difficult for young women to predict the risk of violation and/or limit the probability of being victimized (Koss et al., 1987).

As noted earlier in this chapter, pressure for girls to engage in various forms of sexual behavior (e.g., kissing, fondling, fellatio) is now becoming a normative consequence of dating (Christopher, 1988). There is a fine line between pressure, coercion, and force in many of these interactions. This makes it even more difficult for girls to name the experience of sexual victimization if this happens to them. For example, several of the women in Thompson's (1990) study and some interviewed by Wolf (1997) reported being drunk or stoned when their first experience of intercourse took place.

> So he shows up and I'd been on acid all day. I wasn't prepared, psychologically or any other way. . . . And it's hard to say exactly what I felt when I walked off with him, but I just figured we'd go to sleep. . . . The guy's in the sleeping bag and the next thing I know, it's practically

> like what today would be called date rape. He's on top of me and this is *going to happen*. . . . We were kissing . . . and the next thing I know, my underwear is coming off and I'm being penetrated. And it . . . hurts . . . really . . . a lot. (p. 125)

Despite Katie Roiphe's (1993) arguments to the contrary, the increasing incidence of date and acquaintance rape suggests that the belief in male sexual entitlement and female accountability is very definitely alive and well. Although traditionally,

> sexually aggressive sexual behavior followed after consensual sexual activity, such as kissing, petting, and more intensely erotic behavior . . . [44% of] female college students today report a surprisingly large percentage of both sexual aggression and rape that were spontaneously initiated by their male companions without any antecedent consensual, erotic activity. (Levine & Kanin, 1987, p. 60)

Male-perpetuated sexual assault is most common. However, research suggests that sexual violence and coercion are also reported in some lesbian relationships (Waterman, Dawson, & Bologna, 1989).

The reality of sexual violence and of women's presumed accountability for this violence, is very real for women in North American society, whether or not they exercise "good judgment" and "sexual restraint." Sexual violence occurs; it occurs far too frequently, and the consequences to the victim are often significant (Koss, 1993; Koss & Burkhart, 1989; Shapiro & Schwartz, 1997). The ever-present fear of sexual assault, and the painful reality of being sexually victimized, can profoundly affect girls' experience of themselves as sexual beings (Herman, 1992; Shapiro & Schwartz, 1997). One woman's recollection of being raped as an adolescent girl on her first independent outing from a small rural town to the "big" city, and her attempts to make sense of this experience, reflect the depth of the trauma of rape:

> "For the most part, it was a wonderful heady summer, coming to the big city, chasing sailors, going to the pubs and stuff . . . until one night, we were sitting with these two guys in a pub. I had one drink, only one, and somebody must have slipped me a mickey, because the next thing I know, I'm waking up in the middle of the night in this hotel room with this guy pumping away at me. He was about 45 and ugly as sin. And all I could think about was just pretend that you're enjoying it or you're sleeping, so he doesn't kill you. . . . Then, my period was really late and I sweated and died a thousand deaths as a result of the trauma and the injury. . . . I eventually miscarried, but the message was clear—first freedom trip, going out getting raped, getting

> pregnant—like the message is 'Never leave home, don't dare leave home, . . . and *don't* have sex, don't ever have sex.' "

The way in which society in general responds to sexual attacks on women is also important in the construction of young girls' relationships with their bodies and their experience of sexuality. "Descriptions or accounts of rape and rape imagery appear in various media forms, in film, on television, in advertising, and in the press, as well as within the literary and novel form." They portray rape as "an inevitable consequence of existing relationships between men and women." These descriptions "serve to perpetuate the view that women are unconsciously wanting to be 'taken' " (Smart & Smart, 1978, pp. 93–95). The predominant message in popular discourse and in the media is that the victim of assault is in some way responsible for her victimization. Even subtle questions inquiring into the location, timing, and circumstances of the assault (i.e., "Was she drinking too much?" "Did she lead him on?"), as well as inquiries regarding her clothing or her behavior (prior to, during, or following the attack), infer that something about the girl or the choices she made resulted in this happening to her. The fear passed on by parents in warning their daughters about carefully monitoring their whereabouts, clothing, and behavior implicitly (if not explicitly) reinforces the belief that girls have some control over whether they are sexually assaulted. The underlying message is painfully clear in inferring that the young woman is in some way accountable for the violence.

Presenting another powerful paradox, girls' sexual safety and freedom are placed in opposition to one another (Vance, 1992). Based on the erroneous premise that the demonstration of their sexual desire triggers male passion and lust, girls who are sexually assaulted all too frequently are blamed for unleashing the uncontrollable and insatiable sexual desires of the men who assault them (e.g., "She asked for it," "She deserved it"). Exemplifying this dilemma, Wolf (1997) notes the restraints placed on adolescent girls' freedom of movement and desire at precisely the time in life when their bodies and psyches are ready to step outside of the confines of the family and begin to explore the world. "Awareness that sexual pleasure meant sexual danger and that our own guilt would be held to be a causative factor in whatever harm might come to us was a constant drain on our energy. . . . Perhaps acculturation to the unthinkable is one of the definitions of what it means to become a woman" (pp. 33–34). Within this context, it is difficult for adolescent girls to safely explore the depths and parameters of their sexual feelings and desires when sexual violation may be one of the consequences of doing so. It is difficult for them to comfortably incorporate sexual play into their interpersonal relationships when living under the threat of sexual violence. It is particularly difficult for adolescent girls to develop a sense of sexual entitlement and agency within such a context.

SUMMARY: PROBLEMATIC MEANINGS

Developmental psychologists have long acknowledged the critical importance of the period of adolescence in setting down the foundation for the values, beliefs, and ways of being in the world that are carried into adulthood. These shape the individual's future expectations, choices, and life experiences (Erikson, 1968; Kegan, 1982). Unfortunately, the messages girls receive about their sexuality at this important juncture in their development are highly conflictual. Few reinforce a sense of sexual play and agency. Few reinforce girls' sexual entitlement or erotic pleasure (Fine, 1988). Few messages or images present sexuality distinct from its physical manifestations in heterosexual relationships.

There are few, if any, appropriate expressions within the language of "love" for *self*-love and stimulation. There is an absence of affirming language to represent the range of women's sexual choices and experiences. There is an alarming absence of words in the sexual vocabulary that emphasize choice, mutuality, intimacy, and respect, and a punctuating absence of female desire, spontaneity, and play in popular sexual discourse. There is little social acknowledgment of, or validation for, the experience of girls' embodied sexuality (Foucault, 1978; Vance, 1992). According to Fine (1988), this absence of an acknowledgment of girls' embodied sexual feelings results in their failure to know themselves as the subjects of their own sexuality. "Confused by the contradiction that her own experience makes visible . . . her conflict is about being a girl who gets sexually excited in the context of a culture that says she is not supposed to feel this way" (Tolman, 1991, p. 61). Wolf (1997) underscores adolescent girls' loss of "voice" relative to their own desires. "The culture that surrounds girls signals to them that they must, sexually, forget themselves. They must become passive in relation to the energy of desire, or detached from owning it, even in the face of its increasingly active pressure" (p. 27).

Debold (1991) poses some important questions in response to this pleasure–danger paradigm:

> If women's sexuality is defined by the pleasure and fear aroused by women's bodies which, in turn, may make sexuality dangerous to women themselves, what happens, then, to the play of feelings in girls' bodies as they move into adolescence? If women's sexuality—a powerful part of bodily experience—is constructed as problematic or illicit, then might not this result in women experiencing discomfort or disease in their bodies? (p. 170)

This epitomizes the double bind of the adolescent girl's sexuality. She is presented with the impossible choice of attempting to exemplify the ideals of morality and restraint (being a "good" girl), guarding her virginity at the expense of her own physical pleasure and joy. Or she can act in response to the pleasures and sensations of her body (being a "bad" girl), thereby exposing herself to condemnation and reprisals in daring to act in her own self-interest.

Although this situation is distressing, it is by no means hopeless. It is important to remember that adolescent girls are not passive, sponge-like recipients of their culture, and that sexual meanings are co-constructed. Paradoxical paradigms that juxtapose female sexual pleasure with danger, sexual restraint (being a "good" girl) with sexual corruption (being a "whore"), sexual agency with accountability, and so on, are not in fact, shared fully by girls and women. Rather, social realities are learned and taken in to varying degrees by young women as they adapt to the contextual realities of their lives. As they come to define themselves as sexual and further consolidate the identities they began to develop as children, to varying degrees, girls actively resist or challenge these external messages and passive female sexual scripts. In particular, they challenge those that are inconsistent with their evolving sexual hypotheses.

Actively and passively, adolescent girls assert their resistance to these socially imposed meanings and messages (Gilligan & Brown, 1992; Gilligan et al., 1991; Pipher, 1995). They do so in their refusal to let fear of danger control or circumscribe their actions or relationships. They do so in the bold actions of lesbian or bisexual girls who challenge the orthodoxy and live lives congruent with their needs and desires. Perhaps resistance may even be seen in the more extreme behavior of the anorexic who attempts to deal with the conflicts engendered by social constructions of adolescent sexuality by refusing to embody the characteristics of mature womanhood. Incongruity exists between these externally imposed sexual messages and meanings, and girls' internal, phenomenological, embodied realities. When acknowledged and expressed, this can serve as an important impetus for growth and change (Janeway, 1980). According to Fine (1988), "Diverse female sexual subjectivities emerge through, despite, and because of gender-based power asymmetries" (p. 41). Girls, to varying degrees, attempt to resist these rigid scripts (Wolf, 1997).

CHALLENGE AND CHANGE: CREATING NEW MEANINGS

In our attempts to assist young women to develop a sense of pleasure and joy in their embodied sexuality, it is necessary to "counter the triple-whammy that love, ignorance and guilt already exercise over girls' ability to accept themselves as sexual beings by lightening rather than increasing the load of cultural weight that love must bear." It is important to deal "with sex fully and straightforwardly; giving girls the clues they need to recognize desire" (Thompson, 1990, p. 358). It is important to give adolescent girls the permission and space to experiment and play with their sexuality "in a spirit of lighthearted joy" (Janeway, 1980, p. 18). The exercises presented below are designed to help facilitate this process.

The primary goal of this work is to guide girls to "a different body: a playful woman's body" (Debold, 1991, p. 182). It is important to help them "begin to discover [their] self-defined sexuality" (Kaschack, 1992, p. 87). This work is about helping girls explore their sexuality, connect with their sexual energy, and, ideally, to begin to develop a more self- versus other-defined sexuality. To achieve these goals, it is first necessary for us to examine and challenge our own sexual definitions, assumptions, and paradigms. We need to take account of our beliefs regarding what constitutes "appropriate sexual behavior" for girls and women. It is important to examine critically our assumptions regarding "normal" and "responsible" sexual behavior and expression. In particular, we need to appreciate that adolescent girls today have a different social reality that may serve to both liberate and to constrain how they define and act on their sexual impulses and desires (e.g., more readily available sexual information; more accessible birth control and abortion "for some"; more pressure to engage in the "adult" act of heterosexual intercourse at an earlier age; more exposure to evocative sexual images at an earlier age; the reality of AIDS). There may be similarities between adult women's experiences and theirs of the "heat" of adolescent sexual passion and lust. The threat of sexual violence formed our sexual self-structures, as it no doubt has theirs. However, there are also many differences in women's social realities. These differences must be taken into account and respected in working with young women.

In beginning this work, it is first necessary to assess the extent to which traditional sexual definitions, paradigms, and scripts have been incorporated into clients' self- and belief structures. It is important to assess the way girls have learned to understand and experience their sexuality, individually and in their relationships with others. As noted in Chapter 1, developmental and historical experiences and influences are very important in adolescent girls' sexual self-constructions. It is critical, then, that counselors conduct a thorough review of each client's individual history *before* undertaking any of the exercises suggested below. The *meaning* and *experience* of sexuality will be substantively different for clients who have experienced sexual violence in childhood and/or during their adolescence (e.g., incest, child sexual abuse, rape, sexual assault). Working on issues related to the aftermath of sexual violence is beyond the scope of this book. As such, if counselors determine that sexual violence has been a significant situational or historical factor in a client's life, they should not proceed with the exploratory exercises recommended below. Rather, a referral should be made for specialized work. Also, a list of resources for counselors and clients related to healing from sexual violence can be found in Appendix C.

The following are examples of exercises that may be useful for work with clients who are facing the challenges of trying to develop a comfortable and accepting relationship with their bodies, and with their sexuality. They can assist in identifying the issues, definitions, and meanings that adolescent girls have come to hold about their sexuality and sexual expression that impede the development of a sense of sexual agency and entitlement. However, this may not be an easy undertaking. In North American culture, most people remain untrained in the ability to talk about their own sexual activity or scripts (Gagnon & Simon, 1982). Many adolescent girls may find it difficult to engage in a dialogue or exploration of their sexual feelings and behaviors without experiencing considerable anxiety. For others, even being asked to think about sexual activity in the abstract may be difficult. As such, helpers are encouraged to be aware of the shame and silence that characterize many of our communications about sexuality in North American culture. Talking openly and honestly about their sexual beliefs, feelings, and behaviors is not an easy task for most adult women. We can expect it to be even more difficult for adolescent girls, who are in the early stages of exploring their sexual worlds and consolidating their sexual identities. Counselors are encouraged to help girls inject a sense of play and humor in their explorations as a way of facilitating more in-depth, honest, and meaningful exploration and discussion. It is important to be sensitive to cultural, religious, and ethnic differences in the perceived sexual roles and rights of women, and to respect clients' adherence to more traditional sexual definitions and scripts. Attention to client context is critical in the selection of goals and intervention strategies. These may have far-reaching consequences in terms of challenging their fundamental beliefs and values.

Age is also an important consideration in undertaking and adapting these exercises. There is a world of difference in the emotional and psychological maturity of girls in their early teens and girls in their later teens. Younger girls may not be emotionally ready for some of these activities. Issues related to age of consent are also important. For example, several authors (Anderson & Cyranowski, 1994; Barbach, 1975; Smith, Rosenthal, & Reichler, 1996; Tiefer, 1996) underscore the critical role masturbation appears to play in the development of sexual maturation and self-knowledge for women and men. "Women with masturbatory histories have, in general, a wider sexual behavior repertoire and are more sexually responsive" (Andersen & Cyranowski, p. 1096). Some (e.g., Tiefer, 1996) recommend masturbation training as an important component of sexual education and efficacy for girls and women. Yet this would clearly not be acceptable to the parents of most young adolescent girls. This may also be cause for concern among parents of older adolescents, who adhere to more traditional beliefs regarding their daughters' sexuality and sexual expression. As such, some of the exercises would need to be omitted completely with particular girls or groups of girls, or adapted to reflect the developmental level of the girls in questions. For others, parental permission would be required. On this note, counselors should keep parents of younger adolescent girls informed about the nature and goals of the work that they are undertaking with their daughters. Parents should be included as much as possible in the process of helping girls develop positive sexual self-constructions and sexual agency, as well as a clear sense of sexual responsibility.

Sexual Semantics

When working with adolescent girls, there are a number of activities that can be used to help them explore the beliefs they have come to hold regarding women's sexuality and sexual expression, as well as identifying the sources of these beliefs. For example, in an exercise adapted from Kitzinger's (1985) *Woman's Experience of Sexuality,* individually or in groups, clients can be asked to participate in a word-association activity aimed at identifying both the language and assumptions associated with women's sexuality and sexual expression. First, clients are asked to generate as many words as they can think of that are associated with sexuality. If this exercise is completed in a group, the group leader writes these words down as they are called out by group members. Words that are commonly identified by adolescents during this exercise include "penis," "orgasm," "breasts," "genitals," "horny," "vagina," and so on. Group leaders are encouraged to include words such as "masturbation" and "menstruation" in the list, if these have not been identified by the group members.

Second, when a fairly comprehensive list of "sexual" words has been generated, participants are then asked to write the words down one side of a separate piece of paper. Then, independently, they are asked to work their way down the list, quickly and spontaneously noting the first word or phrase that comes to mind in response to each of the words listed. Their response may be related to a thing (e.g., virginity, bed) or an emotion (e.g., shame, pleasure). Third, having completed this task, participants are then asked to examine their responses and their reactions to these common words, and to attempt to cluster their responses in categories based on whether the response was positive, negative, or neutral. Fourth, each category is then assigned a different color, and participants are asked to color the words in their list according to this assignment. Group members then split up into pairs or triads and discuss and compare the words that elicited a positive response, as well as those that elicited a negative response. They are asked to discuss what their reactions to these words tell them about their perceptions and feelings about the nature of sexuality, about where sexuality is believed to be located (e.g., in the genitals), and about appropriate or inappropriate sexual expression. Large-group discussion of participants' ratings and reactions to the exercise can prove very illuminating in terms of highlighting participants' beliefs and perceptions regarding women's sexuality. This exercise is also useful in helping clients to begin to identify the words commonly used in reference to sexuality, particularly those they associate with anxiety, guilt, or shame.

In extending this exercise, in pairs or small groups, participants can be asked to create a story about women's sexuality and sexual expression, being sure to include each of the words in the list. Reading these stories in the group helps to identify many of the stereotypical assumptions and beliefs girls hold about the nature of women's sexuality, as well as highlighting the way in which language reflects and shapes these beliefs and assumptions.

The "Me Tarzan, You Jane" Approach to Sex

In assessing client needs, it is also important to identify the sexual scripts that guide the beliefs and expectations of young women regarding women's sexual natures and the parameters of "appropriate" sexual expression and behavior. As discussed in earlier chapters, sexual scripts are the products of human interaction. They are like the social norms or rules that guide sexual relationships between individuals. These scripts reflect popular assumptions regarding the sexual rights, roles, responsibilities, and behaviors of women and men (Gagnon & Simon, 1982; Plummer, 1975, 1982; Tiefer, 1995; Weeks, 1985). They differ significantly based on sex—a reflection of the current distribution of power within our patriarchal society. They may be a source of liberation and pleasure, or of considerable pain, guilt, and anxiety. These scripts can be especially problematic when the "rules" of "norms" appear to be contradictory or paradoxical, as in the case of the paradigms discussed earlier in this chapter related to women's sexuality and sexual expression. They can also create problems when they do not reflect or sanction the sexual desires and needs of certain groups of people, as in the case of lesbian or bisexual women. According to Gagnon and Simon (1982), where conflicts exist in the culture, they are inevitably mirrored in the person.

To begin to identify these potential conflicts, it is important for clients to have the opportunity to freely and comfortably explore and examine the sexual scripts that are promoted in popular culture. They need to be able to identify the assumptions and myths that underlie these scripts, and to examine the degree to which these definitions and scripts fit with, or contradict, their own feelings and beliefs regarding their sexuality and sexual expression. As noted in this and other chapters, the media are very strong socializing agents that perpetuate very traditional and limiting notions regarding women's sexuality and sexual expression. Examining media messages, therefore, is a very powerful and useful way to identify popular sexual scripts at "arms length," so to speak, maintaining some emotional distance for the lived realities and beliefs of the participants. To begin this exercise (either individually or in a group), girls are asked to review various magazines, movies, television programs, and romance novels. The purpose is to identify the images and messages that are portrayed in the media regarding what sex is and how is it characterized and expressed. They can select one particularly "sexual" scene or interaction, or a number of different vignettes. Their examinations can be guided by the following questions:

> Where and when do most of these sexual interactions occur?
> What behaviors do they involve?
> What appears to be the goal of these encounters?
> What is the sex of the participants?
> Who initiates these sexual encounters?
> How do the partners appear to feel about each other?
> What is the tone of these interactions?
> Who appears to be in control of these encounters?
> What role(s) does the man play in these encounters?
> What role(s) does the woman play?
> What behaviors do they engage in?
> What do the encounters appear to mean to the man?
> What do they appear to mean to the woman?
> What does he do, and how does he appear to feel when the activity is over?
> What does she do, and how does she appear to feel when the activity is over?

Based on this information, participants are asked to create a script or "sexual narrative" that describes the way in which women's sexuality is defined and depicted in the media, and then the way men's sexuality is characterized.

A discussion should follow about the persistence of sexual myths, such as "Men always want and are ready to have sex," "Women don't need or desire sex as much as men do," "Men should always initiate sex," "Nice girls don't jump into bed right away," "Women can only really enjoy sex if they are in love," "Women often say no to having sex when they really mean yes," and so on. One at a time, participants should read their scripts out loud (accompanied by a particular scene from a video or a magazine advertisement, etc.), and as these narratives unfold, group members should be encouraged to speak out each time they hear a typical sexual "myth." Group leaders then instruct participants to compare the pictures and images they have each selected and encourage an exploration of the *meaning* of these narratives and images. They should be asked to take note of how women's sexual behavior is circumscribed in terms of women's rights, roles, responsibilities, and behaviors. It is also important to highlight biases in these images and myths, based on class, race, attractiveness, and sexual orientation.

Following a discussion of the explicit and implicit messages that are promoted in these sexual scripts, participants should be encouraged to examine and discuss what sex means *to them* personally. They can compare these popular scripts and notions with their own assumptions, beliefs, and feelings regarding their developing sexuality and sexual expression. Areas of potential conflict or contradiction should be identified (e.g., the source, context, or focus of their own sexual interests and desires may be quite inconsistent with the dominant sexual scripts). They should be encouraged to explore the consequences of these contradictions in terms of engendering feelings of shame, guilt, misunderstanding, exclusion, and so on. In identifying their own definitions and assumptions regarding women's sexuality, it is then important to help clients explore the other *voices* in their lives that have contributed, and that continue to contribute, to their sexual self-perceptions and beliefs (see Bell, 1987, for a discussion of the role of different "voices"—such as parents, peers, and religion in girl's sexual decision making). From these discussions, counselors can gain considerable information regarding the degree to which each girl has accepted and incorporated popular sexual definitions and scripts into her own experience of herself as a sexual being. They should take note of the impact of these "normative" constructions on girls' sexual self-esteem and sense of sexual agency.

"Dear Abby"

The goal of this activity is to help explore adolescent girls' beliefs and assumptions regarding their sexuality and the appropriate expression of sexuality for girls and women. Participants are asked to anonymously write letters to "Dear Abby" regarding various sexual dilemmas that they, or someone they know, have experienced, or anticipate (fear) experiencing in the future. These dilemmas frequently involve being physically attracted to someone of the same sex, having erotic fantasies, wanting to masturbate or having masturbated, engaging in intercourse for the first time, having oral sex, being forced into having sex, having a sexual partner who is reluctant to wear a condom, and so on. Once completed, the letters can be put into a bin, and one by one, they can be read aloud, with group members being asked to pretend that they are "Dear Abby" and suggest possible solutions to the dilemmas presented. The types of letters written and the responses generated within the group can provide considerable information regarding participants' issues or concerns. They also serve to highlight girls' sexual beliefs, values, and fears, and to help them develop problem-solving skills. When working with clients on an individual basis, this type of activity can be adapted by having the client take on the role of "Dear Abby" and respond to letters and situations generated by the counselor, or to questions and scenarios the counselor and client have generated together.

"Embodied" Sexuality

Although most of the exercises identified thus far have been fairly cognitive, it is clear from the previous discussion that any study of sexuality must include an exploration of the more embodied aspects of sexuality and sexual expression. Sexual meanings may be social constructions, but the interpretation of these meanings evolves directly out of the experience of living in the developing body of a woman. As such, it is important to help girls get in touch with and explore the way in which sexuality is lived and experienced in their bodies. Guided fantasy can be a particularly useful mechanism to facilitate this type of in-depth exploration. Either individually or in a group, clients are asked to find a place in the room where they can comfortably lie down. When in a prone position, the first part of this exercise begins with progressive relaxation (e.g., clients are asked to contract and release various muscle groups throughout their bodies until they have attained a state of calm and comfort. They should pay particular attention to slowing their breathing and first filling and then fully emptying their lungs—breathing in through their nose and out through their mouth). Once relaxed, clients are asked to allow themselves to float freely and comfortably back in time, to a place where they feel safe and warm, and content, a place where they are able to fully explore their bodies in privacy and comfort. Once in this place, they are directed to try to get in touch with their sexual/erotic energy. They should allow themselves to revel in the power, warmth, and vitality of this energy. They are instructed to just "be" with this energy and to let it envelope them completely. After a time, they are asked to assign this energy a color (usually clients select blue or white) and to visualize this color moving throughout their bodies. The group leader asks them to carefully tune into and be aware of the response of each part of their body as this energy moves throughout them. They are then asked to try to locate the source of this energy within their bodies—the part of their bodies from which it originates. Having located the source of their sexual energy, they are asked to step out of their bodies and observe the way in which this energy effuses and radiates throughout their skin, hair, eyes, and so on.

When the exercise is completed, they are asked to return to the present; are given pastels, paints, and paper; and are asked to portray their experience through a picture or painting. Although this type of exploration is usually experienced as quite pleasant, some clients may have become aware of feelings of discomfort or shame associated with particular parts of their bodies as they moved through the various stages of this fantasy. Facilitators should be aware of the power of this type of activity and be certain to debrief the activity fully with participants. Girls should be encouraged to discuss their experiences (in a group setting, the safest way to debrief is usually in dyads or triads), with their art serving as a vehicle for sharing the sensations and feelings they experienced during the exercise.

They should be encouraged to talk about and share the knowledge they gained during the exercise, related to the embodiment of their sexuality. In a variation on this exercise, clients can be guided through a fantasy of exploring their "sexual treasure chest" (see Bell, 1987), identifying those aspects of themselves that are contained within the chest, and that represent their sexual and erotic selves.

The information gained from these activities can help to guide the choice and direction of subsequent interventions. Activities should be selected based on the extent to which traditional sexual definitions and scripts have been taken in by adolescent girls and have begun to shape their sexual self-perceptions. The focus of these intervention, as with the others presented throughout this book, is on altering the *meanings* that have come to guide young women's understanding of their bodies and their sexuality, and on helping them to deal with the internal conflict generated by the often contradictory and paradoxical social messages regarding the nature of their sexuality and "appropriate" forms of sexual expression.

The following activities are examples of ways counselors can help girls to challenge restrictive notions of male sexual entitlement and female sexual accommodation, and to begin to expand both their definitions and perceptions of the range and realm of sexually appropriate experiencing and expression for women. They are designed to help girls construct *sexual meanings* that serve to free and liberate them from the constraints imposed by restrictive and oppressive sexual norms and paradigms. Ideally, they can help girls to connect with their sexual energy, to assume more responsibility for their own sexual pleasure, and to develop more a self- versus other-defined sexuality.

Self-Defined Sexuality

It is first necessary for clients to understand the degree to which present paradigms regarding women's sexual nature and appropriate sexual expression are social constructions, rather than absolute truths. As aptly stated by Kaschak (1992), "A woman must [learn to] define the boundaries of herself and learn to incorporate men's definitions, sexuality, and needs not as part of herself but as part of the context" (p. 87). This awareness is necessary if adolescent girls are to be free to choose the ways in which their sexuality is experienced and expressed in their lives and relationships. This includes the partners with whom they choose to be intimate, the behaviors they choose to engage in, and the particular circumstances of these interactions (brief encounters, long-term relationships, etc.). It is important to help adolescent girls challenge those paradigms that place men's needs at the center of the sexual equation (i.e., a woman is not considered to be sexually active until her vagina has been penetrated by a man's penis), and that present women's sexuality and desire as dichotomous, deficient, or in some way diseased (e.g., women who are not interested in having sex are labeled "frigid"; those who are interested in having sex with many different partners are labeled "nymphomaniacs" in polite circles, and "sluts" and "whores" in more popular discourse; and those who choose other women as sexual partners are labeled "dykes"). It is also important to expose these young women to literature and information that helps expand the realm of what is considered "normal" sexual expression, and to validate their efficacy and personal readiness to decide when and if they will participate in this "adult" sexual world.

There are several ways in which we can help adolescent girls begin to understand and deconstruct traditional sexual paradigms. One way is through the use of bibliotherapy. In being exposed to the material in books such as Eisler's (1988) *The Chalice and the Blade,* Perera's (1981) *Descent to the Goddess,* Charlotte Gilman's (1973) *The Yellow Wallpaper,* and Germaine Greer's (1971) *The Female Eunuch,* older adolescents can begin to see the importance of power and context in shaping sexual realities. In her book, *Women Who Run with the Wolves: Myths and Stories of the Wild Woman Archetype,* Clarissa Estes (1992) provides some wonderful stories and myths that underscore the power and depth of women's sexual energy and vitality (see Chapter 2, "Heat: Retrieving a Sacred Sexuality"). Books that articulate the joys of loving women, of bisexuality, and of celibacy are also important resources in expanding young women's understanding of the tremendous breadth and diversity of sexual desire and pleasure (e.g., Cline, 1993; George, 1993; Hutchins & Ka'ahumanu, 1991; Loewenstein, 1985; Weise, 1992). Finally, it is important to expose clients to literature that validates self-pleasure and underscores the centrality of women's role in providing their own sexual satisfaction (e.g., Lonnie Barbach's [1975] *For Yourself*).

By placing young women at the center of their own sexuality, we can reinforce a sense of sexual entitlement and agency. Rather then buying into traditional sexual models and paradigms that focus on the role of others in "awakening" the young woman's sexuality (e.g., the "Sleeping Beauty" version of sex), mental health professionals can assist them to explore the depths and range of the sexual and erotic in their experience of their own bodies. A first step in this process is to help educate adolescent girls about their bodies (including their genitals), and about the feelings and sensations that are available to them in response to particular forms of touch and stimulation. It is important not to assume that young women are aware of their own sexual physiology. Rather, girls should first be invited to privately explore their bodies in exercises such as the "Mirror, Mirror" activity discussed in Chapter 5, with the added instruction of sitting in front of the mirror with their legs apart, so that they might fully examine their genitals. Being given permission to examine themselves in an area that for most was "off limits" when they were children, and to "know" their bodies in this way, is critical in taking ownership of their sexuality (Barbach, 1975; Tiefer,

1996). As always, after such an assignment, care should be taken to debrief the girls. Girls can be asked to engage in the fun and informative activity of using clay or plasticine to create a representation of their genitals (this part of the exercises was designed by a colleague, M. Phillips, for her work in training sex therapists). If this medium is not practical or available, girls can be asked to draw their genitals with crayons or pastels, in detail, in the abstract, or even metaphorically (an adaptation of an exercise recommended by Barbach, 1984, pp. 52–54).

Participants should be asked to share and discuss their drawings, while group leaders provide information and clarification of any confusion regarding the location and functioning of particular parts of the genitals (e.g., emphasizing the role of the clitoris in sexual stimulation; responding to questions regarding the "G" spot). Although these parts of the body can be identified using more formal and technically correct language (urethra, labia, etc.), many young women struggle with the clinical nature of this language. Yet they are not necessarily any more comfortable with the slang words that are frequently used in reference to female genitals (e.g., "cunt," "pussy," "box," "clit"). As part of this activity, then, clients should be encouraged to create their own words or symbols to represent their genitals. These words may be euphemisms or metaphors, or they may be names that have particular personal significance. Stephanie Covington (1991) suggests that the flowers in the painting of Georgia O'Keeffe may be particularly appropriate metaphors for women's genitals in that "they carry a powerful message because of this bold connection made by a woman about a decidedly female image" (p. 74). She also recommends that counselors refer to the book, *Language of the Goddess,* by Marija Gimbutas, which "includes photographs and drawings of nearly two thousand symbolic artifacts . . . based on the female form and specific genitalia." Exposing young women to feminine erotic art may also help girls expand their metaphorical repertoire, while underscoring both the symbolic beauty and significance of women's bodies.

Continuing with the theme of self-acceptance and sexual ownership, we should encourage young women to explore their own bodies with the intent of learning about their bodies' responsiveness to various kinds of touch. This also emphasizes the importance of girls taking an active role in their own pleasuring. Within a context of safety and trust, this type of exploration can initially take place through guided imagery. Girls can then be encouraged to continue their explorations within the privacy of their own homes. Several sources are available that can help young women learn the technique of masturbation (e.g., Barbach, 1975; Bell, 1987; Kitzinger, 1985)—an experience that appears to be positively correlated with sexual self-esteem (Smith et al., 1996; Tiefer, 1996). Emphasis should also be placed on the wide range of images and experiences that may elicit sexual pleasure (e.g., books, videos), and on the exploration of this stimuli.

In reinforcing the integration of the erotic, emotional, and physical aspects of sexual experiencing, it is important to underscore the valuable role of fantasy in sexual stimulation and excitement. There is a relative absence of attention in traditional sexual scripts to the significance of fantasy in women's sexual pleasure (Tiefer, 1996). As such, we need to emphasize how fantasies can provide a *safe* and *pleasurable* way for girls to explore and expand the boundaries of their sexuality, on their own terms. Through journaling (Capacchione, 1985), we can ask girls to keep track of the kinds of situations, people, circumstances, and stimuli (e.g., movies, books) that they find sexually erotic and appealing. We might refer them to books such as Nancy Friday's *My Secret Garden* (1973) and *Forbidden Flowers* (1975), and to classic films such as *Women in Love, The Piano, Like Water for Chocolate, Deserts Hearts,* or *When Night was Falling* to facilitate this exploration. A scene that many women I have spoken with find tremendously sensual and erotic is in the movie *Witness* with Harrison Ford and Kelly McGillis. The scene occurs in the barn of an Amish woman's (McGillis) family farm while she and Harrison Ford's character (a police detective investigating a murder witnessed by the woman's son) are dancing to music from the radio. This scene characterizes the unrequited passion that has been developing in this unlikely couple's brief and intensive relationship. Unlike so many Hollywood portrayals of half-naked couples engaged in an orgy of panting and groping, this scene expands the definition of "sexual" activity in presenting a more *emotionally* revealing image of sexual hunger, passion, and desire. Viewing this type of scene from a popular film, juxtaposed next to a more typical, physically sexual scene, can serve as a useful vehicle for the discussion of issues related to sex and intimacy (including differentiating between interactions that are "sexual" but devoid of intimacy, highly intimate but not sexual in a physical sense, and both intimate and sexual).

Being given permission to engage in sexual fantasies may be a quite foreign experience for young women, and as such, they may need assistance in initiating this process. Using the material in their own personal journals, girls can be taken through an activity such as the relaxation and guided imagery exercise discussed earlier (in the exercise "Embodied Sexuality"), during which they can be encouraged to construct a fantasy that stimulates a highly sensual and erotic response throughout their bodies. They may be alone in this fantasy, or they may be with someone else. They should be asked to allow themselves to stay fully and completely open to this experience without imposing values or sanctions, allowing their senses to drink in all that the fantasy offers in the moment. They should be asked mentally to lock these feelings and sensations in a "safe place" in their minds, so that they can return to them again when they desire. In processing this exercise with participants afterwards, counselors should encourage them to continue to explore the boundaries of their sexuality within the safety and privacy of their fantasy world. Girls should be encouraged to stay in touch with this aspect of their sexual experience as an important window to their sexual wants and desires, and to sexual self-satisfaction.

Rewriting Sexual Scripts

It is important to help clients move past strictly heterosexist and phallocentric notions of sexuality and sexual expression. One way in which this can be accomplished is to have clients participate in an exercise that was suggested by Brian McNaught, a gay writer and lecturer, who gave a keynote address at the Human Sexuality Conference in Guelph, Ontario, Canada, in the spring of 1986. To turn traditional notions of sexuality on their heads, so to speak, and to emphasize the power of social norms in constructing our understanding of "essential" sexual truths, clients are asked to imagine a world in which 90% of the people are homosexual. They are asked to imagine that the institutions, laws, and norms reflect the needs and values of same-sex couples, and to consider what their experience of this world would be like *both* as heterosexual women, and then as lesbians. In particular, they should be asked to allow themselves to fantasize what type of woman they would be sexually attracted to, how their sexuality would be defined and acted upon within a lesbian relationship, and what it would mean for them to be sexually involved with another woman in a world where homosexuality was the norm. This exercise can also be done based on the assumption that the world is primarily bisexual. Debriefing is aimed at dialoguing about the boundaries of what is considered normal and acceptable sexual expression in our society, and about the role and meaning of heterosexuality within our culture. In completing this activity, girls can begin to open their minds and lives to the possibility of other ways of experiencing and expressing their sexuality in the world. Those who find a homosexual or bisexual orientation more consistent with their needs and desires can be given assistance to begin to integrate this reality into their sexual identities (see Appendix D for resources on this topic).

The Personals Are Political

Another useful way to explore sexual diversity is to have girls browse through the *personals* section of the local mainstream newspaper. In so doing, they should be instructed to take note of the types of characteristics that are identified in these ads as being most and least desirable, the way in which the men and women placing these ads frame their request for a partner, the desired level of commitment and intimacy implied in the ads, and so on. Based on their review and their identification of the themes that appear in these ads, they should be asked to construct a composite of a "typical" ad that would be placed by a woman, and a typical ad that would be placed by a man looking for a partner. In a group setting, these composite ads should be presented in the large group. They can serve as a vehicle for further discussion of the sexual assumptions, needs, and desires characteristically expressed by the women and by the men who place these ads (e.g., most ads either implicitly or explicitly specify preferences based on sex, race, color, body size and shape, sexual orientation, interests, desire for commitment; some individuals are also explicit about the type of sexual activities they are interested in pursuing). Discussion of these criteria within the group can prove very enlightening in identifying sexual stereotypes and in highlighting the importance placed on physical versus personal characteristics and attributes in defining what is considered sexually desirable by some men and women.

Having completed a review of the personals in mainstream papers, it is also very enlightening to complete a similar review of the personal ads contained in more "fringe" publications. Such a review helps to underscore the diversity of sexual interests and experiences among individuals. It also highlights the importance of context in defining what is normal and acceptable sexual behavior. A review of the personal ads aimed more specifically at meeting a same-sex partner, or at connecting with someone who is interested in a purely sexual liaison (e.g., S & M, group sex) can help to extend the boundaries of what is considered "normal" or "typical" sexuality. This can also be used as a springboard to facilitate clients' personal explorations of their own sexual preferences and desires. In reviewing these ads, it can also be very useful for girls to discuss recreational versus romantic sex and to explore their feelings related to these issues. While it is important to reinforce "responsible" sexual behavior, it is also critical not to disqualify more casual sexual interactions. Adolescent girls are rarely given permission to consider sexual pleasure outside of the context of a committed and intimate relationship. We must exercise care to allow girls to explore their own beliefs and experiences related to more "casual" sex, and to reinforce responsible actions based on their own erotic needs and impulses.

Based on an adaptation of an exercise identified by Joanne Loulan (1990) in *The Lesbian Erotic Dance: Butch, Femme, Androgyny, and Other Rhythms,* girls can then be assisted in identifying the type of partner they are most interested in sexually. They should be asked to construct their own "personal" ad, focused on what they need and would like in a partner with whom they could feel free to express themselves sexually. The emphasis should not be on a lifetime partner or mate per se, but rather on sexual comfort and desire, and on identifying the kind of partner and relationship characteristics that girls feel would allow them more freely and fully to explore and express their sexuality. These ads may be as short or long as each participant wishes. This is an example of an ad developed by a young woman with whom I worked:

> WANTED. Quiet, confident, self-assured male, 18 to 30 years of age, with small ego and big heart, for safe, playful, sexual encounter(s). Must be comfortable with strong young woman and be willing to follow as well as lead. Must also like long baths, sensuous touch, and romantic interludes, as well as wild and spontaneous sexual escapades.

Another young woman wrote the following ad:

> WANTED. Sensitive, caring, older woman, 30 to 50 years of age, to teach and guide 18-year-old, anxious-to-learn virgin into world of sexual ecstasy. The rewards for someone who is gentle, kind, and patient will be worth it.

Consistent with the sexual double standard discussed earlier in this chapter, it is interesting to note that the creator of this ad just assumed that the reader would know the "virgin" being referred to was a woman. In processing this ad, she said that it did not even occur to her that a male might perceive himself in this way, much less have any interest in being "initiated" into the adult sexual world by an older woman. In creating and processing their individual want ads, clients can learn a great deal about their sexual beliefs, desires, and preferences, and about the interpersonal circumstances and personal characteristics required in a partner to make the exploration and expression of their sexuality comfortable and empowering.

"Vavoom" Experiences

Language is a critical vehicle in the interpretation of experience. For example, Loulan (1990) indicts language as the "biggest barrier" to sexual self-acceptance and understanding among lesbians. She goes on to say: "We really don't have words for the sexual aspects of ourselves and each other that make us recognizable, if not yet identifiable. We have the feelings, but we don't have the words" (p. 139). Without the words, the feelings are, in effect, disqualified. Her observations can easily be extended to virtually all aspects of women's sexual experiencing. An important step toward creating a more self-defined sexuality for adolescent girls is first to examine the available language characteristically associated with sexuality, and then to create new language that is less pejorative, conflictual, and oppressive, using words that more accurately reflect their experiences of sexual and erotic pleasure and desire.

This activity (which can be easily adapted for individual work) begins with the group leader briefly discussing the notion of how the language we have available to us both reflects our experiences and influences the way in which we come to understand and make sense of our lives. It is sometime helpful to use the example of Arctic communities, in which Eskimo peoples have dozens of words to describe "snow." Some discussion of the words commonly used in relation to weight (e.g., see Chapter 5) can be useful to underscore the power of language in diminishing self-esteem and instilling a sense of inadequacy. This activity begins with a blackboard or a large sheet of paper on which the words "sex" and "sexual" are written. Girls are asked to think about some of their ideas about how these words apply to women, and then to call out the words that are commonly associated with having "sex" and with being "sexual." Participants should be encouraged to be as broad in their responses as possible, attempting to include as many words as they are aware of that they have heard in reference to these categories (e.g., including references to body parts, sexual acts, and behaviors). It is useful to facilitate the generation of this list by prompting the participants to consider words that are applied to girls who have not yet had intercourse, to those who have had several sexual partners, to those who express themselves sexually with other women, and so on. When a fairly complete list of words has been generated, participants are asked to repeat each of the words and gauge their internal reaction to each word. They are asked to consider the tone of the words and to examine the *meaning* each of these words holds for them (this part of the exercise can be undertaken in the large group or in dyads, or triads, if the group is too large).

If they have previously completed the sexual fantasy exercise discussed earlier, this can be used as a vehicle for examining the limitations of the language related to sex and sexuality that they have generated. They can be asked to recall their sexual fantasy experience and then select words from the list that best capture the sensual/erotic aspects of this experience (or they might recall a very sensual or erotic experience that they have had and attempt to describe this experience using the words from this list). Generally, participants realize that most of the words characteristically used in relation to sex and being sexual are inadequate to describe their experiences. Although some words such as "orgasm" or "passion" may be partially descriptive, most words are far too limiting to fully express the breadth and depth of the phenomena. Girls should be encouraged to move past the constrictions of conventional language and to construct a vocabulary that more fully and accurately reflects their erotic and sensual experiences. They should be encouraged to create new words that more fully capture this aspect of their sexual energy and experiencing. For example, one young woman described the intense, highly sexual reaction she had the first time she laid eyes on her partner as a "*kabong* experience." Another suggested that the word "vavoom" is the best way to describe the passionate intensity she feels when her sexual energy is at its peak. Clients can have a great deal of fun with this exercise if given the poetic license to be creative in their construction of language. The process of creating and sharing new words that more adequately reflect their sexual and erotic desires and experiences can be an empowering and liberating way for young women to begin to take ownership of their sexuality. Reconstructing the language of sex is an important step in claiming a more woman-centered sexuality.

Self-Care

Throughout these activities, it is critical that those working with adolescent girls incorporate discussion and dialogue about the issues of personal choice, readiness, and responsibility. A more self-defined and agentic sexuality necessarily includes the ability to set limits on particular types of behavior that girls are not ready for or with which they feel uncomfortable. It includes being aware of the consequences of certain behaviors (e.g., unwanted pregnancy, sexually transmitted diseases, increased potential for sexual violence). As many philosophers and writers have noted, freedom is not won without responsibility (I recall in particular the existential dictum that the Statue of Liberty on the East Coast should be balanced by a Statue of Responsibility on the West Coast).

Providing information on these issues is critical, particularly during adolescence, when girls are venturing out into the adult sexual world and beginning to explore and engage in behaviors that carry with them some risk. It is important not to withholding access to such information—whether we choose to provide it ourselves (if we are adequately trained to do so) or refer girls to others who can do so in a nonjudgmental manner. In providing the information ourselves, the difficulty is in finding a way not to lecture or become a gatekeeper. One way to potentially avoid this pitfall is to frame sexual/reproductive information as self-care and to encourage girls to respect and stay tuned in to their own values and feelings when engaging in any intimate or sexual interaction. We need to reinforce the fact that girls are entitled to maintain control over the timing and pacing of their sexual explorations, based on their own personal clocks rather than the social clock.

Much like the assertiveness training groups that were so popular in the 1970s, adolescent girls may also need assistance in learning to assert their sexual needs (see Alberti & Emmons, 1995). An exercise that can be very helpful in this regard is to have a group of girls develop a "Sexual Bill of Rights." Among the items on this list, they may include their right to say "no" to unwanted sexual advances, their right to insist that their partner wear a condom, their right to engage in casual sex, their right to be sexually involved with men *and* women, and so on. Another component of this exercise involves having girls also create a "Sexual Bill of Responsibilities." Among the items on this list, they may include their responsibility to themselves not to "go all the way" until they feel they are ready, their responsibility to have "safe" sex, their responsibility to take precautions against an unwanted pregnancy, and so on.

CONCLUSION

These exercises are only examples of the many ways we can help adolescent girls to challenge and reject conflictual paradigms and disempowering sexual scripts, to create language that affirms their sexual experiences and pleasures, and to construct a more self-defined sexuality based on their own needs and urges. Through these and other activities, young female clients can be encouraged to get in touch with a powerful and vital source of their energy; they can start to connect with the pleasures and sensations that their bodies hold; and they can begin the often difficult process of assuming ownership of, and entitlement to, their sexuality in the many ways they choose to express this in their lives.

III

YOUNG ADULTHOOD

7

BIOLOGICAL AND PSYCHOLOGICAL DEVELOPMENT

BIOLOGICAL DEVELOPMENT

Reproductive Health

Young adulthood is generally defined in the developmental literature as the period from 20 to approximately 40 years of age (Stevens-Long & Commons, 1992). For the most part, this period of life is a time of reproductive health and well-being for women. There are relatively few changes in the reproductive functioning of young women, other than a slight decline in fertility and slightly higher risks of complications during pregnancy and childbirth with increased maternal age (Kitzinger, 1985; Mansfield, 1988). The exception to this, of course, is women who experience particular reproductive discomforts such as dysmenorrhea or premenstrual syndrome (PMS). The symptoms associated with both have been reported to have a negative effect on women's sexual desire, comfort, and self-esteem (Golub, 1992). For a more complete discussion of the symptoms and treatment of PMS the reader is referred to Choi (1994) and McNeill (1994), and for an excellent analysis of "media treatment of premenstrual syndrome," the reader is referred to Parlee (1987).

Sexual and reproductive health concerns are also common for women who, as children, were subjected to female circumcision and infibulation, more commonly referred to in the Western World as female genital mutilation (FGM). This practice is still prevalent in Africa, in parts of the Middle East, and in parts of Malaysia and Indonesia. Although illegal in some U.S. states and in Canada, female circumcision and infibulation continue to be practiced by some ethnic and cultural groups (Omer-Hashi & Entwistle, 1995; Toubia, 1993). As adults, most of these women experience serious reproductive health concerns, not the least of which involve chronic bladder and kidney infections, and serious complications during childbirth. Readers who work with women subjected to FGM are referred to Toubia (1993) for a detailed discussion of the far-reaching consequences of this procedure on women's physical, psychological, and sexual health.

Is Biology Destiny?

Women in their 20s and 30s are faced with the reality of a biologically limited reproductive life span. This is also a time when societal pressures to partner and assume a mothering role are greatest for women (Chodorow, 1978). It is difficult to determine the salience of biological realities versus social imperatives in a woman's acceptance or rejection of "the motherhood mandate" (Russo, 1979). However, many of the popular myths and theories purported to explain women's motivations for mothering rest on the assumption that there is a *biological* basis for women's parenting decisions.

The medical and psychological communities have long contended that there is a "maternal instinct," a physiological basis for women's desire to mother. This desire to procreate is assumed to increase in intensity during young adulthood and to make women particularly suited to the caretaking tasks required when raising dependent children (Ehrenreich & English, 1978; Martin, 1987). Based on hormonal and biological structures, women are believed to feel a compelling and sometimes overwhelming *physiological* urge to reproduce. The ticking of their "biological clocks" purportedly propels them into motherhood. Pituitary hormones have been implicated as the source of the biological basis for women's maternal motivations (Anthony & Benedek, 1970).

Women's desire to reproduce, and their "innate" ability to care for young children, are believed somehow to be wired into women's biology in a way that is not so for men. This assumption is implicit in the judgments made about what constitutes appropriate womanhood and adequate mothering (Chodorow, 1978). So strong is this purported link between women and their wombs that those who voluntarily reject motherhood are perceived as rejecting or denying their "essential" natures and conducting themselves in an "unwomanly" fashion (Ireland, 1993; Morell, 1994).

Despite persistent attempts over the centuries to identify a biological link between maternity and the "essential" nature of women, evidence in support of an instinctual or biological basis for mothering has been elusive (Hubbard, 1990; Lisle, 1996; Tavris, 1992; Unger & Crawford, 1992). Following a review of both animal and human research evidence, Chodorow (1978) concludes that "chromosomes do not provide a basis either for the wish for a child or for capacities for nurturant parental behavior" (p. 23). There appears to be "no evidence to show that female hormones or chromosomes make a difference in human maternalness, and there is substantial evidence that nonbiological mothers, children, and men can parent just as adequately as biological mothers and can feel just as nurturant" (p. 29).

Many feminist theorists and researchers point to the salience of gender-role socialization in women's reproductive decision making and commitment to the mothering role (see Chodorow, 1978; Ehrenreich & English, 1978; Hubbard, 1990; Martin, 1987). They suggest that, in all likelihood, women's motivations to parent reflect *social* rather than *biological* imperatives. Ireland (1993) underscores the inconsistency in the contention that there is some sort of hormonal/physiological basis for women's desire and ability to mother. She points in particular to the case of lesbian women who wish to become mothers, or gay men who want to adopt children. The contention of a purely biological basis for reproductive motivations is further undermined by the fact that approximately 5–8% of women voluntarily reject motherhood (Houseknecht, 1987; Veevers, 1980). Hubbard notes the obvious contradictions between stereotypical descriptions of women's biology and the realities of women's lives. She suggests that women's reputed maternal instinct needs to be looked at in light of some women's desperate efforts to avoid having children in the face of considerable social and religious pressure for women to reproduce. Reproductive motives may also be economic, especially for women whose livelihoods and well-being are contingent upon their ability to reproduce. In North American culture, production and reproduction are intimately connected to the economic and political realities of all women's lives (Hubbard, 1990).

Although women are biological organisms like other animals, it is a political exercise, not a scientific one, to try to find a biological basis for our social roles. "Biology and society are interdependent" (Hubbard, 1990, p. 128). To understand women's reproductive choices and motivations, it is critical to examine the context within which these choices are made. The "woman-as-mother assumption [is] . . . closely connected to basic values and beliefs about the proper and normal way of life" (Russo, 1976, p. 148). Social and economic, rather than biological realities, may be more significant factors in directing women's reproductive motivations and actions (Ehrenreich & English, 1978; Ireland, 1993; Rich, 1976).

Infertility and the Medical Pursuit of Pregnancy

Of the women who try to have a child, an estimated 10–15% experience difficulty in reproducing. In the medical literature, "infertility" is defined as the inability to conceive or carry a viable pregnancy to term after 1 year of regular, unprotected intercourse (Mosher, 1988; Thomas, 1989). A woman's inability to conceive may be caused by a number of hormonal or physiological problems, such as blocked fallopian tubes, ovulatory difficulties, endometriosis, or the fertility problems of her partner (Leader, Taylor, & Daniluk, 1984). Medical treatment options range from least invasive to most invasive, with hormone therapy at one end of the continuum and procedures such as *in vitro* fertilization (IVF) and ovum donation at the other. Of the estimated 34 million infertile Americans, approximately 50–60% achieve a viable pregnancy through medical intervention (Leader et al., 1984). Conception rates vary markedly depending upon age, diagnosis, form of therapy, and duration of treatment. Live birthrates range from less than 10% following some forms of tubal reparative surgery, to 80% after 6 months of hormonal therapy for an uncomplicated ovulatory disorder. More complex technological procedures such as IVF reportedly have a 20–25% pregnancy rate and a 16–20% delivery rate (commonly referred to as the "take home baby rate") per cycle of treatment (Medical Research International, 1992).

Contrary to the contention that infertility is indicative of a woman's ambivalence toward femininity and maternity (Benedek, 1952), no evidence has been accumulated to support psychogenic factors in the etiology of infertility (Sandelowski, 1990a). There is substantial evidence, however, to support the link between medical intervention and considerable psychosocial distress for infertile individuals (Abbey, Andrews, & Halman, 1991; Berg & Wilson, 1991; Daniluk, 1988; Mahlstedt, 1985; Wright, Allard, Lecours, & Sabourin, 1989). Considerably more is known about women's reproductive biology than men's. It should not be surprising, then, that women currently endure most of the medical infertility investigations and treatments (Crosthwaite, 1992; Stanworth, 1987). The invasiveness of these procedures has been reported to wreak havoc on a woman's relationship with her body, and on her experience of her sexuality (Daniluk, 1991a; Leiblum, 1997). Of particular importance in this discussion are the powerful medications commonly prescribed to treat infertile women. Although the side effects of many of these drugs are generally downplayed by the pharmaceutical companies, women on "fertility" drugs frequently report a wide range of psychological and physiological symptoms when taking these medications (Daniluk & Fluker, 1995). Pharmacological agents commonly used in the treatment of infertility have been reported to cause psychological reactions ranging from minor mood swings and depressive symptoms to psychotic reactions and severe personality disturbances. Hot flashes, night sweats, weight gain, excessive hair growth, memory loss, and headaches are among some of the more common and noxious side effects of these drugs. Some women report substantially decreased sexual desire while undergoing medical treatment for infertility. It is difficult, however, to separate the effects of these reproductive medications from the well-documented toll that prolonged medical intervention appears to take on the sexual functioning, satisfaction, and self-esteem of infertile women (Daniluk, 1996). Follow-up studies are currently under way (e.g., the National Institutes of Health–sponsored study, Health Surveillance of Women Treated for Infertility by IVF) in response to concerns about the long-term safety of these hormonal medications for infertile women and their children (e.g., Klein & Rowland, 1988). Readers who work with infertile women are referred to Daniluk and Fluker (1995) for a more detailed discussion of the physical and psychological side effects of the most commonly prescribed medications for impaired fertility.

Pregnancy and Motherhood: Are They Good for One's Health?

Medical practitioners have long contended that pregnancy is a necessary step in the process of physical maturation, and one that is important for women's reproductive health (Ehrenreich & English, 1978). Pregnancy and its concomitant hormonal changes have been considered a treatment, if not a cure, for everything from dysmenorrhea (painful periods/menstrual cramps) to premenstrual tension (Golub, 1992). Some physicians promote pregnancy as insurance against the risks of certain types of cancer (e.g., cervical and uterine cancer). These beliefs are based on the assumption that pregnancy is a natural state of being for a woman. In their support of the importance of pregnancy in maintaining or increasing a woman's reproductive health, gynecologists and physicians have pointed to the "increase in uterine vascularity and blood supply . . . a change in pain-sensitive nerves in the uterus . . . [and] dilation of the cervix that allows for unobstructed menstrual flow" (Golub, 1992, p. 161).

In reality, there appears to be little evidence in support of the contention that pregnancy is either necessary or even desirable for maintaining women's reproductive health (Golub, 1992). Few, however, would debate the fact that pregnancy, childbirth, and mothering precipitate a number of physiological changes in a woman. Some of these changes have implications for a woman's experience of her body and her sexuality. Although few studies have been conducted to examine the relationship between hormonal and psychological changes in pregnant women, it is important to note that hormonally, the changes of pregnancy are considerably *greater* than those experienced during the menstrual cycle (Unger & Crawford, 1992). With fertilization of the ovum, the pituitary continues to release luteinizing hormone, and large quantities of progesterone are produced by the placenta throughout the pregnancy. The production of estrogen is considerably greater during pregnancy than at any time in the menstrual cycle. Increases are reported in the levels of stress-associated adrenocortical hormones, whereas levels of norepinephrine are characteristically lower during pregnancy (Unger & Crawford, 1992).

These dramatic hormonal changes are implicated in a number of characteristic changes during pregnancy. These include feelings of enhanced health and well-being, as well as symptomatic complaints related to nausea, fluid retention, changes in appetite, weight gain, loss of energy, and, in some cases, diminished sexual desire in the first and last trimester of pregnancy (Kitzinger, 1985). Kaplan (1986) notes the relationship between hormonal changes and mood fluctuations experienced by pregnant women. Many of these parallel the symptoms of depression. Given the difficulties in differentiating between the physical and the social consequences of pregnancy, however, she suggests caution in making any definitive assumptions about the relationship between depression and pregnancy.

Pregnant women must also adjust to the dramatic bodily changes that accompany pregnancy and childbirth, not the least of which include substantial increases in size and weight. These increases may be experienced as liberating by some and as frighteningly out of control by others. According to Ussher (1989),

> With the growth of the child the abdomen will grow and the genitals will change in texture and color, the labia becoming engorged like that of a sexually aroused woman. Depending on their attitude to these changes, women will look on their changing bodies with enjoyment and delight, marvelling at their growth, or view themselves with horror. (pp. 98–99)

Reactions to pregnancy include "feeling temporarily free from cultural demands to be slim, feeling awe and wonder, feeling afraid and disgusted by their size, or feeling alienated and out of control" (Unger & Crawford, 1992, p. 409). Some women report feeling "fantastic," "beautiful," "outstanding," and "incredibly sensual," during pregnancy. For others, loss of control over their bodies leaves them feeling "fat," "gross," and "disgusting."

The pregnant woman must also come to terms with the unique experience of having a living organism growing inside her body (sharing her body with another living being). This may be experienced as "comfortable, exciting, wondrous and enjoyable" or "uncomfortable, unpleasant, invasive and hard to tolerate" (Hawkins, 1990, p. 85). Referred to by Bergum (1989) as a sense of "embodied responsibility . . . in pregnancy, the woman shares her body with the growing child, an experience bound by fatigue, weight gain, nausea, flatulence, shortness of breath, vulnerability, and clumsiness that can be only partially controlled" (p. 89). There is increasing medical and social pressure on pregnant women to monitor what they eat, reduce their intake of alcohol, and eliminate smoking to ensure an ideal prenatal environment for the child. It is important to note that this sense of "embodied responsibility" (Bergum, 1989, p. 89) begins not when the child is born, but rather when the child is conceived, with pregnant women being admonished to make their bodies like temples, eating only what is nutritious for the developing child and avoiding smoking, alcohol, excessive stress, and sometimes sexual activity for fear that harm may come to the fetus. According to Kaplan (1990), the fetus "displaces the woman altogether"; the woman's body "is now to be in the service of the fetus, . . . an entity in its own right, . . . rendering [the woman] irrelevant to what is going on in the womb" (p. 417). This leads some women to become excessively vigilant during pregnancy, and to feel tremendous guilt if their child suffers any abnormalities or ill health at birth. Fear of doing damage to the developing child is commonly cited as a reason for avoiding intercourse during pregnancy (Kitzinger, 1985).

During childbirth, the experience of embodiment may be even more extreme, with each woman's labor having its own rhythm and progressing at its own pace. Kitzinger (1985) discusses the potential power of this experience. Herself a midwife, she notes how, for some women, childbirth is experienced as highly erotic:

> A woman who is enjoying her labor swings into the rhythm of contractions as if her birth-giving were a powerful dance, her uterus creating the beat. She watches for it, concentrates on it, like an orchestra following its conductor. . . . The uterus, the vagina, the muscles enfolding the vagina and rectum, the lower back, the rectum itself and the anus, the buttocks, tissues around and between the vagina and anus, and the clitoris are all suffused with heat as if with liquid fire or as if brimful and pouring over with glowing color. It can be the most intensely sexual feeling a woman ever experiences, as strong as orgasm, even more compelling than orgasm. (pp. 209–210)

Unfortunately for women in the Western World, the medicalization of childbirth has resulted in many being largely disconnected from their bodies' rhythms and the intense sensuality of childbirth. Despite efforts by midwives and licensed practical nurses to return the birthing experience to a more "natural" and welcoming environment, many births in North America still occur in sterile and antiseptic medical environments. Women are hooked up to monitors (e.g., fetal heart monitors) and their perineums are still frequently cut to avoid possible "tearing." They may attempt a "natural," unmedicated labor, but many are encouraged to turn to medications to reduce the pain. Unfortunately, these medications also dull the sensations of women's bodies during childbirth (Hyde, 1990). Ironically, Canada and the United States, two of the more "developed" countries of the world, boast some of the highest rates of cesarean section. Approximately one out of every five births occurs by cesarean section (Bergum, 1989), leaving the mother completely disconnected from childbirth. Women's birthing experiences are still frequently co-opted in the service of "safety" (Bergum, 1989; Ehrenreich & English, 1978; Kitzinger, 1985; Ussher, 1989).

A woman's experience of childbirth will in all likelihood influence her experience of her body and her sexuality as she embarks on motherhood. A particularly traumatic birthing experience may leave women feeling like strangers to their bodies. Women may feel like failures if their birth results in undesired medical intervention or medication. According to Kitzinger (1985), "It can be a long, painful journey to get on good terms with your body after such an alienating experience, to begin to like it and allow sexual passion to sweep through every pore" (p. 219). There are also significant physical changes that accompany the postpartum period. As hormonal levels drop dramatically, the reproductive organs alter in size and shape, and the woman must adjust to her postpartum body. "Sadness and emotional instability . . . settle on 50 to 70 percent of women three to four days after they give birth and lifts of its own accord within a week to ten days" (Partridge, 1996, p. 87). Approximately 10–20% of women experience a more protracted period of depression, lasting for a period of up to 6 weeks following the birth of a baby. A smaller percentage (estimates range from 3% to 9%) experience more significant, long-term postpartum depression (Gruen, 1990; Kleiman & Raskin, 1994). There is considerable debate in the literature regarding the definition, etiology, and symptom profile of these postpartum mood changes. It is especially difficult to tease out the contribution of hormonal shifts, physical exhaustion, sleep deprivation, and role changes that occur for women following the birth of a child, and to distinguish postpartum depression from "the blues" (Bergum, 1989; Kitzinger, 1994; Kraus & Redman, 1986).

Finally, in terms of the link between motherhood and sexuality, the experience of feeding and mothering an infant and young child can be physically taxing as well as being highly sensual and erotic. Few experiences parallel the intensity or physical intimacy of caretaking a child during the first few years of life. Breast-feeding, in particular, is a very sensual experience for some women.

> It is not just that the mammary glands are organs of sexual arousal, but that the rhythms of breast-feeding—the buildup to breast fullness as the baby gets hungry, the speed with which the breasts respond with warmth when the baby cries, the erection of the nipple as the baby seeks it with an urgent, searching mouth—have an intensely sexual quality. (Kitzinger, 1983, p. 225)

Unfortunately, North American society neither acknowledges or sanctions the sensuality and eroticism inherent in the experiences of birthing and caretaking a child. This can engender feelings of shame and guilt for many women who do find this experience stimulating (Adler, 1994; Oberman & Josselson, 1996; Ussher, 1989). According to Rich (1976), "since there are strong cultural forces which desexualise women as mothers, the orgasmic sensations felt in childbirth or while suckling infants have probably until recently been denied even by the women feeling them, or have evoked feelings of guilt" (pp. 179–180).

It is clear from this discussion that the biological and physiological changes that accompany pregnancy and motherhood, as well as the medical treatments characteristically employed in the treatment of impaired fertility, necessarily have an impact on women's experiences of their bodies and of their sexuality. From this discussion, it would appear that biological factors cannot be dismissed in attempting to understand women's reproductive experiences. However, we must also consider the very powerful role of psychosocial factors in any woman's experience of her sexuality, whether or not she experiences pregnancy and motherhood.

Other Bodily Changes

From the standpoint of biological development, women in their 20s and 30s are generally in relatively good physical health (Kimmel, 1990; Stevens-Long & Commons, 1992). This fact is reflected in the lack of information in most books on the physical and biological changes experienced by women during this period of the life cycle (e.g., Boston Women's Health Collective, 1992; Unger & Crawford, 1992). Much is written about the dramatic physical changes experienced by girls during childhood and adolescence, and about the challenges involved in adapting to the physiological and biological changes characteristic of middle age and later life. However, attention in the literature to women's health concerns during young adulthood is limited to the issues related to fertility and reproductive health discussed earlier.

The exception to this is literature that pertains to coping with physical disabilities such as rheumatoid arthritis, multiple sclerosis, paralysis, and so on, and research examining the sequelae of breast and reproductive cancers. The incidence of these cancers appears to be on the rise for women in their 20s and 30s. Estimates of breast cancer are now one in eight. Of women who are diagnosed with breast cancer, 80% have no family history of the disease (Caldwell, 1994). Ovarian and uterine cancers occur more frequently in mid- and later life (Gross & Ito, 1992). Although cancer crosses all economic boundaries, "poorer women who do not have access to healthful living and working conditions" appear to be especially at risk for cervical cancers at an earlier age than middle-class women (Boston Women's Health Book Collective, 1992, p. 573).

Whatever their age or life stage, women diagnosed with cancer face not only concerns about their mortality and feelings of bodily betrayal, but also such physically mutilating surgeries as radical mastectomy and hysterectomy. Despite more conservative approaches to the diagnosis and treatment of breast cancer (e.g., lumpectomy, radiation), every year, thousands of women in the United States and Canada lose their breasts because of cancer (Love, 1990; MacPhee, 1994). "Each year about 650,000 women in the United States have a hysterectomy" (Boston Women's Health Collective, 1992, p. 598). It is interesting to note that "prior to 1981, hysterectomy was the most common surgical procedure performed in the United States, and today, it ranks as the second most performed major surgical operation" (Leiblum, 1990, p. 500). Equaled only by Australia, the rate of hysterectomy in Canada and the United States is double that of England and Wales, three times that of Sweden and Norway, and four times that of France and Japan (Kjerulff, Langenberg, & Guzinski, 1993).

The loss of a breast or uterus will no doubt have a profound impact on a woman's experience of her body and her sexuality (Boston Women's Health Collective, 1992; Gross & Ito, 1990, 1992; Kitzinger, 1985; Johnson, 1987). As Kitzinger (1985) notes, "Losing any part of the body in a mutilating operation, however necessary and however life-saving the surgery, involves grieving. This process is long and painful for some of us. It can profoundly affect our view of ourselves and our sexuality" (p. 297).

Noting the psychosocial difficulties of coping with the loss of a breast, Kitzinger (1985) reports that "25 percent of women who have mastectomies eventually need some kind of psychotherapy, and for some women sex comes to a stop" (p. 305). The consequences of a hysterectomy are also far-reaching, leaving many women feeling "empty," "neutered," and in need of emotional support (Bernhard, 1992; Kitzinger, 1985).

The specific concerns of women with disabilities and of women who have been diagnosed with cancer cannot adequately be addressed in this book. The reader is referred to Appendix F for a list of resources that may be useful for mental health professionals in their efforts to help women cope with physical disability, chronic illness, or cancer.

From Biologically Inferior to Multiply Orgasmic: Sexual Functioning

In terms of the sexual functioning and physiology of women in young adulthood, it is safe to say that our knowledge of the breadth, range, and texture of women's sexual experiences and desires is still in its infancy. If we rely on more traditional definitions of sexual functioning, young adult women appear to experience few physical barriers to the expression and enjoyment of their sexuality. Certainly, the studies by Masters and Johnson (1966), although not beyond reproach (as discussed in Chapter 4), have provided useful evidence to dispel the myth that women's sexual responsiveness is inferior to that of men. Quite the contrary, based on their detailed laboratory examinations of the bodily responses of men and women to sexual stimulation, Masters and Johnson concluded that the sexual response cycles of males and females are actually more similar than different. Adequate sexual stimulation during the excitement phase produces vaginal lubrication and swelling for women, which is analogous to penile erections for men. What constitutes "adequate stimulation" for any woman, however, is very much an individual issue. There is wide variation between women and men, and between women, as to what contextual, situational, relational, and psychological factors elicit sexual excitement for any individual. It would appear that for most women, *physical* stimulation of the genitals is only one source, albeit an significant source, of stimulation for maintaining sexual excitement. "The exact area and type of genital stimulation needed for orgasm depends upon the physiological make-up and learned response patterns of each individual woman" (Barbach, 1976, p. 59).

As noted in Chapter 4, Masters and Johnson (1966) propose that both men and women progress through the four phases of the sexual response cycle (excitement, plateau, orgasm, resolution) in roughly the same manner, with orgasm resulting in urogenital spasms every 0.8 second during this phase of the cycle. Contrary to Freud's belief in the superiority of vaginal orgasms for women, their research data suggest that the sexual response cycle remains the same "whether the orgasm occurs through clitoral stimulation alone, through manual masturbation, through use of a vibrator, through love-making with another female, as the result of intercourse with a male partner, or fantasy alone" (Barbach, 1976, p. 63). In fact, research evidence confirms that "every orgasm manifests itself in the whole pelvic region regardless of the part of the body that has been stimulated" (p. 64).

This research also found that the vasocongestive responses that produce an erection in the male are much more vulnerable to disruption and interruption (i.e., impotence, premature ejaculation) than the female response (Golden, 1988). The time period required between orgasms (the refractory period) also appears to be shorter for women than for men (Masters & Johnson, 1966). And finally, these findings confirm that women are capable of multiple orgasms, and these orgasms "tend to be more intense when self-induced by clitoral stimulation than when achieved through heterosexual intercourse" (Ehrenreich et al., 1986, p. 67).

Some writers (e.g., Tiefer, 1987, 1995, 1996) have rightly argued that Masters and Johnson (1966, 1970) have reduced women's sexuality to a discussion of mechanics and hydraulics, presenting a linear, decontextualized vision of sexual behavior based on male norms. However, it is also important to acknowledge how the technical information provided by Masters and Johnson has served to quantify the physical aspects of sexual expression and dispel some of the persistent myths regarding women's diminished physical capacity to experience sexual desire and satisfaction. Surveys by sex researchers like Kinsey et al. (1953), Hite (1981, 1987), and Wyatt, Peters, and Guthrie (1988a, 1988b) have also been influential in legitimizing the wide range of activities that women engage in and find sexually stimulating.

Certainly, it is problematic to reduce women's sexuality to a goal-oriented focus on physiological functioning and orgasm, placing limitations on an experience that clearly involves much more than the stimulation of a woman's breasts and the function of her genitals. Women's sexuality is more than just the sum of particular body parts. What this work does do, however, is underscore the fact that women's biology is not what limits them from exploring the depths of sexual expression. Although some women may be unable to experience orgasms, in most cases, it would appear that these difficulties have less to do with biological limitations and more to do with the psychosocial realities of women's lives.

PSYCHOLOGICAL DEVELOPMENT

"Essential" Womanhood

Just as the medical community proposes a maternal instinct (Hubbard, 1990), many in the psychological community believe that the desire for and the attainment of motherhood is essential to the psychological development and sexual maturity of adult women. Sigmund Freud (1969) theorized that woman's desire for a child, in particular, a son, represented compensation for the loss of a penis. Helena Deutsch (1945) contended that women develop charm and beauty only after they have given birth. Eric Erikson (1968) proposed that women need to fill their "inner space" with a child. These theories imply that women who desire autonomy and independence over maternity are psychologically immature, neurotic, and infantile. They suffer from "incomplete feminization" (Ehrenreich & English, 1978, p. 276).

Other theories of women's psychological development have been proposed that emphasize the importance of both *psychological* and *social* factors in the reproductive roles women assume and in their satisfaction with these roles (e.g., Gilligan, 1982; Jordan et al., 1991; Kaschak, 1992; Miller, 1986). But the assumption that motherhood is somehow essential to women's development is both implicitly and explicitly reinforced in North American culture, and is even more strongly reinforced by certain religious and ethnic mandates. For example, despite considerable evidence to the contrary (Houseknecht, 1987; Ireland, 1993; Morell, 1994; Veevers, 1980), voluntarily childless women are still perceived by others as being somehow psychologically deficient in their rejection of the motherhood role. They are repeatedly faced with questions and doubts regarding their selfishness and personal adequacy based on their apparent "refusal" to reproduce.

Because the desire to mother is assumed to be "natural" for women, relatively little attention has been paid in the psychological literature to the complex host of psychosocial factors that motivate women's reproductive choices (Baruch, Barnett, & Rivers, 1983; Gerson, Alpert, & Richardson, 1990). Our knowledge is also limited regarding the way in which the experiences of pregnancy and mothering, voluntary childlessness, or infertility shape women's perceptions of themselves and their sexuality. We turn, now, to a brief review of this literature.

Mothering

Despite the purported significance of mothering in women's psychological development, most of the research on mothering has been focused on the impact of mothers on their *children's* development (see Caplan, 1989, for a critique of this literature). Emphasis has been placed on the adequacy or inadequacy of mother's efforts to rear their offspring, particularly mothers who also work outside the home. For example, in their book entitled *Motherhood and Mental Illness,* Brockington and Kumar (1982) identify and expound upon the many "neurotic disorders in childbearing women" that have "undesirable effects upon the psychological development of the newborn child" (p. 71); a perspective that continues to be promoted in Brockington's 1996 version of this book.

More recently, however, researchers have begun to employ both quantitative and qualitative methods to examine the experience of mothering from the perspective of mothers themselves. They have begun to examine women's lives and sense of self as their mothering roles evolve and change through the various stages of their children's development (e.g., Bergum, 1989; Gieve, 1989; Kaplan, 1992; Knowles, 1990; McMahon, 1995). Based almost exclusively on examining the experiences of heterosexual women who mother their own biological children, this literature supports the contention that the assumption of a mothering role has a formative impact on women's physical and psychological experience of themselves. It is difficult, however, to distinguish between the social realities of mothering in terms of roles and expectations versus the realities of being engaged in a unique relationship with an*other.* In the words of Adrienne Rich (1976),

> Nothing had prepared me for the intensity of relationship already existing between me and a creature I had carried in my body and now held in my arms and fed from my breasts . . . the psychic crisis of bearing a first child, the excitation of long-buried feelings about one's own mother, the sense of confused power and powerlessness, of being taken over on the one hand and of touching new physical and psychic potentialities on the other. . . . No one mentions the strangeness of attraction . . . to a being so tiny, so dependent, so folded-in to itself—who is, and yet is not, part of oneself. (p. 17)

Referred to by McMahon (1995) and Bergum (1989) as a transformative experience, one that is shaped by culture and class, women who become mothers report significant changes in their sense of themselves as women, in their intimate relationships, and in their relationships with significant others (especially extended family members and, in particular, their mothers). These changes often begin when a woman becomes pregnant. In her hermeneutic–phenomenological study of six women in their transition to motherhood, Bergum was struck by the "transformative experience of having a child on one's mind" (p. 101). She notes the ever-present "sense of responsibility" (p. 83) that is involved in mothering a child in North American culture. She speaks of the struggle in balancing the needs of the child with women's own needs, as mothers attempt to answer the question: "How can one lose oneself to another, and yet be oneself?" (p. 40). She also points to the transformative effect of mothering in shaping a woman's life path and sense of self. For many, assuming the responsibility for another compels them to take responsibility for their own lives. "What has been a self-regulated, self-defined, and self-contained life is now suddenly broken by the experience of the Other, the child. And in taking responsibility for the child as Other, we are forced to be responsible also for ourselves" (p. 84).

The power of assuming responsibility for the life of another to shape the experiences of women who mother was expressed by one of my clients when she said,

> "I think women do a lot of healing through having their own child. We heal the child in ourselves by taking care of our children and loving them. . . . I didn't even know how to love. I had to open that whole part of me up again. . . . Like when I had my daughter, I just looked at her and I thought, you know, I have all these aspirations for her, but she'll never be any of them unless I become them."

Price (1988) talks about what motherhood "does to your mind." Rich (1977) and others (e.g., Chodorow & Contratto, 1992; Gieve, 1989; Hawkins, 1990; Phoenix, Woollett, & Lloyd, 1991) expound upon the power and tyranny of the "institution of motherhood" in shaping women's understanding and experience of mothering and of themselves as mothers. Nicolson (1986) refers to the psychological reintegration that is required of women who mother. Women must grieve the loss of self and attempt to adapt to the major changes in their lives, relationships, and identities as they negotiate this transition. This perspective is also underscored by Oberman and Josselson (1996) in their identification of the "matrix of tensions" that characterizes the mothering experience for women.

While mothering a child may indeed transform a woman's experience of herself and her relationships, it remains to be determined how mothering affects a woman's experience of her sexuality. Almost no attention has been paid in the literature to the sexual needs, desires, or experiences of women once they make the transition to motherhood (Kitzinger, 1985; Rich, 1977; Unger & Crawford, 1992). This is consistent with the contention that motherhood and sexual agency cannot coexist. There are only token references to the sexuality of mothers in the literature, and these tend to focus on physical exhaustion and the fear of becoming pregnant, two factors that make it difficult to maintain a "quality" sex life. Much is left to be learned about women's experiences of their sexuality at each stage of mothering.

Infertility

An infertile woman is unable to assume a role that she has been socialized to pursue for a lifetime. She is incapable of achieving what so many other women appear to achieve with relative ease. This necessarily has an impact on her sense of competence and self-esteem (Llewelyn & Osborne, 1990; Menning, 1988; Woollett, 1991). The terminology used in reference to their fertility status, words such as "barren" and "sterile," and the pity invoked in others at the knowledge that they are unable to fulfill their maternal role, leaves many infertile women feeling like sexual and reproductive failures. They often feel like failures as women (Daniluk, 1997; Ireland, 1993; Sandelowski, 1993). The words "woman" and "infertile" often seem mutually exclusive (Menning, 1988).

So strong is the belief in women's responsibility for reproduction that women frequently blame themselves when the diagnosis is exclusively male-factor infertility (Abbey et al., 1991; Nachtigall, Becker, & Wozny, 1992). Women often attribute the cause of the infertility to their own biological failure, to perceived transgressions such as relinquishing a child for adoption or having had an abortion, or to an extramarital affair (Berg, Wilson, & Weingartner, 1991; Daniluk, 1991a, 1997; Greil, 1991; Mahlstedt, 1985). Women report a decrease in sexual satisfaction with prolonged infertility treatment, and perceive their inability to conceive as a direct assault on their sexual self-image and self-esteem, and on their sense of themselves as complete and competent women (Berg et al., 1991; Greil, 1991; McGrade & Tolor, 1981). Women who experience fertility problems are more sensitive to fertility-related stimuli (pregnant women, babies, etc.) (Berg et al., 1991; Daniluk, 1991a, 1997) and tend to be more distressed by the comments of others regarding their childless status (Mahlstedt, 1985; Menning, 1988). In the words of one infertile woman with whom I worked,

> "Every week, I seem to hear about someone else who's pregnant, and each time I hear someone is pregnant, I feel like I've died inside. . . . No one will ever understand this, but it's like every time they give life, in my mind, it's like giving death."

Having been socialized to believe that to be fulfilled they must reproduce, when faced with obstacles to their fertility, women frequently become even more committed to the goal of having children, and to the pursuit of medical options to achieve this goal (Greil, 1991; Ulbrich, Coyle, & Llabre, 1990). They often find it difficult to get off the medical merry-go-round, irrespective of the physical, psychological, social, and financial costs involved in the continued pursuit of treatment, even when faced with very remote probabilities of a successful outcome (Braverman, 1997; Sandelowski, 1993). A poignant example of this difficulty in letting go is apparent in the story of a colleague, herself a psychologist, who came face-to-face with the extent of her desperation in pursuing infertility treatments and was forced to confront the futility of her efforts to conceive a child:

> Following several years of investigations, my physician informed me that extensive surgery would provide my only hope of conceiving a child. My immediate response was "book it." "But don't you want to know what it involves," said the physician, to which I responded "book it." "But don't you even want to know the probability of success or the risks," said he. I implored him, "Please, just book it." At that moment I realized that had the physician told me women with one leg had a better chance of conceiving a child, I would have unhesitatingly offered to have my leg cut off. I knew then that it was time to quit . . . that it wasn't making sense anymore. (Daniluk, 1997, p. 119)

This anecdote underscores the level of anguish and desperation experienced by many infertile women as they attempt to make "informed decisions" about the continued pursuit of medical intervention.

Reflecting the strong social link between femininity, motherhood, and value for women in North American culture (Chodorow, 1978; Rich, 1977; Ussher, 1997), both intentionally and involuntarily childless women experience and perceive greater pressures to assume a motherhood role, and more negative sanctions in response to their childlessness (e.g., they are often considered selfish, unfulfilled, unwomanly) (Ireland, 1993). Involuntarily childless women in particular feel stigmatized by their inability to produce a child. They experience a profound sense of personal failure when their efforts to reproduce are unrealized. As stated by Nachtigall et al. (1992), "Any failure to fulfill the motherhood role negatively affects a woman's perception of herself because the failure to biologically reproduce represents a failure to meet gender role expectations" (p. 119). The personal and social consequences are even greater for women from cultures where the inability to procreate presents a serious threat to their marital relationships and their economic survival. In the words of one highly educated professional Muslim woman, whom I interviewed prior to her *seventh* round of IVF, "If I cannot produce a child in the eyes of my husband, my family, and my culture, I am nothing."

Even though some women ensure their adult status in the eyes of others by becoming mothers through adoption, they must live with having never experienced pregnancy and childbirth. These are two very significant social symbols of sexual success and mature womanhood in most cultures of the world. It should not be surprising, then, that the inability to bear a child and the medical investigations involved in treating infertility are important factors that shape women's experiences of their sexuality, their sexual identities, and their sense of sexual agency.

Voluntary Childlessness

If the infertile woman is perceived as somehow psychologically deficient and unfulfilled—someone to be pitied—the voluntarily childless woman is viewed at best as a psychological aberration, and at worst as a traitor to her sex. "Maternal ambivalence is seen in some way as pathological, as a woman's denial of her 'natural' impulses and inability to come to terms with her 'real purpose' " (Ireland, 1993, p. 13). Much of the research on women who have refused childbearing has focused on identifying demographic and personality variables that are correlated with intentional childlessness. Some of these include advanced educational achievements, being firstborn, having assumed caretaking responsibilities in childhood, having high career aspirations, and having strong needs for autonomy, freedom, and independence (see Houseknecht, 1987, for a review of this literature).

Women who reject the motherhood role appear to come to their childlessness in different ways, some knowing from an early age, and others arriving at the decision through a series of postponements and delays (Houseknecht, 1987; Ireland, 1993; Morell, 1994; Veevers, 1980). Whatever route they take in their reproductive decision making, current research supports the psychological health and well-being of these women. Despite attempts to identify an underlying psychopathology that would explain their rejection of mothering, the available literature suggests that the psychological health and well-being of voluntarily childless women appears to be no different than that of mothers (Baruch, 1984; Baruch et al., 1983; Ireland, 1993; Mercer, Nichols, & Doyle, 1988; Morell, 1994; Veevers, 1980). In fact, in their study of the developmental transitions in women's lives, Mercer et al. (1994) report that in comparison to women who were mothers, "a larger number of *non*mothers . . . achieved integrity, the last developmental stage defined by Erikson" (p. 185). Based on her research with voluntarily childless women, Landa (1990) "suggests that the ego and moral development of voluntarily childless women . . . is highly evolved, but that their paths to maturity are atypical, starting with precocity in childhood and adolescence, proceeding through a long developmental moratorium in early adulthood, and accelerating again at midlife" (p. 143). This and other research (e.g., Ireland, 1993; Morell, 1994) confirms that, contrary to social expectations, voluntarily childless women appear to have contented and fulfilled lives. Even those who select to terminate a pregnancy appear to suffer few long-term psychological consequences if the decision is freely chosen and legally sanctioned (Dagg, 1991; Kushner, 1997; Lemkau, 1988).

This research would suggest that the problems most frequently reported by the voluntarily childless do not appear to be related to a sense of "absence" or "loss" in having not experienced pregnancy and motherhood. As with all life decisions, they may have some sense of sadness or loss at "the road not taken," but few appear to experience serious regrets at having chosen to forego motherhood (Lisle, 1996; Morell, 1994; Safer, 1996). Instead, it would appear that "something is missing in our definitions of 'woman' because there is no valid place for [the voluntarily childless] in existing psychological theory" (Ireland, 1993; p. 135). The difficulty comes in attempting to "consolidate and construct their own atypical adult female identities—as women, but not as mothers" (p. 16). To do so requires a rejection of the deficiency model of childlessness and the creation of more expansive beliefs about women's lives and the value of women's other "creative labors."

Body Image Changes

Little attention is paid in the psychological literature to young women's experiences of their bodies and to the development and maintenance of positive body image. This situation exists despite the importance of the body in defining women's value and worth within our culture. Other than the books and articles focused specifically on eating disorders and weight preoccupation, there is relatively little discussion of the relationship between identity, self-esteem, and the experience of living in a woman's body during this period of the life cycle. Yet at the time when many women are establishing themselves in the world of work, and are continuing to negotiate the challenges of intimate relationships, the body still plays a significant role in their experiences. When women enter their 20s they do not leave all of the bodily insecurities of adolescence behind. Rather, the body images women developed in childhood and adolescence form the foundation for their adult bodily self-perceptions (Hutchinson, 1994).

Women's feelings of bodily inadequacy and insecurity continue to be reinforced throughout young adulthood, within their intimate relationships, following the birth of children, and by the realities of the world of work, where women are clearly discriminated against based on their weight and "attractiveness" (Brown & Rothblum, 1989). As articulated in the books of Wolf (1991) and Faludi (1991), young adult women are primary consumers of "beauty" and health care products and programs. Many young adult women continue their efforts to tone, trim, and shape their bodies to meet the relentless cultural ideals. Many still experience feelings of inadequacy about their bodies and engage in dieting, exercise, or cosmetic surgery to alter their physical "flaws" (Friedman, 1993; Seid, 1989; Smith, 1990; Thompson, 1994). It would appear that during young adulthood, when women are usually at the height of their physical strength and prowess, many continue to treat their bodies like battlegrounds upon which they wage self-destructive wars (Bartky, 1990; Faludi, 1991; Seid, 1994; Ussher, 1989).

From Fig Leaves to Fruit Flies

Just as myths and misinformation abound in the area of women's physical sexual adequacy and responsiveness, so too are there a host of equally unsubstantiated fallacies regarding women's sexual natures and what constitutes normal and abnormal adult sexual identity, functioning, and desire. Psychoanalysts contend that women's "renunciation of sexual agency and . . . acceptance of object status are the very hallmark of the feminine" (Benjamin, 1988, p. 87). There is no question from a psychoanalytic perspective as to "Who's on top?" (Buchbinder, Burstyn, Forbes, & Steedman, 1987), who the players should be in the sexual drama, and what their respective roles are. Many neo-Freudian theorists (Clara Thompson, Karen Horney, Nancy Chodorow, Jessica Benjamin, etc.) have cogently repudiated Freud's contention regarding the existence, much less centrality, of penis envy in the psychosexual formation of the female. They have argued that the major sexual dilemma for women is not penis envy but one of acknowledging their own sexuality in this culture. However, as I have discussed elsewhere in this book, the beliefs and assumptions that permeate psychoanalytic theory are still highly influential in informing many of the current myths regarding the sexual needs and expression of adult women.

Where psychoanalytic theory has failed the requirement of scientific verification, sociobiology has stepped in to reinforce the barricades of male sexual privilege. Based on the behavior of creatures as phylogenetically incompatible to humans as the common fruit fly (Bateman, 1948), and drawing on animal research, primarily from the fields of evolutionary biology, anthropology, and primatology, sociobiologists like Symonds (1979) and Wilson (1978) have attempted to support the "naturalness" of the current sexual arrangements. Their theory is based on the Darwinian premise that both men and women have an innate drive to reproduce their genes, although males and females adopt quite different strategies to do this. In a nutshell, sociobiologists suggest that "males compete with other males for access to desirable females, and their goal is to inseminate as many females as possible. Females, in contrast, are motivated to attach themselves to genetically 'superior' males because of the female's greater 'investment' in terms of time and energy in her offspring" (Tavris, 1992, pp. 214–215). The recent popularity of sociobiological explanations of the sexual natures of men and women serves to further maintain the sexual double standard and sexual status quo.

In response to these phallocentric theories, some writers (Katie Roiphe's 1993 book aside) have attempted to free women's sexual expression from the constraints of passivity, submission, and procreation. They propose instead a vision of women's sexual expression as a wellspring of sensory and erotic possibilities, limited only by the imagination and creativity of the individuals involved, and by the dictates of a society that perceives the "unleashing" of women's sexuality as dangerous (Vance, 1992). Others (e.g., see Kitzinger, 1987; Loulan, 1987; Rich, 1980; Plummer, 1975, 1992; Weasel, 1996) have posed strong arguments against the "naturalness" of heterosexuality, underscoring the centrality of male power and domination in our current sexual arrangements. Still others (e.g., Jordan, 1986, 1987; Jordan et al., 1991) have attempted to highlight the importance of connection and mutuality in women's psychological development and sexual interactions, emphasizing the inseparability of relational intimacy and sexual pleasure for women. Commenting on the interpersonal nature of sexual desire, Jordan (1987) contends that while men may focus their sexual feelings in their genitals, for women, it is the "relational context in which these acts and responses occur [that] provides meaning and joy" (p. 14). Based on her research with 50 women, Gina Ogden (1985, 1994) underscores how sexual ecstasy for women is not limited to the genitals, but rather includes "what they sense in their whole bodies—fingers and toes and ears as well as clitoris and G Spot" (1985, p. 47). According to Ogden, the involvement of the mind, heart, and soul is as important as the body in defining what is pleasurable for women.

Despite these recent efforts, it is still difficult to say with any authority what we really know about the psychology of adult women's sexuality. According to Lewis (1980), "The psychology of female sexuality is nearly as poorly formulated now as it was in Freud's time" (p. 35). While we have learned more about the capacity of women's bodies to respond in a pleasurable way to particular stimuli, our current theories have evolved out of a particular set of assumptions. They are inadequate to fully explain the wide variance in women's sexual desires and experiences (e.g., how some women can separate sex and love; how celibate women express their sexuality; why some women are sexually attracted to other women, some to men, and some to both; how some women can [learn to] express their sexuality without shame or guilt). Many myths have been debunked, but our theories are still sorely lacking. As noted by Webster (1988) in reference to the state of our knowledge regarding women's sexuality, "My hardest questions come when I find the theories and the words cannot help me in trying to work with women who are in pain" (pp. 298–299).

CONCLUSION

Sexuality is "a construct that emerges in interaction as a result of expectations and negotiations, not something 'inside' each of us" (Tiefer, 1987, p. 88). As such, in our attempts to understand the diverse sexualities of women and how these may become problematic during young adulthood, it may be more useful to look outward rather than inward. As Person (1980) states, "Even sexuality, so clearly grounded in biology, is embedded in meaning and cannot be understood without reference to culture. Individuals internalize aspects of their interpersonal world. . . . This internalization shapes both their experience of desire and expression of sexuality" (p. 644). In the next three chapters, we turn our attention to the larger social context within which young adult women negotiate their sexuality. Specific attention is paid to women's reproductive choices, bodily comfort, and sexual expression during this life stage.

8

CREATING A LIFE

In another
life, dear sister, I too would bear six fat
children. In another life, my sister, I too
would love another woman and raise one child
together as if that pushed from both our wombs.
In another life, sister, I too would dwell
solitary and splendid as a lighthouse on the rocks
or be born to mate for life like the faithful goose.
Praise all our choices. Praise any woman
who chooses, and make safe her choice.

—MARGE PIERCY,
"The Sabbath of Mutual Respect"

I did not know the woman I would be
nor that blood would bloom in me
each month like an exotic flower,
nor that children,
two monuments,
would break from between my legs
two cramped girls breathing carelessly,
each asleep in her tiny beauty.
I did not know that my life, in the end,
would run over my mother's like a truck
and all that would remain
from the year I was six
was a small hole in my heart, a deaf spot,
so that I might hear
the unsaid more clearly.

—ANNE SEXTON, "From Those Times . . . "

A woman's experience of herself as a sexual person is profoundly shaped by the reproductive choices she makes and roles she assumes. Does she create her life as a childless woman? Does she attempt to have children but find she is unable to? Does she become a mother? Whatever procreative choices a woman makes, and whether she even perceives that she has a choice, will be shaped by the powerful pragmatic and symbolic cultural link between women's sexuality and reproduction (Greer, 1984; Ireland,

1993; Martin, 1987). The belief that women should want to mother and that motherhood represents women's ultimate personal and sexual fulfillment is firmly embedded in history and culture. It has become a basic "truth." This socially constructed truth is internalized to varying degrees by women and necessarily shapes their understanding and experiencing of themselves as women and as sexual persons, in whatever reproductive roles they assume.

In her book, *Of Woman Born: Motherhood as Experience and Institution,* Adrienne Rich (1977) underscores the way in which the social construction of mothering informs and shapes the experiences and self-conceptions of all women, those who mother as well as those who do not. "Pregnancy, childbirth, and motherhood are an intrinsic part of women's experience, regardless of whether or not we decide to give birth to children" (Ussher, 1989, p. 76).

Attention to the social context within which women make and live with their reproductive choices is critical if women are to begin to comprehend the meaning they make of their sexuality as mothers, as infertile women, and as voluntarily childless women. Social communications about the meaning and significance of procreation and mothering in women's lives necessarily influence women's reproductive choices. They inevitably shape women's sexual self-conceptions as they live with the consequences of these choices.

SEXUAL INVISIBILITY: MESSAGES TO MOTHERS

Motherhood is an experience that purportedly "transforms" a woman's sense of herself and her relationships (Bergum, 1989; Rich, 1977). Birthing, breast-feeding, and nurturing a child are highly physical and emotional experiences that necessarily shape and change a woman's sense of herself as a sexual person (Kitzinger, 1992, 1994). Rich (1977) suggests that the unique sexual, erotic, and intimate aspects of pregnancy, childbirth, and mothering are an important part of women's more varied heritage of sexual enjoyment. If validated, these experiences have the potential to expand and strengthen a woman's sexual self-conceptions. If not acknowledged, women may well be left feeling guilty, ashamed, and confused about these experiences (Llewellyn & Osborne, 1990; Ussher, 1989).

Women may turn to the popular or academic literature on mothering to understand their erotic feelings when breast-feeding their child, or to make sense of the changes in their intimate relationships and levels of desire during the early years of parenting. However, in so doing, they will find few answers to their queries. While there are dozens of books filled with advice on how to care for children at each stage of their development, there is virtually no attention in the literature to the sexual desires and sexual experiences of mothers. The work of feminist theorists and researchers related to mothering (e.g., Bergum, 1989; McMahon, 1995; Phoenix et al., 1991) also exclude any discussion of the sexual and erotic aspects of mothers experiences in their adult relationships or in their relationships with their children. Even books that specifically address women's sexuality and sexual development (e.g., Covington, 1991; McCormick, 1994) pay little or no attention to the changes in women's sexual self-conceptions and intimate relationships when they become mothers. The few notable exceptions include the work of Kitzinger (1985, 1992, 1994), Rich (1977), and to a lesser degree, Hyde (1990).

If women turn to the popular media, they will find no shortage of highly sexualized images of young adult women. However, from advertisements for maternity clothing through representations of mothers at all stages of the family life cycle, images of women as mothers *and* as sexually interesting and desirable people are rare. Apart from Demi Moore's naked, pregnant profile for the cover of *Vanity Fair,* sexuality and motherhood do not appear to coexist in the popular media. In her review of "current representations of sex, work and motherhood, in select recent films and women's science fiction" (p. 409) Kaplan (1990) notes how, in depictions of "female sexuality" within these sources, mothers are "excluded or marginalized" (p. 422). The implicit message appears to be that, with maternity, women lose their sexual desirability and appeal.

Changes in women's intimate relationships are inevitable when couples make the transition to parenthood (Cowan & Cowan, 1992; Kitzinger, 1985; Schnarch, 1991; Stiglitz, 1990). Some heterosexual couples report enhanced sexual intimacy following the assumption of parenting roles. More frequently, however, dissatisfaction is expressed by men and women. In particular, couples complain of the decreased frequency of lovemaking and the lack of time, energy, and opportunity for intimate interaction (Cowan & Cowan, 1992). Women, especially, report less interest in sex after their children are born. It is difficult, however, to determine whether this reported decline in sexual interest is related to the physical and social demands of parenting young children (e.g., sleep deprivation; being "on call" 24 hours a day; increasing financial responsibilities), or to changes in the relationship dyad with the inclusion of a new and highly dependent family member. Certainly, fatigue is a major barrier to sexual intimacy for many women. Also, the experiences of pregnancy, childbirth, and breastfeeding leave many women feeling like their bodies are not their own (Kitzinger, 1985; Rich, 1977). In lesbian relationships, the presence of a child can upset the balance of power and precipitate changes in the merger–separation dynamic within these relationships (Crawford, 1987; Stiglitz, 1990). It would appear that however sexual and erotic a couple's relationship may have been before the arrival of a child, accommodations must be made for both heterosexual and lesbian couples in response to the realities of parenting.

How women and their partners understand and make sense of these changes has implications for their sexual and relationship satisfaction. Unfortunately, there is also little public attention to, or acknowledgment of, the changes in the sexual experiences and needs of women and their partners over the family life cycle. Books and articles on parenting generally do not address changes in the sexual relationships and desires of couples once they become parents. A similar lack of attention exists in the popular literature directed at enhancing relationship satisfaction (e.g., Gray, *Mars and Venus in the Bedroom: A Guide to Lasting Romance and Passion,* 1997) or facilitating communication (e.g., Tannen, *You Just Don't Understand,* 1991). As such, women and their partners are faced with the absence of realistic sexual paradigms by which to reconstruct their sexual lives and renegotiate their sexual expectations once they become parents. There are few representations available to them in terms of the varied expressions of sexual passion and intimacy within the context of a changing and evolving family constellation (Schnarch, 1991, 1997). There are even fewer for women who parent without partners, and women who partner with other women.

The virtual absence of attention to the sexuality of women who mother is striking. This is not because pregnancy or child rearing result in women no longer being interested in, or capable of, sexual and erotic feelings and experiences. It is because of a host of social factors that perpetuate the distinction between maternal and sexual feelings and behaviors, and depict a narrow range of appearance and behaviors that are believed to constitute acceptable erotic feelings and sexual expression.

SEXUALITY AS LOSS: MESSAGES TO INFERTILE WOMEN

The link between fertility and sexuality is reinforced by the larger culture early in a woman's life. Adolescent girls are admonished to "be careful" when engaging in sexual interactions and to assume the primary responsibility for preventing unwanted pregnancies. Adult women are charged with the responsibility of selecting the "right" time to have children, and are held accountable for the outcome of their reproductive efforts (Menning, 1988; Rich, 1977).

Most women assume, then, that they are fertile. They believe they need only throw away the contraception and have intercourse (or in the case of lesbian women, their inseminations) at the right time of their cycles, and they will become pregnant. When a pregnancy does not occur after repeated efforts, women are confronted with the reality of infertility and all that this means, personally and socially.

Socially, women who desire to produce a child but find they cannot are confronted with a number of explicit and implicit messages from others that call into question their sexual and personal adequacy. Most organized religions support motherhood as the ultimate realization of feminine worth and value (Letson, 1987). Some religions permit a man to have several wives, so that he might realize his procreative potential, and encourage him to relegate his wife to the level of servant if she is unable to bear him children (Menning, 1988). In the Judeo-Christian tradition, children are viewed as heavenly blessings, whereas a woman's barrenness is considered to be a punishment for spiritual and/or moral transgressions. These religious messages powerfully shape the self-perceptions of infertile women and can instill feelings of tremendous guilt, inadequacy, and failure.

The medical community may also contribute to the infertile woman's feelings of sexual and personal inadequacy. Medical treatment has traditionally been based on the conceptualization of infertility as a disease, the cure for which is a viable pregnancy (Martin, 1987). For many infertile women, menstruation comes to symbolize this disease. It is a monthly reminder of the infertile woman's "failure" to conceive. The language commonly used in reference to the problems experienced by infertile women (e.g., "hostile cervical mucus," "incompetent cervix," "tubal disease") infer deficiency. Also, the primary focus of medical testing and intervention is on the female partner of the infertile couple. It is not uncommon for women to undergo years of painful and humiliating medical investigations and treatments in pursuit of a child. During this time, every intimate aspect of their lives and bodies are subjected to medical scrutiny. Physical and emotional depletion, and feelings of sexual inadequacy, are frequently the aftermath of the medical management of infertility (Daniluk, 1996).

The messages infertile women receive from many others in their worlds also reinforce this connection between infertility and inadequacy. In their attempts to help and be supportive, others often proffer "advice" and solutions to help the infertile woman conceive (i.e., "Quit work," "Take a holiday," "Adopt a child," "Abstain from having sex for awhile," "Lift your legs after intercourse," "Try a particular sexual position," etc.). This advice implicitly infers that she is somehow responsible for her inability to achieve a viable pregnancy in terms of her personal or sexual inadequacy. Ironically, the assumption underlying these frequent communications appears to be that to be fulfilled, all women should *want* to have a child. The infertile woman either *wants* it too much (i.e., she is trying too hard to get pregnant and is getting too "stressed out"), or she *doesn't want* it badly enough to do what is necessary to get pregnant (e.g., give up her job or career). In either case, the deficiency is hers in being unable to achieve what so many other women appear to achieve with relative ease.

The link between sexual intimacy and failure is also inescapable in the case of infertility. Unsuccessful efforts to procreate necessarily put considerable stress on a couple's sexual relationship as the emphasis of physical sharing (interactions) turns from "making love" to the goal of "making babies." Most infertile couples say it takes literally years to regain the levels of pleasure, spontaneity, and excitement that characterized their intimate interactions prior to experiencing infertility (Greil, 1991; Leiblum, 1994, 1997). This stress in infertile relationships is also exacerbated by attributions of responsibility. For example, it is not uncommon for men to assume that it is their partner's fault that they are unable to get pregnant. Women, too, appear to share this assumption. The belief that the woman must somehow be at least partially to blame for the couple's inability to conceive often persists, even when men have been identified as having a serious fertility impairment (Daniluk, 1997; Nachtigall et al., 1992). As Greil (1991) points out, irrespective of the source of the problem, it is the woman who fails to become pregnant, and who must live with the monthly reminders of her failure that play themselves out within her body.

INCOMPLETE SEXUALITY: MESSAGES TO THE VOLUNTARILY CHILDLESS

The social stigmatization experiences of infertile women are shared somewhat by women who choose not to reproduce or become mothers. Voluntarily childless women do not experience the sense of biological failure and punishment that is so prevalent among infertile women. However, they are confronted with a host of subtle and overt messages supporting the belief that in not realizing their procreative potential, they are denying their "womanliness." As Safer (1996) notes,

> No matter how content she is with herself or how sensual she feels, every voluntarily childless woman must contend with the virtually universal perception that her behavior brands her as selfish and deficient in the capacity for unconditional love, the womanly virtue most traditionally associated with mothering. . . . Deeply ingrained is the assumption that any real woman ought to possess limitless reserves of altruism, which are manifested in the desire to care for children. (p. 159)

Perhaps even more than the woman who desires to have a child but is unable to do so, the sexuality and sexual adequacy of voluntarily childless women are also called into question by their apparent refusal to accept their biological destinies. Part of the problem seems to stem from the fact that childless adult women do not quite fit the available social or sexual paradigms. In rejecting the role that most define as mature and fulfilled womanhood, these women are socially and sexually an enigma.

> As long as a female is young and unmarried, her childlessness is unquestioned, even honored, since she represents the virgin archetype. When it is a matter of considered choice, however, the reaction is often different. The attractive lover of man, the Aphrodite or mistress type, is usually tolerated. But a nullipara who is old, isolated, or angry, or who is not sexual or maternal, runs the risk of being regarded as an anti-mother or

> an imperfect male and being cast out of the human family. (Lisle, 1996, p. 235)

These women present a threat to the status quo (Ireland, 1993; Safer, 1996).

In the media, childless women are often represented as attractive and sexually alluring until they secure a male partner. Then they are expected to become mothers (e.g., the popular sitcom *Mad About You*). Even the necessity of having a partner is overlooked, as in the case of *Murphy Brown* or *Grace Under Fire*, as long as women choose to become mothers. Motherhood is portrayed as bringing out the best in these women—taking the edge off and making them softer. When they do not become mothers, however, they are often portrayed as embittered and angry. These women pose a threat to home and family [as in the case of the Glenn Close character in *Fatal Attraction* (Kaplan, 1990) or Demi Moore's role in *Disclosure*]. The implicit message is that, even more than marriage, motherhood is essential to fulfilled womanhood.

We have no words or language in our common vocabulary to express and validate the identities, sexuality, and reproductive choices of women who live outside of the socially sanctioned role of mother that do not infer inferiority (Lisle, 1996; Morell, 1994). Women who do not have children are commonly referred to by words that position them in relation to motherhood. Words such as "child*less*" or "*non*mother" implicitly communicate a sense of absence or deficiency.

SUMMARY: PROBLEMATIC MEANINGS

Reproductive choice is relative; it expands or constricts depending on what a woman perceives is possible. If women equate sexual adequacy and womanhood with motherhood, then procreation can be experienced as an imperative. The only choice will be when, not whether, to become a mother. For a heterosexual woman, this choice may be seriously confounded by the availability of a desirable partner. Many women in the current cohort reach their mid-30s not having found a man with whom they want to partner or who is ready to parent (Anderson & Stewart, 1994; Jacob, 1997; Mattes, 1997). Lesbian women may find it difficult to access an appropriate donor (Jacob, 1997). There are also biological limits on the time available to produce a child. As such, the pressure to fulfill this social mandate and personal desires can be great. Ethnic norms and religious beliefs can make this pressure even more intense. For example, a professionally successful, unpartnered woman from Mexico reflected on this. She said,

> "I am an anomaly within my family and culture. . . . While some people understand my marital status, they can't appreciate or accept my parental status as a childless woman, irrespective of my other accomplishments."

At 37 years of age, she is contemplating donor insemination as her only "viable" option to reduce the stigma and sense of failure she feels in having not become a mother. For lesbian women, the imperative may well be experienced as even more conflictual, given the lack of social sanctioning for mothering within a homosexual relationship (Leiblum, Palmer, & Spector, 1995; Pollack, 1990; Tasker & Golombok, 1997).

Many factors are involved in a woman's acceptance or rejection of the motherhood mandate. These include past and present life circumstances, family of origin, cultural and religious beliefs, personality characteristics, needs and values, parenting motivations, opportunity, and so on (Collins, 1987; Houseknecht, 1987; Veevers, 1980). Depending on their class, religion, and ethnic background, for some women, their economic and social well-being is contingent upon their ability to procreate and assume a mothering role (Ferguson, 1986; Rich, 1977; Ussher, 1989). Societal messages and limited role options significantly influence the reproductive choices of all women.

Perhaps more than any other adult role, motherhood confers a "built-in identity" for women (Safer, 1996, p. 143). However, the lack of a comfortable coexistence between motherhood and sexuality within our culture makes it particularly challenging for women to integrate their experiences of themselves as mothers into their identities as sexual persons. The literature suggests that "it is almost inevitable that many women will suffer a major crisis in sexual identity" once they become pregnant, and when they assume a mothering role.

It would appear that many women have internalized the culturally perpetuated notion that "sexuality is inconsistent with [the] image of woman as mother" (Ussher, 1989, p. 93). This makes it difficult for women to incorporate a new identity as both a mother and a sexually viable person into their self-structure. According to Ussher (1989), "Defining sexuality as linked to reproduction, yet simultaneously denying the existence of sexuality in the pregnant woman or the mother, perpetuates the split between body and self which we first identified in the adolescent girl" (p. 92). Women who mother are left with the task of attempting to define and carve out some space for a legitimate sexuality, which includes their experiences of themselves as mothers, and as sexual persons.

Conflicts regarding their sexual adequacy and femininity are particularly pronounced for women who experience infertility (Daniluk, 1996; Leiblum, 1997). Loss of sexual self-worth, self-esteem, spontaneity, and desire is the price paid by women whose repeated efforts to produce a child result in failure. Reproductive failure and sexuality become inextricably linked in the experiences of these women. Infertile women are faced with having to come to terms with the sense of inadequacy and feelings of sometimes profound grief that accompany these reproductive losses. They also face the formidable challenge of having to redefine themselves as competent, complete, and sexually vital women, despite their inability to produce a child.

Maternal instinct and desire are believed to be part of every woman's experience. These are supposed to be wired into women's reproductive biology (Lisle, 1996; Safer, 1996). Women who do not desire children need not be specifically told by others that they are odd or different in their apparent absence of "maternal drive." It is inevitable that they will question their normalcy and womanhood in light of their socially aberrant lifestyle choice (Anderson & Stewart, 1994).

Childless women's reproductive choices are admonished. They are left with little or no guidance as to how to maintain valid and agentic sexual identities and self-perceptions. Irrespective of how many other satisfying life roles women may be engaged in,

> In the absence of alternative perspectives from which to view herself, the childless woman . . . may identify with the ideas of emptiness or deviancy and make them her own . . . feeling somehow damaged and not fully women in their own minds because they had not had a child. . . . However, to the degree that a childless woman has internalized a different and more positive perspective, she will not accept these view or projections, and will be a source of disorientation to others. (Ireland, 1993, pp. 131–132)

CHALLENGE AND CHANGE: CREATING NEW MEANINGS

Current conceptualizations of women's sexuality leave all adult women in a *no-win* situation. In so closely linking sexuality with fertility, and fertility with womanhood, there is no place for true reproductive choice. They leave no room for women to explore the full range of their sexual and erotic potential in whatever reproductive roles they assume. As counselors, we need to help women identify the contradictions and gaps inherent in these conceptualizations of women's sexuality. It is important to begin to create more inclusive sexual paradigms that affirm the full range of women's reproductive choices. We need new paradigms that acknowledge the sexual and erotic potential of the mothering role as well as the many other roles women engage in throughout their lives. As Lisle (1996) points out,

> A body that has never been pregnant can be regarded as potent, still in anticipation, invested with self-potential and self-possession. . . . Whatever the many ways we use our bodies, . . . for lovemaking, dancing, running, or other forms of bodily exertion, . . . it is important for those . . . who have never given birth to experience them as womanly, sensual, strong, energetic, and even eloquent. (pp. 180–181)

In working with women who are struggling with the decision of whether to have children, then, it is important to help them explore the extent to which they have internalized these narrow and restrictive gender-role expectations. As much as possible, it is important to help them separate these external expectations from their own internal needs and desires. It is necessary to help clients construct identities as women and sexual persons, irrespective of the reproductive choices they eventually pursue.

For women who choose to mother, we need to validate the erotic intensity and intimacy that is often experienced by women in caretaking an infant or child (Kitzinger, 1992, 1994). The potential of the mothering role in deepening and expanding a woman's sexual expression and experience needs to be supported. Women and their partners may also need information on incorporating the role of parent into their lives. They may need assistance in renegotiating their intimate expectations in light of the realities of their new obligations, and support for exploring new ways to keep their passion and eroticism alive and vital.

Women without children may need help to create identities based on a rejection of the deficiency model of child*less*ness, and on the acceptance of more expansive beliefs about the depth and scope of women's lives and creative labors. In particular, women who had hoped to become mothers but are unable to do so need assistance in separating their sexuality and womanhood from their reproductive status, so that these "failures of biology" are not perceived as personal and sexual failures. It is important to help infertile women let go of their "identification with [their] womb[s] as the place to nourish a child so another kind of creative child can be born" (Ireland, 1993, p. 154). We need to validate the many and varied ways in which women's "creativity" and sexuality takes form and gives richness and meaning to women's lives and the lives of others in their worlds. We need to support life without maternity as an equally moral and valid life choice and path.

Given the dearth in the available clinical literature on motherhood and sexuality, creativity will be required in our work with women around these issues. We need to draw from our clinical repertoires and personal experiences in developing activities and interventions that promote and reinforce the maternal and sexual self. We must be careful not to implicitly or explicitly reinforce oppressive and contradictory beliefs regarding the sexuality and reproductive choices or functioning of women. It is important to remember that we, too, have grown up with the madonna–whore sexual paradigm as our primary model for understanding women's sexuality. We must be cognizant, then, of the degree to which we have internalized these dichotomous notions, creating confusion and discomfort in our experiences of our own sexuality as mothers or as childless women. We need to be aware of how these notions and assumptions shape our perceptions of clients and influence our ability to work in an accepting and expansive way with women as they attempt to create congruent identities that are inclusive of their reproductive choices and the sexual aspects of their lives.

Not only in our selection of interventions, but also in our use of language, we need to be cognizant of our own implicit beliefs and assumptions about the centrality of motherhood—and in particular, biological motherhood, in women's lives. A rather striking example of this type of implicit bias is apparent in the common practice of referring to the biological parent of an infertile woman's adopted child as the child's "real" or "natural" mother. In our own lives, and in our work with clients, we need to honor female desire, eroticism, energy, and creativity in its many forms of expression. When working with young adult women, we can play an important role in validating the reproductive choices and sexuality of all women—those who have children and those who do not. The following exercises and interventions are examples of ways we may begin this process.

To Have or Have Not: Reproductive Decision Making

There are many ways to help facilitate the process of reproductive decision making. Since the emphasis of this book is on women's sexuality, I will limit my discussion in this section of the chapter to helping women work through issues related to the link between sexuality and women's reproductive roles and choices. However, I would recommend that those who are uncertain about *if* and *when* they want to pursue motherhood be directed to books such as Elizabeth Whelan's (1980) *A Baby? . . . Maybe?*, Merle Bombardieri's (1981) *The Baby Decision*, and Diane Elvenstar's (1982) *Children: To Have or Have Not?* These books provide useful activities that women can undertake to begin a personal examination of the costs and benefits of both options. Working through these exercises can help women sort out their own parenting needs and desires and how these may best be met. These books give guidance on dealing with the formidable social pressures to procreate and help readers explore the short- and long-term consequences of pursuing motherhood or choosing to remain child-free. Jeanne Safer's (1996) book, *Beyond Motherhood: Choosing a Life without Children*, is an especially good resource for helping to validate the choice to forego motherhood and for exploring the child-free option and lifestyle. I would also recommend Mardy Ireland's (1993) book, *Reconceiving Women: Separating Motherhood from Female Identity*. Although this book is more theoretical and somewhat less accessible to a general audience, it provides an excellent discussion of the creation of valid identities for women who, by choice or circumstance, are not mothers. For a list of these and other resources related to reproductive health and decision making, motherhood, reproductive losses, and voluntary childlessness, the reader is referred to Appendix E.

Birthing the Self: Guided Imagery

A guided imagery exercise can begin to help women with the more difficult task of deconstructing the "woman equals mother" equation. It can facilitate the inner exploration of clients' needs and desires. Counselors can ask clients to envision themselves living in a world in which women are not primarily responsible for having and raising children. In this world, motherhood is not central to the identity of women. Rather, it is considered normal for both men and women to rear and care for children. Healthy development is symbolized by the realization of individual potential and abilities, so that the needs of the family and larger social community are better met. From childhood on, the birthing of the self is considered the goal of healthy psychosocial development.

Once involved in the visualization of such a world, where all people are encouraged to become whatever they truly desire to be, irrespective of their sex or relationship status, participants should be asked to follow the growth and development of their own lives as members of this world. Beginning in early childhood, and progressing into adulthood, they should try to imagine how their lives would have unfolded. What choices would they have made, based on the realization of their strengths, abilities, and desires? What *self* would they have birthed into adulthood? In this world characterized by freedom of choice, would motherhood have been a part of that self or not? If so, how much of their identities would have been composed of mothering? If not, how would their identities have been realized in this world?

In processing this visualization, the use of a pie diagram representing the various parts of the "self" can be a useful visual representation of the relative proportion of each component of a woman's identity. It is helpful to point out the restrictiveness of the acceptable representations of adult women in our culture. With maternity and motherhood being so strongly reinforced as the only psychologically and socially acceptable role options for women, the difficulty for many women in freely choosing to have or not to have children should be underscored. It is important to explore with women what their reproductive choices might be if these choices were to be based on what they know about their own needs and desires. What might their decisions be if they were based on what they believe is right for them? In facilitating the exploration of the ways in which clients' lives and identities can be represented other than through mothering, the many avenues for the expression of women's other "creative labors" can be legitimized and reinforced.

Another exercise that can be used to begin to tease out women's perceptions of the link between motherhood and sexuality is to ask women to explore their perceptions of the sexual vitality of women who have children and women who do not. One way to facilitate this exploration is to direct them to think about two women they know personally who are in their 50s or 60s, whom they perceive as exuding a strong and vital sense of their sexuality. One woman should be a mother and the other should be child-free. They should consider what it is about these women that contributes to this impression of sexual vitality. Is it their appearance, their manner of being in the world, their self-assuredness, and so on? Then, they should consider whether there are differences between the sexual self-presentations of these women based on their respective reproductive statuses. It can be very enlightening for clients to realize that the sexuality of these women is something inherent within them—a reflection of the way they feel about themselves as women—rather than being associated with whether they are mothers. This activity can also be useful in helping women to consider the possibility of the healthy coexistence of sexuality with motherhood, since these images are rarely reinforced in our culture.

The Decision to Mother

Shared Intimacies: The Gift of Life

Women who have made the transition to motherhood may need assistance to maintain a sense of their own sexual agency as they deal with the physical and psychological changes characteristic of pregnancy and mothering. They may need support to deal with the sexual and erotic sensations that often occur in women during pregnancy, childbirth, and the caretaking of their babies and young children. Integrating the social and emotional realities of motherhood into their sexual self-constructions may also prove challenging for some women.

Beginning with pregnancy, female clients may need assistance in dealing with the often dramatic physical changes in body size and shape, as well as the discomfort that frequently characterizes the first and third trimesters of pregnancy (Kitzinger, 1985). Only a small percentage of women appear to become severely ill or incapacitated during pregnancy. Many report an enhanced sense of physical well-being while pregnant. However, "the changes in a woman's body which take place during pregnancy have a considerable effect on personal identity and image of self" (Ussher, 1989, p. 98). Women may be particularly fearful about losing control over their size and weight. This can be especially stressful, given cultural messages suggesting that to be beautiful, women must be thin. The "contradictory discourses which say 'attractive woman = slim' and 'woman = mother' mean that a woman cannot be attractive and be pregnant, or a new mother, at the same time" (p. 99). Depending on a woman's relationship with her body, she may perceive the bodily changes of pregnancy as exciting and wondrous, or she may feel alienated from her body and bodily sensation. To assist in facilitating bodily comfort and connection, readers are referred to the exercises in the next chapter on body image, which can be adapted for work with women during pregnancy.

Mothering a child "transforms" the boundaries of the self for all women (Bergum, 1989), including the sexual self. With a host of cultural messages suggesting that sexuality and motherhood cannot coexist on the same plane, it can be especially difficult for women who mother to find their way to a valid sexuality (Chodorow & Contratto, 1992). In working with women who have selected to mother, it is necessary to help them to construct their "own discourses about mothering, which will allow these experiences to be viewed positively and realistically" (Ussher, 1989, p. 102).

There are few examples in the clinical literature on how we might work with women on these issues. As noted earlier in this chapter, even the most woman-centered, progressive, and feminist literature on mothering largely ignores the issues of sexuality and sexual agency (e.g., Bergum, 1989; Gieve, 1989; Price, 1988). It may be helpful to refer women to several of the books by Shelia Kitzinger (1974, 1978, 1983, 1992, 1994) on women's sexuality and mothering. The link between women's sexual and maternal experiences are not the explicit focus of these books, and these issues are not fully explored. Shelia Kitzinger is a midwife, however, and is one of the few authors who acknowledge the sexual and erotic side of many aspects of women's mothering experiences (e.g., pregnancy, childbirth, breast-feeding). Her books are particularly rich because of her anthropological fieldwork examining the birthing practices of women of many diverse cultures. She liberally infuses her writing with the customs and birthing rituals of women of other, diverse cultures, many of whom perceive "life outside the uterus" as a "continuation of life inside it" (Kitzinger, 1992, p. 176). Drawing on the experiences of these women, she helps the reader to reconnect with a significant aspect of women's experience that has been lost in the medical co-opting of the birthing process. Through her work, she is able to enhance and expand our limited knowledge of the ways in which women's sexual and maternal realities can and do coexist. She offers suggestions on how these can be nurtured and respected throughout the reproductive changes and experiences of women's lives. A list of other excellent resources on the pregnancy, birthing, and mothering experiences of women is included in Appendix E.

When working with pregnant women and mothers of young children, counselors should provide information on the physical and psychological realities of pregnancy and mothering. Women often need encouragement to caretake themselves and to ensure that their own physical and psychological health needs are met. They may need support to know that in caretaking themselves, they are acting responsibly toward their children. Pregnant women can also be assisted to explore the possibilities of less sterile and invasive approaches to childbirth (home births, birthing rooms in hospitals, midwifery, etc.) while still availing themselves of the benefits of medical technology, should their particular situation warrant this type of intervention. They can be encouraged to appreciate that there is no one "right" or "correct," or more "womanly" way to labor and birth a child.

Whether they give birth with or without medication to ease the pain, whether or not they require medical intervention, the act of giving life is a remarkable female accomplishment and a precious gift (Kitzinger, 1992, 1994).

Through their exposure to the stories and experiences of other women, new mothers can be encouraged to see pregnancy, childbirth, and mothering as experiences that women have shared in for centuries. Only recently have these been co-opted by the medical profession and turned into a medical malady (Ehrenreich & English, 1978; Kitzinger, 1983). Clients can be encouraged to tune in to the changes in their bodies, and open themselves up to the new feelings and sensations that are a part of pregnancy, birthing, and the intimate act of mothering young children. These should be reinforced as part of a unique and intimate journey that women can choose to share with significant people in their lives (e.g., their children, their partners, their mothers). Clients should be encouraged to maintain an accepting relationship with their changing bodies during the various stages of their maternity and mothering experiences. When confronted with new physical and visceral sensations and experiences, they should be encouraged to explore and accept these as a potentially exciting dimension of their sexuality.

Women can be assisted in consolidating identities that are inclusive of their mothering experiences as well as their erotic and sensual feelings and experiences. Through the use of such expressive techniques as art therapy, body work, metaphors, guided imagery, and visualizations, clients can be asked to envision these aspects of themselves, first as two discrete entities, and then as parts of a symmetrical whole. If clients can envision both aspects of their lives and selves existing on the same phenomenological plane, the parts of themselves as mothers and the sexual aspects of their identities, then these can be symbolically joined (through dance, art, writing, etc.) to create a complete gestalt. For example, in a simple exercise, counselors can ask clients to draw a picture or create a metaphor that symbolically represents their perceptions of themselves as mothers (or as pregnant women). Following this, they should create another that represents their perceptions of their sexual selves. Having completed this task, clients can engage in a process of self-exploration, discussing the nature of these images/metaphors, the feelings they evoke, and the degree to which each encompasses a part of themselves and their identities. Through this exploration, clients can be encouraged to find ways to envision *both* important aspects of their experiencing, motherhood and sexuality, coexisting in harmony. Emphasis can be placed on the way both maternal and sexual energy are important sources of growth and renewal, each complementing and nourishing the other in ways that serve to enrich women's lives and experiences.

Sometimes it is necessary for women to reconsider their images of their own mothers and grandmothers as sexual people. Many adult children have difficulty conceiving of their parents as being "sexual" or engaging in sexual activities. And yet, as several writers (e.g., Chodorow, 1978; Lisle, 1996; Rich, 1976) have acknowledged, our mothers are the primary role models of what it means to be a woman, a mother, and a sexual person. Women learn what it means to be maternal from their mothers (or another primary female caretaker, e.g., grandmother). Their ability or inability to see their mothers as sexual people can be an important conduit to envisioning themselves as both maternal and sexual. To facilitate this link, it can be useful to use biographical interviews and genograms to help women expand their knowledge and perceptions of their mothers. In an exercise described by Howe (1990), women are asked first to chart their family relationships using a genogram. In this way, they can situate themselves relative to their family lineage and, in particular, their maternal lineage. Then, clients should be asked to conduct a biographical interview of their mothers. Besides learning about their mothers' early hopes, dreams, and aspirations, including reproductive aspirations, daughters should ask their mothers to focus on their relationship histories. If a mother is no longer alive, a daughter can interview a close friend or family member (e.g., a sister) about her mother's life. A review of photo albums can also be a useful adjunct to this process. In undertaking this exercise, women are often surprised, moved, and enlightened to learn about the many other dimensions to the life of this woman whom they have only seen and known as "mother." In putting on different lenses to examine their mothers' lives, they are often able to see them as women, mothers, and as sexual persons. In envisioning them in this way, they may be able to begin to envision themselves in this way as well.

Information and assistance may also need to be provided so that women and their partners might find stimulating and creative ways to continue to have their sexual needs and desires met despite the demands of caretaking children. While most of the available popular literature does not address typical changes in couples' patterns of intimacy and sexual expression during the various stages of the marital and family life cycle, helpers may find the work of David Schnarch useful in this regard. In particular, Schnarch's recent book, *Passionate Marriage: Sex, Love and Intimacy in Emotionally Committed Relationships* (1997), provides suggestions on how to assist couples in keeping the passion and intimacy alive throughout the various stages of their relationships. Lonnie Barbach's 1984 book, *For Each Other: Sharing Sexual Intimacy*, is also recommended. Lesbian couples may find Joanne Loulan's work (e.g., *Lesbian Sex*, 1984; *Lesbian Passion: Loving Ourselves and Each Other*, 1987) useful. Women who are solely responsible for parenting often find it especially difficult to have their sexual needs validated and fulfilled. These women may benefit from an exploration of how they might satisfy this important part of their lives on their own (e.g., self-stimulation, fantasy, erotica) and in their intimate relationships, without feeling like they are compromising their parental responsibilities (Barbach, 1976; Bennett & Rosario, 1995; Cline, 1993).

Reproductive Losses

Empty Wombs

Whatever the source of women's motivation to mother, be it cultural mandate or personal desire, the inability to mother or the loss of a child is a profoundly painful experience. This requires compassionate intervention on the part of the counselor. Grief work is a significant part of the therapeutic process when working with women who suffer reproductive losses. They must cope with a multitude of losses associated with their inability to bear a child (i.e., loss of a child, loss of fertility, loss of a dream, loss of self, etc.). According to Menning (1988), "Failure—or, more accurately, inability—to grieve is the single most common presenting problem" (p. 104) for women who experience fertility problems. For more detailed discussions of ways in which the grief work associated with reproductive losses might be facilitated, the reader is referred to Appendix E. In particular, the book, *Never to Be a Mother,* by Linda Anton (1992), is an excellent, step-by-step guide to resolving the pain of childlessness. Constance Hoenk-Shapiro's books (1988, 1993) are also useful resources in helping women work through various reproductive losses. I find Ellen Glazer and Susan Cooper's (1988) book, *Without Child,* to be a particularly good resource for infertile women and their partners. This book is filled with short personal essays and poems by women and men who share their struggles in attempting to resolve their infertility and to fulfill their desire to parent. Sandra Leiblum's (1997) recent edited book, *Infertility: Psychological Issues and Counseling Strategies,* is also an excellent resource for mental health professionals on how to help women and their partners make informed treatment decisions, work through the pain and losses associated with infertility, and consider their other parenting and nonparenting options.

When reproductive losses occur within the context of a relationship, it is important whenever possible to include both members of the infertile couple in the counseling process. The inability to realize their love and caring for each other in the creation of a new life is a pain shared by both members of the infertile couple (this includes lesbian couples). When couples can share their mutual grief over this loss, it can be a significant step in removing the stigma of failure from the infertile woman and in cementing the emotional bond between the members of the couple (Daniluk, 1997; Greil, 1991; Leiblum, 1997). As the member of one infertile couple stated,

> "Infertility has tested us. It has taken us to the edge of despair and has brought us to a new understanding and depths; new tightness together as a couple. . . . I wouldn't wish this experience on anyone, but in some ways, its made us so much stronger. . . . If your relationship can survive infertility, it can survive anything."

Often, after women have had an opportunity to complete some of the grief work involved in healing from a reproductive loss, the issue of sexual failure becomes a critical focus of counseling. Women who are infertile, and women who experience other reproductive losses (e.g., miscarriage, stillbirth), may feel like sexual failures. Being unable to bear a child, or losing a child through miscarriage or stillbirth, is often experienced not only as a significant personal loss, but also as a loss of womanhood. As Kitzinger (1985) notes, "The death of a child can strike at the root of sexuality and at a woman's own sense of herself as a person . . . when a baby dies a woman may feel that the grieving is centered in her gut, uterus and entrails and as if these organs have been torn from her living body" (p. 292). These women may need help to begin separating their feminine identities and sexual adequacy from their reproductive status, so that these failures of biology are not perceived as personal failures.

Unfortunately, however, as with the clinical literature dealing with women's experiences of motherhood, with few exceptions (e.g., Leiblum, 1994, 1997), the literature on infertility and reproductive losses provides little guidance in this regard. We know little about how to help clients deal with the damage to their sexual spontaneity, sexual desire, and sexual self-worth that results from repeated unsuccessful attempts to produce a child. We know even less about helping women integrate their fertility status into their sexual self-structures in a way that allows women to maintain their sexual agency and sexual esteem. Creativity on the part of the helping professional is required to find ways to assist the these women (1) to heal from the sexual trauma that is often a part of the invasive medical procedures employed in the treatment of infertility; (2) to define their sexuality as separate from their fertility and parenting status; and (3) to reconnect with their bodies, with their partners, and with their sexual selves.

When clients have been involved in the extensive pursuit of medical solutions to their infertility, there is virtually no aspect of their bodies or their lives that have remained untouched—literally or figuratively. Following repeated pelvic examinations (sometimes with several people in the room); the injection of multiple probes, dies, and instruments into their vaginas, uteri, and tubes; and the examination of the most intimate details of their sexual activities (both past and present), women often feel violated. Many infertile women with whom I have worked express shame and humiliation over what has been done to their bodies. Not unlike victims of sexual assault, they frequently blame themselves for having allowed this to occur. Working through this sense of violation, taking back ownership of their bodies, and beginning to set appropriate boundaries around physical contact are important components in the healing process. This is also critical to sexual healing.

When working with infertile women, it is important first to acknowledge the sexual trauma that is characteristic of the medical management of infertility. Like other trauma victims, infertile women need to work through these issues before they are ready to begin working on issues of sexual pleasure and intimacy (Leiblum, 1997). They may need help to direct their anger, not at themselves for having done everything they could to fulfill their desire for a child, but rather at the insensitivity demonstrated by some members of the medical community in not respecting their personal boundaries and needs (Sandelowski, 1990b). Even if they have been treated with compassion and respect by the medical personnel who managed their investigations and treatment, the invasiveness of the procedures involved in an infertility workup may still leave emotional scars (Daniluk, 1997; Menning, 1988; Nachtigall et al., 1992). Journal and letter writing can be effective ways for clients to process some of their anger and pain at these boundary violations. This type of affective expression can help them to begin to reclaim some of the power they had to relinquish when involved in the medical pursuit of a pregnancy. Letters written to a particular practitioner or clinic can be quite cathartic, whether or not they are actually sent. Journals provide a benchmark for women to look back and realize how far they have come in working through and letting go of their anger and grief (Daniluk, 1991a). Other affective and expressive techniques, such as body work and art therapy, can also provide an outlet for the expression of these feelings.

Infertile couples often spend years having sexual intercourse "on demand," based on the menstrual cycle rather than on any feelings of intimacy and desire. During this time, the meaning of sex changes from "making love" to "making babies." Not surprisingly, many infertile women report a complete lack of spontaneity and playfulness in their sexual interactions (Leiblum, 1997). Many experience an overwhelming sense of disconnection from their own sexual desire (Mahlstedt, 1985; Menning, 1988). Finding ways to help clients reintroduce intimacy, pleasure, and joy into their sexual lives is another important component of the healing process. Infertile women frequently need validation of the fact that, after years of having timed and planned intercourse, sexual desire and spontaneity necessarily suffer. They need assurance that these losses are contextual and usually temporary. Most frequently, they begin to subside once women have gained a certain amount of distance from the pursuit of medical solutions, and once they have had an opportunity to grieve the many losses involved in being unable to produce a child. After years of intercourse being linked to procreation rather than pleasure, coitus becomes associated with failure for many infertile women. It is important to help clients abandon the notion of intercourse as the goal of sexual expression and to reduce performance pressure by helping women to expand the possible alternatives for erotic and intimate pleasure. Women and their partners may need to abandon intercourse completely for a time and focus their energies on other ways to regain a sense of intimacy, and slowly rekindle their erotic desire (Leiblum, 1997). For example, sensate focus exercises (see Barbach, 1984) can be effective in helping clients begin to reconnect with the sexual and erotic aspects of their bodies after the trauma of medical intervention, without the pressures of the expectation of intercourse.

A number of affective techniques can be used to help women define their sexuality as separate from their fertility and parenting status, and to facilitate an exploration of the other ways their sexuality is represented and expressed in their lives, and in their bodies. For example, using relaxation and visualizations, clients can be encouraged to consider the notion of sexual energy as a vibrant force, a bright, white light that is contained inside each of us. Some particularly visual and expressive clients may select their own, different symbol to represent their sexuality, one that has particular significance to them. Whatever symbol they elect to use, clients can be asked to envision the source of this light or symbol representative of their sexuality, and to picture from where in their own bodies this light is emitted (eyes, face, stomach, etc.). What point is the warmest and brightest? Where is this light the dimmest? When they move toward the source of the light, what feelings are elicited for them? While some clients will identify the uterus as the source of their sexual energy, clients who have experienced reproductive losses often report their souls, spirits, or hearts as the source of their greatest erotic energy. Many report that when they open themselves to this energy, it infuses their bodies with warmth. Women can be asked to picture harnessing this light and allowing it to warm their bodies. As they begin to heal from their reproductive losses, they can begin to redirect this energy throughout their entire bodies. Clients who are uncomfortable with guided imagery, or who find visualizations difficult, can be encouraged to use art, dance, or movement as a vehicle to begin to envision their sexuality as distinct from their ability to reproduce.

Because of the bodily betrayal that is often experienced by women who have reproductive losses, clients may need assistance in working through their feelings toward the parts of their bodies that they believe have betrayed them. For example, several infertile women I have worked with feel very let down by their uteruses. They often feel "duped" by the fact that they have been forced to endure years of monthly cycles of bleeding, inconvenience, and sometimes discomfort, only to find out that the organ that has been responsible for these experiences is somehow faulty or defective in its inability to carry a pregnancy. For some, this sense of betrayal precipitates a demand for a hysterectomy, since the organ "serves no useful purpose." For others, it results in a sense of profound alienation from this part of their bodies, resulting in feelings of being "cut off" from the waist down.

It may be important to help women work through their feelings of anger and alienation toward the parts of their bodies that represent their failure and yet are often most representative of their womanhood. For example, through the use of a two-chair technique, a dialogue can be facilitated between the client and her reproductive organs. During this exercise, the woman should be encouraged to express her anger and disappointment at having to live forever with an "empty womb." Women should be encouraged to reframe their understanding of the meaning of these organs as more than a place just to nurture a child. They may come to appreciate that this is the source of their bodily rhythms and cyclicity. It may also be significant in their experience of sexual stimulation and orgasm. They may find comfort in the fact that this organ is representative of their connection with nature and with other women.

In time, women who have experienced reproductive losses can begin to regain a sense of acceptance of, and comfort in, their bodies. They can construct complete and integrated identities, irrespective of their parental status. Once they have grieved the losses associated with their inability to bear a child, made peace with their bodies, and found a way to feel whole and complete, irrespective of their reproductive status, these women can again experience passion, spontaneity, and delight in their sexuality and its expression in their lives and intimate relationships.

Nonbiological Procreation: The Decision Not to Mother

Women's Other Creative Labors

According to the literature, and in my clinical experience, while others may question their sexuality, few women who choose to remain voluntarily childless express conflicts about their sexuality per se, in light of their lack of maternal desire. More often, the questions that are raised have to do with their normalcy as women (Ireland, 1993; Lisle, 1996; Safer, 1996). This uncertainty about their normalcy, combined with their natural concerns about later having regrets, can make the reproductive decision-making process very difficult and protracted (Safer, 1996). This is particularly true for the current cohort of young adult women who are being led to believe that with the advancements in reproductive technologies they can delay the pursuit of a first pregnancy into their late 30s and even into their 40s (Crosthwaite, 1992; Klein & Rowland, 1988; Rothman, 1989; Stanworth, 1987). For many young women, closure is not reached on this decision until menopause makes the choice irrevocable (Veevers, 1980).

An important part of assisting women to bring closure to this decision involves validating a child-free life as a legitimate and responsible option. Women may need help to expand their definitions of womanhood to include the wide range of women's creative labors. Counselors need to reinforce the fact that there are many valid avenues to creativity and many paths to a rich and meaningful life—with maternity and motherhood being only one role option. As Lisle (1996) points out, throughout history women have been "procreative in nonbiological ways" (p. 65). Women who are considering remaining childless can be asked to consider childless women throughout history who have made important contributions through their other labors (e.g., their political actions, their writing, their art). To bring this exploration closer to home, women can be asked to review their own lives and to consider older friends and women in their own families who are, or have been, procreative in ways other than through mothering. This exploration should include a personal exploration of how they, too, can lead fulfilling and creative lives other than through mothering.

If women without children are to be free to choose childlessness as an option, they need to be able to envision femininity, womanhood, and sexuality as coexisting without the prerequisite of procreation and mothering. They need to be able to identify themselves and other women without children as vital and sexual and womanly. Counselors should encourage young adult women who are considering childlessness or who are committed to a child-free life, to identify other childless women they know who exemplify these characteristics. They may benefit from seeking out and talking with older women who are not mothers, who may act as role models of ways to construct meaningful lives and female identities without becoming mothers (Ireland, 1993; Noble, 1990).

It is also important to deal with the physical connection between women's reproductive organs and their fertility. Ireland (1993) stresses the importance of women without children being able to perceive their wombs as a source and site of creativity, irrespective of their reproductive status. Rather than being an empty "inner space," this distinctly female organ, the uterus, can be reinforced as an important source of physical and sexual sensations and energy. In her book, *Without Child: Challenging the Stigma of Childlessness,* Lisle (1996) underscores the importance for women who have never given birth to experience their bodies as "womanly, sensual, strong, energetic, and even eloquent" (p. 181).

> Instead of living with the idea of an empty inner space, all women—especially childfree ones—can hold it as a symbol of internal fecundity, inner richness, and the possibility of renewable life whether we are sexual or celibate, with or without child. A body that has never been pregnant can be regarded as potent, still in anticipation, invested with self-potential and self-possession. (p. 180)

Body work and dance can be especially good nonverbal vehicles for helping clients explore the creative and sexual energy that emanates from within their female bodies (Rush, 1975; Simonds, 1994; Turner, 1990). This type of work can also be very therapeutic for women who have experienced hysterectomy and other reproductive losses.

Lisle (1996) notes the importance of women who do not assume the role of mother to find a way to work through and make peace with their rejection of a role that was assumed by the long line of women in their families (i.e., their mothers, their grandmothers, their great grandmothers)

"Even though not all women are mothers, and all mothers do not have daughters, every woman is born a daughter" (p. 86). For some women, it is the memories of an angry and embittered mother that motivate their choice to remain childless. Their work involves ensuring that they are not rejecting an experience that they may really desire out of their fear of becoming like their mothers. For others, it is the lack of desire to replicate the apparent constrictions of their mothers' lives that fuels their desire to construct lives outside of the mothering role. These women may need assistance to escape from the tyranny of the role of the all-giving, selfless mother, and to envision mothering in a more expansive way. And for still others who came from homes where they were well loved and nurtured, and their mothers appeared to delight in the mothering role, the difficulty may come in feeling as if they are not capable of replicating the kind of mothering they felt fortunate enough to have experienced. Or they may experience difficulty in rejecting the valid and desirable adult role of mother to pursue lives that are more consistent with their needs, values, and desires. Women who do not desire to mother often struggle to reconcile their decision to reject a role, however desirable or undesirable, that centrally defined their own mothers' lives, and that defines the lives of most adult women (Ireland, 1993; Lisle, 1996; Safer, 1996). These women may need assistance in finding ways to validate their own life paths without invalidating the life paths of their mothers. They may also need assistance in dealing with the inevitable sense of loss in terms of the "road not taken" (Ireland, 1993; Morell, 1994). As Lisle so accurately points out, whether women become mothers or not, "there are no lives without limitations, no choices without losses" (p. 169).

9

IN THE PRIME OF LIFE

Living in Our Bodies

I've been in many
rooms, and have come to realize
the fullest room was empty. To
get there you must sass back
God and fight him for the door.
And when you enter, you must
laugh at the empty fullness,
greet your perfect self in the
corner—and when she, the Goddess,
asks you what you see, as clouds,
thin air, float by: you must
answer: I see the
freedom. She isn't pleased
or displeased—she's been expecting
you forever. She knows what
you had
to do
to love
your
self.

—ALMA LUZ VILLANUEVA, "Sassy"

As Valverde (1985) states, "To think and talk about sexuality is first of all to think and talk about bodies" (p. 29). Sexuality is lived and expressed in many diverse ways by women. The sensations of the body are an important avenue for the experiencing of erotic pleasure and sexual vitality. As women adjust to the common (e.g., slowing of the metabolic rate, pregnancy) and unique (e.g., mastectomy, physical illness or disability) bodily changes and experiences that characterize their progression through this stage in the life cycle, their ability to maintain a positive relationship with their bodies will be a significant factor in their ability to enjoy and delight in their sexuality.

The development and maintenance of intimate relationships is considered to be a primary task for women and men between the ages of 20 and

40 years (Erikson, 1968). Such intimacy requires self-disclosure. The ability to appropriately self-disclose requires a strong sense of self (Kegan, 1982; Stevens-Long & Commons, 1992). How a woman feels about her body is a significant component of any woman's experience of self. The maintenance of body-image satisfaction in young adulthood involves a two-way interaction between women's phenomenological experience and perceptions of their bodies, and the messages they receive from lovers and other significant people in their lives (e.g., friends, colleagues) regarding their physical attractiveness and desirability. As discussed in the Chapter 1, the impact of the feedback women receive about the adequacy of their bodies from those who are important to them will be especially significant in informing their self-perceptions (Tantleff-Dunn & Thompson, 1995). Correspondingly, how any woman feels about her body will influence the degree to which she is able to share herself, and her life with others, in terms of physical and emotional intimacy.

As women enter young adulthood, they bring with them the psychological baggage of the past in terms of their sexual and bodily self-perceptions and their ability to feel at home and comfortable in their own skin (Fisher, 1986; Jaggar & Bordo, 1989). The experiences of childhood and adolescence form the foundation for women's adult bodily perceptions (Fisher, 1986; Hutchinson, 1985, 1994). For some women, this foundation may well lack the structural integrity necessary to sustain the weight of other sources of influence that shape their experiences and perceptions of their bodies in adulthood. These include the acceptance or rejection of intimate partners, the beliefs and values of the members of each woman's reference and normative groups (such as religious, ethnic, occupational, lifestyle—e.g., homosexual), and the powerful influence of the popular media (Bartky, 1990; Gagnon & Simon, 1982; Kilbourne, 1994; Seid, 1994). We turn, now, to a closer examination of these influences.

HAVE YOU GAINED A LITTLE WEIGHT LATELY?: MESSAGES OF FRIENDS AND LOVERS

The acceptance and approval of their bodies by their current partner is especially important in the development and maintenance of positive body image for women in young adulthood. Comments or behaviors that are perceived as critical or rejecting are incorporated into women's self-structures, shaping their assessment and perceptions of their bodies, and ultimately of their relative worth. For example, a woman may enter adulthood feeling at home and grounded in her body. Yet this may slowly be eroded over time as a consequence of being in relationship with a lover who persistently makes overt or subtle comments about the inadequacy of her body (e.g., "Is it that time of the month or are you putting on a little weight?"; "Does everyone in your family have saddle bags?"; "Are you sure you should have that dessert?") (Freedman, 1988; Friedman, 1993). Another woman may experience feelings of physical inadequacy and shame as a consequence of being in relationship with a partner who makes continual comments about the physical attractiveness and desirability of other women's bodies, but never reinforces her desirability. For women who enter young adulthood already feeling negative about their bodies, these types of comments may indeed "cut to the core." They may undermine any vestige of self-respect and esteem women managed to salvage from their childhood and adolescence. "If you are naked and having sex, someone saying you have a little surplus can be devastating to young women" (Damrosch, cited in Schneider, 1996, p. 68). Even a discrepancy between a woman's self-rating of her body and her perceptions of her partner's ideal female body image seems to affect negatively a woman's body image, irrespective of whether the partner directly communicates dissatisfaction with her appearance (Tantleff-Dunn & Thompson, 1995).

On the other hand, some women are fortunate to have partners who reinforce their physical desirablility and adequacy. These interactions serve to strengthen the positive self-perceptions of women who already feel comfortable in, and good about, their bodies. They can also be a significant source of validation and support in altering the negative self-perceptions of women with poor body image (Hutchinson, 1985). Lesbian relationships are noteworthy in this regard. Research suggests that lesbians in general appear to place less emphasis on the importance of physical attractiveness in their intimate relationships. While there are appearance norms in lesbian communities, these appear to serve the purpose of assisting "members of an often oppressed group to identify one another." They also help to "provide a group identity" (Rothblum, 1994, p. 92). These norms are more inclusive of a diverse range of women's body shapes and sizes.

Friends, too, can be influential in their comments or deafening silence regarding a woman's size, weight, or appearance. For example, women who are considered overweight are subjected to a range of both overt and subtle aspersions. This appears to be especially true for large women and those considered obese (Tiggemann & Rothblum, 1997). Women who are considered overweight by today's restrictive standards are stigmatized and stereotyped. They are subjected to discrimination in the workplace and are frequently the focus of public ridicule (Greaves, 1990; Harris, 1990; Rothblum, 1992). Based on the "widespread presumption that fatness is always pathological" large women are subjected to "relentless pressure to lose weight" (Burgard & Lyons, 1994, p. 212). Even the language used in reference to large women (e.g., "overweight") implies that there is an ideal or correct weight that these women are clearly over. Erdman (1995) notes how the word "obese" is commonly used by physicians as an indicator of disease, and the word "fat" is often used in a "derogatory and shame-inducing way" (p. xvii). As in the case of women without children, discussed in Chapter 8, there is no available language that does not imply judgment or position women in relation to a standard of appearance that is difficult, if not impossible, to attain. In her book *Such a Pretty Face: Being Fat in America*, Marcia Millman (1980) underscores the subtle negative judgment implicit in such a backhanded compliment. It infers that if only the woman would exercise self-control and lose some weight, she could be really beautiful. This appears to be especially true for white women. Within black and Latino ethnic groups, there appears to be greater cultural acceptance of larger size among women (Root, 1990).

Meanings are based on women's perceptions, which in turn have been shaped by their particular history. Depending on the strength of her bodily self-perceptions and esteem, even a well-intended comment such as "You're looking great. Have you lost weight lately?" by a friend or acquaintance may be interpreted by a woman as inferring that the sender previously perceived her as being fat. What is not said by significant others in terms of validation of their attractiveness and desirability may also be perceived by women as implicitly communicating disapproval. By default, friends and lovers can unknowingly reinforce feelings of bodily inadequacy, irrespective of their benign or benevolent intentions.

ONE STANDARD OF BEAUTY—TIGHT, LIGHT, AND WHITE: MEDIA MESSAGES

As noted throughout this book, the cultural messages perpetuated through the media are also highly formative in shaping young adult women's perceptions of female attractiveness and desirability. They frequently generate and reinforce feelings of personal and physical inadequacy (Bartky, 1990; Hutchinson, 1994; Kilbourne, 1994; Seid, 1994; Unger & Crawford, 1992). According to Seid (1994), "Values, which in the past were shaped at a community level and transmitted slowly from parent to child, have now been replaced by media versions of the world" (p. 154).

And what are the values currently communicated by the mass media regarding the bodies of women in their 20s and 30s? The average weight of North American women has increased over the past two decades. However, the ideal female weight promoted in the media, and "represented by actresses, models, and Miss Americas, has progressively decreased to that of the thinnest 5–10% of American women." A statistical deviation has been normalized, "leading millions of women to believe that they are abnormal" (Seid, 1994, p. 8). In the early 1980s, the average model weighed 8% less than the average American woman. She now weighs 23% less (Wolf, 1991). "In the past 30 years, the voluptuous size-12 image of Marilyn Monroe has given way to the size-2 likes of *Lois & Clark* star Teri Hatcher" (Schneider, 1996, p. 67).

Images of women of normal weight and appearance are relatively absent in the media, making it difficult for most women not to judge themselves as somehow deficient (Kilbourne, 1994; Ussher, 1989). Unger and Crawford (1992) note how "overweight women are also symbolically annihilated by the media. They have virtually disappeared as models in women's magazines over the last 35 years" (p. 586). Reflecting our "fatphobic" attitudes in modern America (Seid, 1994), when large women are portrayed in film or television, their weight is frequently a continual focus of jokes and jeers (e.g., Rosanne Barr's struggles with food and weight). With the exception of those in traditional nurturing roles (e.g., mother, grandmother), women in roles of power, authority, or adventure are characteristically portrayed in the popular media as thin and attractive, irrespective of their socioeconomic status or color (Wolf, 1991).

"Both on TV and in magazines, we are exposed to images of women who are anorexic, surgically altered, and airbrushed or computer-altered" (Hutchinson, 1994, p. 154). More and more often, children of 13 and 14 are being dressed up to represent young women in the popular media (Kilbourne, 1994). Their tall, thin, waif-like images are seductively presented as both real and attainable if women exercise the appropriate self-control over their appetites and their bodies. The message is that to be considered attractive, a woman must force her body to conform to a female ideal that virtually "violates the anthropomorphic reality of the average female body" (Seid, 1994, p. 8). Indeed, Blood (1996) notes how the women in her study on dieting motivations consistently cited the media "as a key factor in maintaining [their] preoccupation with body size and shape." In the words of one of her participants: "There's a lot of media imagery in magazines and on television that totally portrays an ideal that I'm not. . . . I just don't look like they do in those [fashion] magazines. I don't look like people on TV look. Just being confronted constantly with what's appropriate and that this [indicating self] isn't" (p. 116).

The act of creating and recreating ourselves by altering our natural appearance is a phenomenon that has occurred throughout recorded history. "Dress and adornment are basic to all human cultures. Even the most primitive tribes find ways to decorate the body." Altering our physical appearance is a game we engage in "from the moment we slip out of the womb to the moment of our deaths" (Seid, 1994, p. 9). It may be highly pleasurable in the celebration of beauty and individuality. It may be painfully oppressive, as in the case of current media representations, in its demands for further and further refinement. Depending on the values being perpetuated and the degree to which young adult women feel free to adhere to, or reject, cultural standards, the game may be impossible to win. With the virtual absence of realistic images of adult women, media messages allow the seeds of physical inadequacy and discontent that were sewn in adolescence to flourish for many young women, irrespective of their size, weight, class, color, or sexual orientation (e.g., Bartky, 1990; Bordo, 1993; Burgard & Lyons, 1994; Cash, 1990; Fallon, 1990; Friedman, 1993; Plous & Neptune, 1997; Striegel-Moore, Tucker, & Hsu, 1990).

SUMMARY: PROBLEMATIC MEANINGS

Despite the advances made by the women's movement over the past 25 years, considerable evidence exists that feeling comfortable with and at home in our bodies is still a difficult achievement for many women (Wooley & Wooley, 1984). However accomplished we may be in the other areas of our lives, it is virtually impossible for any woman not to internalize to some extent cultural messages regarding the standards of bodily acceptability for women (Bartky, 1990). Current estimates suggest that "85% of American women diet chronically and 75% feel humiliated by their body size and shape" (Bloom, Gitter, Gutwill, Kogel, & Zaphiropoulos, 1994, p. xi). Certainly the available statistics from the diet industry and cosmetic surgeons underscore the extent of this "normative discontent" (Rodin et al., 1984). The number of cases of aesthetic surgery performed by board-certified plastic surgeons in the United States increased from under 400,000 in the early 1980s to over 600,000 by the end of the decade (Hesse-Biber, 1996). Canadian statistics for 1988 indicate a correspondingly high rate (40,000) of "elective" surgeries for cosmetic reasons.

The serious concerns about the safety of silicone implants notwithstanding, breast augmentations are again on the rise in the United States. Certainly, more men than ever are also choosing to go under the surgeon's knife to correct "flaws" of nature or indulgence. However, Canadian and American statistics confirm that 87–90% of those choosing cosmetic surgery are women (Gillespie, 1996; Wolf, 1991). Statistics from the burgeoning diet industry are similar, with $8.4 billion in revenues being recorded by weight-loss clinics in the United States in 1991. A corresponding threefold increase in the number of franchised diet clinics was reported in Canada between 1987 and 1991 (Faludi, 1991). Women between the ages of 20 and 60 are the primary consumers of these services. As well, women spend literally billions of dollars on creams and cosmetics to improve or enhance their looks, and on dyes and shampoos to eradicate any signs of aging.

Cultural messages that prescribe an unrealistic, ideal appearance for women based on the physical attributes of increasingly younger (prepubescent) adolescent girls are pervasive. As such, it should not be surprising that few adult women are able to honestly say that they are happy with their bodies and with how they look. In a large survey of over 30,000 women in *Glamour* magazine, Wooley and Wooley (1984) found that women pervasively experienced dissatisfaction with their bodies, particularly the fat-bearing areas of the thighs, hips, and waist. Forty-two percent of the respondents in the study reported that losing weight would make them the happiest (over work success, a date with a man they admired, or hearing from an old friend).

These results are obviously based on data from a biased sample (those who read *Glamour*—and as such are interested in a beauty-tips magazine).

However, they are consistent with the observations of several researchers and clinicians (e.g., Bordo, 1993; Rodin et al., 1984; Seid, 1994; Striegel-Moore et al., 1990). In her book, *Lesbian Passion,* Joanne Loulan (1987) recounts how she "often asks audiences, 'Who absolutely loves her body?' The last time [she] did that, there were 400 women in the audience and thirteen of them raised their hands" (p. 41). As Rothblum (1994) and others (e.g., Beren, Hayden, Wilfley, & Striegel-Moore, 1997) note, regardless of our sexual orientation, socioeconomic status, or race, all women are bound to be "affected" to some degree "by society's emphasis on physical appearance for women" (p. 84). The words of a feminist colleague underscore the process of struggle and reconciliation, common to the experiences of so many women:

> "I was unhappy with my appearance and unsuccessfully tried a number of diets over the years. At one point I decided to be like Ghandi and fast one day a week. At another, I decided that if my dog only needed to eat once a day, that was all I needed. On still another occasion, I joined (and quickly dropped out of) an expensive weight loss clinic, which required that I follow a 500 calorie a day diet. Once I tried to throw up after overeating, but could not bring myself to complete the act. I felt I should not indulge in such an easy way out, but should live with the consequences of my actions. I attempted the infamous Scarsdale Diet at another point. During one of my more sane moments, I joined Weight Watchers. Nothing worked. I could not stand being told what to do: when to eat, what to eat and how many times to chew. In time, I gave up, and at 23 I decided that I might as well live with my large sized body and get on with the rest of my life. . . . I am now left with the difficult task of trying simply to accept and perhaps even like my body."

The statistics presented here suggest that even a woman in young adulthood who has successfully traversed the tumultuous waters of adolescence is not free within North American culture to enjoy the experience of living fully in her body with a sense of pleasure, entitlement, and self-acceptance. Rather, to varying degrees, all women, as well as their partners, are responsive to the unrealistic demands of the standards of physical appearance that are perpetuated within our culture. As a result of the internalization of these cultural messages, many young adult women, like contortionists, are left attempting to force their bodies into submission through weight-loss programs, fitness regimens, cosmetic creams, and, in some cases, the surgeon's knife. Failure to meet these unrealistic standards frequently engenders feelings of personal failure (Kaschak, 1992; Seid, 1994). This body image dissatisfaction is not limited to white, heterosexual, middle-class women. Rather, body image dissatisfaction has been reported for women of color and, to a lesser extent, for lesbian women (Beren et al., 1997; Striegel-Moore et al., 1990; Thomas & James, 1988; Thompson, 1992). An apparently indiscriminate predator, body image dissatisfaction appears to have no class boundaries, affecting socioeconomically advantaged and disadvantaged women alike (Faludi, 1991; Wolf, 1991). This dissatisfaction may be even more severe for women who are physically disabled and those who are subjected to such mutilating surgeries as mastectomy or hysterectomy (Campling, 1981; Cunningham, 1992; Gross & Ito, 1990, 1992; Johnson, 1987).

According to Wolf (1991), "To live in fear of one's body and one's life is not to live at all." She suggests that the requirements for physical beauty imposed on the present generation of women can leave us "materially and psychologically poor" (p. 52). In reinforcing feelings of insufficiency, they can eat "away at energy and self-love and reduce women's abilities to act powerfully" (Brown, 1987, p. 63). They can diminish spontaneity and pleasure, leaving many women feeling hypervigilant and in fear of losing control over their "appetites." These fears are apparent "in the woman who can never enjoy a meal, who never feels thin enough, or that the occasion is special enough, to drop her guard and become one with the moment. They are in the woman whose horror of wrinkles is so great that the lines around her eyes shine with sacred oil, whether at a party or while making love" (p. 130). In reference to the gains made by women over the past two decades, Wolf suggests that "it profits women little if we gain the whole world only to fear ourselves" (p. 130). By internalizing a dominantly negative appraisal of their bodies, and by learning to depend on the "mirrors of other peoples' eyes" rather than on their own, women have difficulty in "establishing a coherent and stable sense of self" and, in some cases, of "valuing the self at all" (Ling, 1989, p. 310). Brownmiller (1984) concurs in suggesting that "unending absorption in the drive for a perfect appearance . . . is the ultimate restriction on freedom of mind" (p. 51). The resulting states of guilt and shame stand in the way of "the emergence of an authentic delight in the body" and prevent women from discovering "the beauty, character, and expressiveness" (Bartky, 1990, p. 42) of their bodies.

Roberta Seid (1994) talks about the "treacherous polarities that dominate our thinking" (p. 13) in reference to our bodies. Women come to believe that in rejecting the tyranny of thinness, they are doomed to a life of fatness. They worry that in rejecting starvation, they are embracing gluttony. They fear that in refusing to whip their bodies into shape on the aerobic's floor they are choosing lethargy, that in rejecting the ascetic rituals of beauty and youth, they are embracing ugliness and old age. She argues that women need to "find a saner middle ground where our bodies can round out with more life, flesh, and health; where we can relish the fruits of our prosperity without self-punishment; and where we understand that the nourishment that is one of life's greatest pleasures is also one of its most basic necessities" (p. 13). In finding this middle ground, women are freer to delight in their embodied sexuality.

CHALLENGE AND CHANGE: CREATING NEW MEANINGS

A woman's relationship with her body is an important component of her ability to be in relationship with others (Chernin, 1986). In working with young women on issues related to their sexuality and sexual expression, it is important first to assess their current feelings toward, comfort in, and perceptions of, their bodies. Seeing through the eyes of each woman, however accurate or inaccurate her self-perceptions appear to be, can provide a point of reference from which to help clients begin an exploration of the sources of their physical and sexual self-perceptions (Blood, 1996). Exploration of clients' current intimate friendships and relationships often proves to be fertile ground for identifying potentially powerful sources of negative body perceptions, as well as sources of validation and empowerment.

Because current bodily self-perceptions are built upon earlier experiences, this work also frequently requires a retrospective focus. Counselors may need to help clients unpack the baggage of the past. In particular, it may be necessary to explore the messages they received from significant others in their lives about their bodies, and the meanings they incorporated into their self-structures related to their physical adequacy.

The goal of this work is to help women become "embodied . . . to experience the body as the center of existence—not as focus, but as reference point for being in the world" (Hutchinson, 1994, p. 155). It is to help them connect with the power and vitality of their bodies, and to begin to set their own standards for beauty and health. This work requires helping women learn to trust and depend on their own eyes rather than the internalized perceptions of others in evaluating their bodily appearance. It involves working through feelings of insufficiency and failure, which leave many women walking in "frozen bodies"; disconnected from their sexuality and an important source of sensual and erotic pleasure (Kasl, 1989). As Tiefer (1996) notes,

> In order to achieve a lasting therapeutic transformation, women need to move from experiencing their bodies as primarily the focus of comparison-based appearance appraisal to experiencing their bodies as ever-changing individualizes sources of sensations and competencies. This requires a massive reframing . . . "affirmative body work." (p. 58)

Affirmative body work can be undertaken individually or in groups. However, many authors (e.g., Daniluk, 1993; Friedman, 1993; Hirschmann & Munter, 1995; Hutchinson, 1985; Seid, 1989) note the power of women sharing the personal accounts of their lives with other women. Groups decrease isolation, normalize women's struggles with body image, and help women create more agentic narratives. As Heilburn (1988) notes in her book, *Writing a Woman's Life,*

> We must begin to tell the truth, in groups, to one another. Modern feminism began that way, and we have lost, through shame or fear of ridicule, that important collective phenomenon. . . . As long as women are isolated one from the other, not allowed to offer other women the most personal accounts of their lives, they will not be part of any narrative of their own. (pp. 46–47)

Counselors should consider group work whenever appropriate and possible. Group work can be especially transformative when client's concerns are related to the "normative discontent" of living in an adult woman's body in a culture that engenders feelings of shame and inadequacy. Groups can also be a powerful source of strength and support for women as they attempt to live comfortably in their bodies. The information and support received from others can help women to cope with the unique physical changes and realities of their lives.

It is also important to remember that as women growing up in a patriarchal world, we, too, have been and continue to be subjected to myriad messages that suggest that our bodies are inadequate. Consequently, many of us have also struggled (and perhaps continue to struggle) with feelings of bodily shame and insufficiency. Many have dieted, relentlessly counted calories, or pursued thinner thighs and a flatter stomach through fitness and even cosmetic surgery. Many have spent, and continue to spend, money on facial creams and hair dyes in an attempt to "correct" our deficiencies and hide the signs of aging. As counselors, we take this baggage into the counseling room. We carry with us into our work with clients our own set of beliefs and expectations about desirable and appropriate standards of beauty and attractiveness. Without awareness and care, we may inadvertently impose these on clients. We may do so by our focus on the importance of nutrition when working with large or thin women, or by our excessive attention to the risks involved in cosmetic surgery, and so on (Agell & Rothblum, 1991). It is important to be aware of our values and beliefs. We must take care not to make judgments about our clients in their adherence to, or rejection of, the standards of beauty promoted in their ethnic, cultural, or socioeconomic group.

The activities discussed here are only examples of the types of exercises counselors might employ when working with female clients. Readers are also referred to the books by Hutchinson (1985), Borysenko (1988), Freedman (1988), and Hirschmann and Munter (1995) for many other excellent examples of assessment and intervention strategies to improve women's relationships with their bodies. Other useful resources may be found in Appendix B.

Finally, impaired body image is often a long-term consequence of sexual and physical violation (Golding, 1996). Body hatred and feelings of estrangement are common experiences for adult survivors of child sexual abuse (Courtois, 1988; Maltz, 1991; Simonds, 1994). Internalized perceptions of the "body as 'dirty,' 'nasty,' 'bad,' 'evil,' 'out of control,' or 'untrustworthy' can be very difficult to overcome for many women" (Westerlund, 1992, p. 52). Before proceeding with any of the following exercises, counselors need to be sure to ascertain that women have not experienced this type of victimization. If they have, their healing will require more specialized work (Maltz, 1991; Maltz & Holman, 1987; Westerlund, 1992). The specific needs of these women are beyond the scope of this book. As such, the reader is referred to Appendix C for a list of recommended resources for working with survivors of sexual violence.

The Pencil Test: Pass, Fail, or Draw

However confident and self-assured a woman may be in other aspects of her life, the body is one area of particular discomfort and vulnerability for many women. As such, it is often useful to begin this assessment of body image with exercises or activities that are less threatening. For example, the "Mirror, Mirror" exercise described in Chapter 5 is an excellent tool for helping women of any age to identify and confront their feelings and perceptions regarding their bodies. For some women, however, standing naked in front of a mirror (literally, or in a guided fantasy) may prove to be too difficult in the early stages of this work.

Other ways of engaging in this type of exploration include the use of more expressive and affective techniques such as letter writing, metaphors, and drawings. For example, individually, or in a group setting a woman can be asked to write a letter to a stranger who will be meeting her in the future, and who will be faced with the task of having to identify her among a group of other women. In this letter, the woman is asked to introduce herself and describe her appearance in as much detail as possible. A woman should be encouraged to describe her height, weight, coloring, and bone structure, from head to toe. She should include any particular physical characteristics that she feels might help the stranger to differentiate her from other women in the group. While she may make references to such distinguishing characteristics as hair color, she should be encouraged to focus more exclusively on the characteristics of her body.

If this exercise is undertaken in a group, when the letters have been completed, all participants should place their letters in a box. The group leader then reads each letter, and the group members are charged with the responsibility of identifying the author of each letter based on the descriptions contained within it. Participants should be encouraged to provide feedback to each other as the letters are read. Emphasis should be place on reinforcing the accuracy of each individual woman's self-perceptions, reinforcing her individuality, and gently challenging perceptions that appear to be unnecessarily harsh or critical. This exercise serves the purpose of helping women gain considerable information about their own self-perceptions. They also learn about the perceptions of others regarding their physical characteristics and appearance. In an attempt to help women begin to focus on the importance of the observer in women's body image perceptions and comfort, group members should also be encouraged to speculate on how their letters might differ based on the characteristics of the stranger who will be meeting them (e.g., sex, age). Similar processing can occur in individual sessions, with the counselor helping to verify or challenge the accuracy of the woman's self-perceptions. She should be encouraged to explore the way the characteristics of the stranger (observer) influence her comfort in describing specific aspects of her physical appearance.

Metaphors can also be used to assist women in identifying and exploring their perceptions of their bodies. These can describe their current or desired perceptions of their bodies, feelings toward their bodies, and/or relationship with their bodies. Such metaphorical descriptions can provide considerable information about women's real and ideal body image perceptions. For example, one woman in my research group described her perceptions of her body as like "being in a house of mirrors." In this metaphor, she emphasized her sense of distortion regarding her body and the importance of the "other" (friends, lovers, family members, society in general) in shaping her experience of herself as too fat or too thin, inadequate or attractive. In processing this metaphor, she was able to identify how removed she felt she was from being the author of her own experience of her body. She subsequently used an eagle metaphor to describe her desired goal of coming to a place where she could perceive her body as vital and powerful, and experience a sense of freedom and ease. Another woman in this group brought in the following poem to articulate her relationship with her body and her struggles in being able to see herself/her body more clearly and in a more accepting and loving way: "She did suffer, the witch, trying to peer round the looking glass, she forgot, someone was in the way." She went on to proclaim,

> "When I stand in front of the looking glass, looking at my body, he is in the way, he, man, and he's saying 'those thighs, that bum, those breasts, those shoulders, that face' . . . I can't stand it, I want him out of there. . . . The reason this verse just bumped me on the head is because I always have to remember someone is in the way of seeing me as I am and valuing me as a woman. As long as men's standards are in our head, how are we ever going to peer around and get a glimpse of ourselves? Because they're in the way."

In response, another group member lamented: "I've stood in front of the mirror a hundred times and said out loud, 'I can't see, I can't see.' " Similar to the concept of double consciousness discussed earlier, the comments of these women reflect the experiences of many women. Many experience profound difficulty in being able to really see themselves as they are, rather than seeing themselves through the critical eyes of others.

In assessing the adequacy of their bodies and their appearance, women tend to be especially critical about particular parts of their bodies. Frequently, the body parts they identify are the ones most associated in our culture with women's sexuality and femininity (breasts, thighs, hips, stomach). Women also come to hold particular emotions in their bodies, emotions that are associated with various body parts (e.g., women who have been sexually traumatized often hold tremendous tension and anger in their jaws and stomachs) (Maltz, 1991; Maltz & Holman, 1987; Westerlund, 1992). Drawing can be a very facilitative mechanism to help women identify specific areas of bodily discomfort. For example, following a relaxation exercise, women can be progressively guided through a fantasy in which they are asked to focus on each discrete part of their body, from the head down to the feet. Rather than thinking about the particular body part, women should be encouraged to be attuned to the feelings that surface for them in association with each part of their bodies. When the exercise has been completed, they can draw a picture of their bodies. They can color the various body parts with colors that reflect the feelings that surfaced in association with each body part during the guided fantasy. For example, women often associate the color red with anger and find that they carry much of their anger in their stomachs, so they color their stomachs red. The color black is often used to reflect feelings of shame or disgust. It is a color that serves to "cover up" or "hide" the disowned body part(s) in question. Some women will color their genitals black, or their hips, or thighs. It is also important to encourage women to identify the areas of their bodies that are associated with feelings of joy and pleasure. In time, these feelings can be generalized to other parts of their bodies with which they are less comfortable. Considerable information can be gained in processing these colored drawings. Counselors can learn about women's feelings toward, and relationship with, the various parts of their bodies. This information can be very valuable in helping to gauge the pacing of counseling and to determine the most appropriate interventions (e.g., having clients give voice to the body part that is most associated with shame, guilt, pain, stress, joy).

Clothing also serves as an important indicator of women's comfort with, and perceptions of, their bodies and body parts. Exploration of how women dress, the types of clothing they wear, the colors, the textures, and so forth can be a significant source of information about their relationships with their bodies. For example, women often attempt to wear clothing that "covers up" the parts of their bodies that they are most ashamed of (e.g., stomach, hips, thighs, breasts). As noted in Chapter 5, women can be asked to take a critical walk through their wardrobes (literally, or in a fantasy). They can explore the purpose various types of clothing serve in attempting to accentuate or cover up particular parts of their bodies. This can help them to identify particular areas of pride, as well as those areas and body parts associated with discomfort and vulnerability. Specific types of clothing have different meanings for individuals as well. It is important, therefore, to explore with women the messages they are attempting to send out to others regarding their feelings about themselves and their bodies, based on the clothing they characteristically wear. Dramatic changes in clothing can provide women (and counselors) with important information regarding significant experiences or turning points in women's self-perceptions.

How comfortable women feel in their bodies can also be assessed, individually or in a group, through movement. Women can be asked simply to walk around the room, taking note of their step, their gait. They should take note of the way they hold their shoulders, their heads, their bodies, and of their needs for personal space. This information can reveal a great deal about how they live in, and experience, their bodies. In adding movement to this simple exercise, they can gain even more information from the rhythm and sway of their hips, the looseness or tightness of their shoulders and chest, the movement of their feet. Women should be encouraged to be aware of the various parts of their bodies as they move. They should be sensitive to areas that are resistant to uninhibited and easy movement, as well as those areas that flow effortlessly and freely. This information can be used as a beginning point of reference as they attempt to extend this sense of comfort to other areas of their bodies.

The language women use in relation to the various parts of their bodies can also be quite telling in terms of their self-perceptions. For example, when women refer to themselves are "hippy" or "chunky," a judgment is inferred by these words. These words often reflect their perceived lack of adequacy in meeting some internalized standard. Alternately, adjectives such as "reliable," "useful," "resilient," "comfortable," "agile," or "strong" suggest a very different relationship with the body. Certainly, the word "fat" is a loaded word for many women in our culture. This word is commonly associated with feelings of failure and inadequacy (Erdman, 1995; Friedman, 1993; Seid, 1994).

Underscoring the salience and power of the *word* "fat" in popular discourse, Friedman (1993) discusses how women "learn to encode their feelings in the 'language of fat' " (p. 288). The word "fat" serves as a more acceptable vehicle for expressing feelings of anger, fear, and powerlessness for women in our culture. Consistent with the notion of "woman as body" (Greenspan, 1983, p. 181), "fat" and its corollary "thin" take on a multiplicity of meanings in the lives of women. When women perceive themselves as "fat," it is important to help them examine what this means in terms of their self-perceptions.

Several writers (e.g., Brown & Rothblum, 1989; Chernin, 1986; Goldenberg, 1990; Orbach, 1986) note the way in which weight is used by some women to maintain a degree of psychological distance and physical safety from others. Excessive weight provides a way to avoid intimacy and the corresponding risks associated with close relationships (e.g., pain, loss, rejection). For some, being far outside the ideal range of weight may actually represent freedom from having to be hypervigilant in terms of food. On the other end of the continuum is the woman who is never "thin" enough to consider herself desirable, or whose rituals around food and weight keep her safely preoccupied, so that there is little room in her life for intimate relationships (Seid, 1989).

The connection between weight and voice is also well documented in the literature. Some women appear to use their bodies to communicate their experiences of being devalued, objectified, and silenced within our patriarchal culture (e.g., Brumberg, 1989; Hirschmann & Munter, 1995; Jacobus, Keller, & Shuttleworth, 1990; Orbach, 1985). Others suggest that women's struggles over weight and attempts to maintain "control" over their bodies, is actually a metaphor for their feelings of having so little control over other aspects of their lives (e.g., Bartky, 1990; Orbach, 1985). While being thin may appear to enhance women's power and status in their ability to attract men, increased size can actually be a method of avoiding being rendered powerless by avoiding being sexualized. "Fat is about protection, sex, nurturance, strength, boundaries, mothering, substance, assertion and rage" (Orbach, 1978, p. 6). Weight clearly has multiple meanings in women's lives. It is important to fully explore these meanings and to be sensitive to the words clients characteristically use as they describe their bodies (e.g., "fat," "thin," "good," "bad," "pretty," "ugly," "gross"). The development of a repertoire of language and alternate meanings that reinforce bodily acceptance and comfort is also an important part of affirmative body work.

Never Good Enough: Examining the Sources of Bodily Shame

Many women have learned to depend on the mirrors of other people's eyes rather than on their own in their self-assessments. This frequently results in feelings of shame and inadequacy being associated with their bodies. Part of the process of attempting to change negative self-perceptions and build on women's more positive self-evaluations involves helping them to identify the source of these messages. Women need to eliminate the perceptions of people in the mirror who prevent them from seeing and valuing themselves and their bodies. The exercises that follow are useful in facilitating this type of exploration of the many sources of women's discomfort with their bodies, some of which date back to earlier periods in their development.

Women who have struggled with body image dissatisfaction often have very painful and conflicted relationships with their bodies. Counselors should proceed with great care in exploring past histories, being certain to ensure that women are emotionally and psychologically ready to undertake this type of exploration. Participants must maintain control over the timing and pacing of these activities. Helping them first construct a "secure container" for any overwhelming feelings that surface during this type of exploration can be a useful mechanism to ensure psychological safety (e.g., see J. Ellis, 1990, pp. 249–250, for an excellent example of this technique). Women may also find it difficult to access some of their early memories and feelings related to their bodies. Reviewing family photographs from childhood and adolescence, or engaging in psychodrama or family sculpting, can help to increase awareness of bodily messages and experiences.

In helping women to begin to identify the sources of the messages they received regarding the inadequacy of their bodies, it is useful first to guide them through a progressive relaxation exercise. Next, counselors can walk them through an *early recollection* of the first time they remember hearing there was something wrong with their bodies (that they were too fat, too thin, too tall, too short, too hairy, knock-kneed, etc.). Women can be asked to take note of how old they were when they received this message, and of who made the comment. Was the comment made directly to them, or was it something they overheard? What did they do with this information? How did they respond? What did they say? How did they feel? Where in their bodies was this feeling located? Can they feel it now? What would they like to have said to the person who made the comment, if they had the words and power they now have as adults to respond in an assertive way?

When the exercise has been completed, clients should be asked to spend some time debriefing the experience. They may wish to keep a journal and write down their reactions and reflections. They may also process this verbally or through an expressive medium such as art or movement. As a follow-up, women can be asked what other messages they recall hearing about their bodies as they grew up. How did these messages shape their experience of, and relationships with, their bodies: as children, as adolescents, and now as adults?

Given the tremendous significance of families in constructing girls' early experiences of their bodies (Gagnon & Simon, 1982; Laws, 1980), it is helpful to explore women's recollections of the perceptions of significant family members toward their developing bodies. One way to engage in this type of exploration is to use the following exercise adapted from Rita Freedman's (1988) book *Body Love: Learning to Like Our Looks—and Ourselves: A Practical Guide for Women.* First, ask participants to identify the people in their childhood and adolescence who they feel were most influential in their development. Then ask them to answer the following question: "When you were 5, what would your _____ (mother, father, sister, brother, etc.) have said about your body if they were talking to a friend?" This questions can be asked repeatedly, with the age being changed in 5-year increments (5, 10, 15 years). Other significant sources of influence can also be identified by participants at different ages (specific friends, a gym coach, a dance teacher, etc.). Women should be encouraged to identify both those whom they experienced as very supportive of their looks and appearance, as well as those who were harsh or critical. In working through this exercise, women are able to identify the people whose perceptions were most influential in shaping their early experiences of their bodies. They can begin to identify the negative and positive messages they received. They can take note of the particular periods of development when these messages changed in response to changes in the shape and size of their bodies. They should also take note of the messages they have received about their bodies from lovers. The impact of these messages should be examined in terms of their current enjoyment of their bodies and their freedom of sexual expression.

Lifelines can also be quite useful tools in helping women assess changes in their perceptions and experience of their bodies over time. Using age as the bottom axis (from birth to the present), the side axis can include "level of bodily comfort," or "degree of bodily satisfaction." Lifelines can provide visual representations of particular struggles (with weight, disability, etc.) and successes (in athletics, dance, etc.) clients have experienced related to their bodies at various times in their lives. They can serve as a vehicle for contextualizing these experiences relative to particular developmental or personal events that were influential in shaping their relationships with their bodies. Guided autobiography is also an excellent technique for use in affirmative body work. Using sensitizing questions to elicit autobiographical recollections, women can be assisted in identifying the salient themes related to their relationships with their bodies over the course of their lives (see Birren, 1987, and de Vries, Birren, & Deutchman, 1990, for examples of using and applying this technique).

It is also important to examine the impact of media messages on women's experiences of their bodies. There are many ways in which this might be accomplished, including the use of collages. I have found it particularly useful to ask women to browse through various magazines in search of three particular photos: (1) one of the body of a woman that is most similar to their own, (2) one of a body of a woman that they would most like to resemble (emulate), and (3) one of a body of a woman that they most fear becoming. Finding a photo of their desired image usually poses no challenge. However, finding a photo that they believe is most similar to their own bodies frequently proves to be a difficult task for women. This fact alone is often instrumental in eliciting some awareness on the part of women that the images of women's bodies portrayed in the media do not reflect the reality of most women's lives and bodies. Interestingly, finding a photo that represents an image they most fear becoming can also be quite challenging. These are usually taken from the covers of tabloids. The pictures are often accompanied by headlines criticizing some famous personality for letting herself go (the recent debate over the weight gain of the 1997 Miss Universe comes to mind). The pictures that are identified prove to be an interesting focus of discussion, particularly within a group setting. Women can discuss why they selected the pictures they did and how these relate to their perceptions and fears about the adequacy of their own bodies. They can also receive feedback from others, gently challenging the accuracy of their self-perceptions and confronting their fears.

Women may have special needs based on their personal histories that require specific emphasis in counseling. For example, clients who have undergone a mastectomy for breast cancer may need help to integrate this loss into their body image and sexual identities. Prior to this work, however, they may need to work through their fears of coping with a life-threatening illness. Readers are referred to Appendix F for a list of excellent resources for working with women who are coping with illness and disability.

Exorcising the Demons

The following exercises can help clients begin to work through and reject some of the messages that have contributed to their negative self-perceptions and feelings of physical inadequacy. Building on the activities discussed earlier, through a guided fantasy, women can be taken back to their *earliest recollection* of the first time someone said something critical about their bodies. Prior to reliving the fantasy, they should be instructed to bring their adult selves along in the fantasy, so that their child selves can have an advocate to stand up for them on their behalf. Once engaged in the fantasy, women should return to the earlier scene and attempt to relive it. They are to put themselves back into the scene in as much detail as possible. This time, after the negative comment is made about their bodies, they are to "freeze frame" the scene and begin a dialogue with their adult selves about how the comment makes them feel, and what they might like to say to the person making the comment. The adult should encourage the child to stand up to the person making the comment, or, if necessary, speak on the child's behalf. The adult should discount the accuracy of the comment and highlight the child's physical strengths. Various hurtful scenes from the woman's life can be replayed in a similar manner. In each case the child/adolescent (with the support of the adult) should refute the comments, identify their impact, and conclude with an emphasis on her positive physical attributes.

It can be helpful to follow up this type of exercise with psychodrama or family sculpting. These techniques can be used to facilitate catharsis, insight, and a sense of personal mastery in responding to and rejecting the negative messages of others that women have internalized. Some women may have difficulty visualizing scenes or relinquishing control. In these cases, corrective endings to painful and shaming experiences can be constructed through the use of letter writing, narrative, or Gestalt two-chair techniques.

Bibliotherapy is also another excellent way to help clients begin to recognize the extent to which societal standards of feminine beauty serve contribute to their feelings of inadequacy. Certainly books such as Susan Faludi's (1991) *Backlash: The Undeclared War Against American Women,* and Naomi Wolf's (1991) *The Beauty Myth* help to identify the problems experienced by women in attempting to conform to these unrealistic cultural standards. They identify the economic and political motivations that motivate and perpetuate women's insecurities. Clients may also benefit from Cheri Erdman's (1995) *Nothing to Lose: A Guide to Sane Living in a Large Body* and Judith Rodin's (1992) *Body Traps* in challenging internalized stereotypes related to women's bodies.

Another short and powerful example of the cultural construction of beauty is an article entitled "They Called Me 'Chicken Hips': Adding Weight to an Image of Beauty." In this brief essay, Catherine Pigott (1991) talks about her experience as a North American white woman who spent a year teaching in a village in Gambia. In the article, she speaks of the Gambian women's reactions to her thin body and of her body's difficulty in filling out and holding up her *lappa* (the traditional Gambian women's dress). She talks of the beauty of the traditional dances, which came alive as "women swivelled their broad hips and used their hands to *emphasize* the roundness of their bodies"; how, in fact, "one needed to be round and wide to make the dance beautiful" (p. 17). She goes on to speak of how her perception of beauty and her body altered during her time in Gambia. She came to accept the fact that in Gambia, "it is beautiful—not shameful—to carry weight on the hips and thighs, to have a round stomach and heavy, swinging breasts." Powerfully underscoring the cultural construction of women's physical insecurities, she indicates how in Gambia "women do not battle the bulge, they celebrate it" (p. 17). She also notes the absence of guilt and shame in Gambian women's relationships with food. In Gambia, "fat is desirable," rather than being "feared and despised" (p. 17). In stark contrast to North American culture, there, the natural curves of women's bodies "hold beneficial meanings of abundance, fertility and health." Exposing women to this type of story and helping them explore cultural differences in images of beauty can be instrumental in underscoring the role of context in defining beauty and perpetuating insecurities.

It is important to acknowledge the difficulty women in mainstream cultures experience in trying to reject the baggage heaped upon them from every billboard, magazine cover, and television program. Books and articles such as those described earlier can help women step back and see their feelings of physical insufficiency as not being their own failures. Rather, these can be framed as the failures of a culture that is unwilling to appreciate and celebrate the strength, character, and beauty of diverse female forms.

The "Scales" of Justice

Another important part of affirmative body work involves helping women to let go of their desire to achieve a standard of bodily acceptability that is neither healthy or realistic, given their particular genetic history and endowment, their lifestyle, and their age and life stage. One way to begin this process is to have clients review and bring in photographs of various members from both sides of their families (e.g., mothers, fathers, grandmothers, aunts, uncles). As women review the various pictures of their family members, counselors should engage them in a discussion of their ethnic and cultural histories, asking questions such as "Which side of your family do you think you most resemble in terms of your body shape, size, and appearance?" They should be encouraged to identify the characteristics they find most attractive about their family members (bright eyes, beautiful hair, strong hands, etc.). This should be followed by an exploration of their own physical characteristics that they see they have inherited from their families (both those with which they feel most satisfied and those with which they feel least satisfied). It is useful during this exploration to reinforce the characteristics about which women feel good. Those they are most critical of should be reframed (e.g., women who are critical of their rounded stomachs or broad shoulders can be encouraged to think and speak about these attributes in more affirming ways: "strong" broad shoulders, "warm, nurturing" stomach, etc.).

In dealing with genetic endowment and issues of weight, some clinicians (e.g., Freedman, 1988) suggest that it is useful to discuss the concept of "set point theory." Set point theory is based on the assumption that "the body has a natural weight and that all people, fat or thin adjust their metabolism to maintain that weight" (Erdman, 1995, p. 17). Others support the use of the Body Mass Index, a measure based on weight and height, used by physicians and dietitians to determine "healthy" weight ranges. In an attempt to determine what is a realistic weight range for them, Freedman suggests that women first attempt to take a weight history. They should determine their weight patterns from puberty (approximately 15 years old) until the present. Photos and special events may be helpful cues in completing this exercise. A lifeline can be used to plot and track this information (with age on the bottom axis and weight on the side axis). Women should be encouraged to examine the range of weight fluctuations over time. On the basis of this information, they should calculate their average weight and their weight range (the range in which they seem to vacillate when they are not actively dieting). Attention to dramatic fluctuations in women's weight can provide important information regarding their relationship with food and the types of life events that have triggered weight loss or gain for them. Based on a review of their weight history, their activity levels, and their genetic backgrounds, women can usually calculate a set-point range that is reasonable for their body and metabolism.

Having calculated their set-point range, it is useful to have women design a ritual to psychologically and emotionally "let go" of their desire to obtain or return to a weight that is not realistic for their bodies or their lifestyles. For example, often women have a very conflictual relationship with their weight scales. They hate to get on the scales for fear of having put on a few pounds. And yet they feel compelled to continue to weigh themselves on a daily or weekly basis to ensure that they do not allow their weight to "get out of control." In rejecting the "tyranny" of her scale (and symbolically rejecting the tyranny of oppressive cultural standards), one client took her scale to a local park and ceremoniously threw it off the bluff into the ocean below. As it crashed against the rocks, she repeated to herself the following affirmation: "In celebration of the woman that I am." In what she referred to as "a liberating move," another woman dropped her scale down her apartment garbage chute from the 10th floor. Another had kept a pair of size-8 jeans that she had worn several years before when she was involved in a rigorous exercise and weight control regimen. Now, at the age of 36, it became apparent to her that she likely would never again fit into these jeans. She also realized that she no longer had any desire to force her body into such conformity. Her "freedom ritual," as she called it, involved bringing the size-8 jeans to her women's group and presenting them to another group member with the instructions to pass them on to her 13-year-old daughter. Affirming her acceptance of her adult woman's body, she said, "These are young girl's jeans, and I am a woman, not a girl." In carrying out a ritual that is personally significant, women can make a powerful statement to themselves and to others about their acceptance of their bodies, and about their lack of willingness to accept the judgments of others regarding their physical adequacy.

It is also important to help women give voice to their own bodily pleasures, needs, and desires. To do so requires a level of self-acceptance that includes embracing the comfort and joy that comes from living more wholly and fully in their skin. The following words of a colleague who spent years struggling to live more fully and comfortably in her body exemplify the hard-earned achievement of physical self-love:

> "Recently, I have come to realize that I have been using my body as a political symbol, that with it I am making a social statement. I am deliberately taking up space. . . . I refuse to try to be small. I no longer want to be a little wisp of a thing, who eats like a bird. I deliberately eat in public, and large amounts, if I want. This is in direct challenge to the ideal of woman as small and a delicate eater. I enjoy food, and endeavor to celebrate eating, rather than fearing food. I no longer pretend I am not hungry and then go home to binge in private. I am not going to let society dictate my behavior in this arena. I wear

comfortable, solid shoes, rather than teetering around on heels. Never a woman of delicate mannerisms and voice, I am celebrating my very lack of socially defined femininity. My gestures are often large, and I have never been described as a delicate walker. I can command attention because of my height and size, and I delight in being able to see in a crowd and reach the highest cupboard."

Affirming the Self

There are many other exercises that can be used to help women become more comfortable in, and accepting of, their bodies. For example, Burgard and Lyons (1994) discuss the usefulness of dance and movement in helping women "reoccupy" and feel more grounded in their bodies. Through such kinesthetic and creative modalities, women can begin to get in touch with their bodies. They can become more aware of where in their bodies they feel most alive, and where they do not feel anything. Women can be helped to redraw the boundaries of their awareness to include more of their bodies. They can begin to have access to the full range of their physical and erotic senses. Shelia Richards, a feminist teacher, artist, and counselor in Stockbridge, Massachusetts, conducts body casting workshops for women. The goal is to help participants transform their relationships with their bodies and rediscover and reclaim the sacredness and essence of the female spirit. In these workshops, women learn to celebrate the female form in all its diversity. Joan Turner (1990) provides some excellent examples of the power of therapeutic massage and body work in helping women begin to live more fully in their bodies and in the world. Some native healing rituals such as sweat lodges can also be powerful experiences in facilitating bodily awareness and acceptance (Achterberg, 1985; Allen, 1986).

Some women experience considerable difficulty in identifying the characteristics about themselves about which they feel good. They can be encouraged to ask a woman that they respect and trust to tell them what she finds most attractive about their appearance and body. If there are few characteristics that women can initially identify as desirable, then they can focus on the traits they appreciate. Emphasis should be placed on making a concerted effort to add a new characteristic each week to their list. Repeating verbal affirmations such as "My body is powerful" and "I am a uniquely beautiful woman" can be effective ways to counter the negative and critical self-statements that women are inclined to make about themselves. They should be encouraged to take time to nurture their bodies and selves.

In my own clinical work, I have found guided fantasy to be especially useful in helping women feel more at home in their bodies. For example, following a basic relaxation exercise, women can be asked to take themselves in their minds to a place from their past where they felt tremendous calm and peace. Once there, they should be encouraged to drink in the scene fully with all their senses, taking note of the sounds, smells, and feel of this place. Then, they should be asked to picture themselves there without clothing, comfortable in their nakedness. They should try to allow their bodies to languish in the warmth and comfort of the place, being fully accepting of their bodies and how they fit perfectly in the contours of the scene. When they are able to connect with a feeling of profound well-being and self-acceptance, they should be encouraged to attempt to contain this feeling within a special container that they construct in their minds. This container should be placed in a safe psychological place, so that they can later return to it as they desire. The power of this simple exercise becomes apparent as women attempt to process and debrief the experience. For example, in a workshop that a colleague and I recently conducted, one woman in the group referred to herself as "a woman of size." This woman reflected on how she was able to experience a deep sense of acceptance of her body during this guided fantasy. She noted how this experience was a "gift" for her. It was the first time in years that she recalled feeling comfortable about the size and shape of her body.

Another powerful guided fantasy that I sometimes use in my work with women is an inner-child activity. This activity is aimed at helping women reconnect with a time earlier in their lives when they lived more fully and freely in their bodies. For many, this is a time prior to adolescence. It involves an initial relaxation exercise, followed by a guided fantasy. During the fantasy, women are asked to return in their minds to a time in their youth when they felt free and at home in their bodies. They are to take their adult selves into this fantasy and observe the child as she is engaged in whatever activity she is involved in (swinging on a swing, biking, climbing a tree, etc.). I ask them to be cognizant of their lack of self-consciousness and freedom of movement as the child plays. Then, they are asked to approach the child and have a conversation with her about how she feels about her body. They are to consider how this has changed over time and contemplate when this feeling of bodily contentment was lost to them. The adult should ask how the child perceives and experiences living in this body now that she is grown. They are to ask the child when she feels most connected to the adult in terms of a sense of embodiment. When does she feel most shut down and rejected? The exercise concludes with the adult making a plan with the child to connect with her more frequently in the future. It ends with a commitment to the child to be more accepting of this body that they share.

Another tool to correct negative self-perceptions involves asking women to identify the part of their body toward which they feel most negative. Typically, this might be their hips, their thighs, or their stomachs. Questions that can facilitate this exploration include the following: When you are with a lover or in a situation where you are undressed in front of other people (e.g., in a shower room at a gymnasium), what part of your body are you most self-conscious about and most reluctant to have others see? What part of your body do you have the most difficulty looking at when you stand in front of a full mirror? Once a particular body part is identified, women should try to imagine giving that part of their body a voice. They should be guided to have a conversation with this body part. This may be done using a two-chair technique. It may be undertaken as a written dialogue. Women should be encouraged to express their feelings of disdain or disgust toward the part in question. In turn, the body part should be given a "voice" to respond in terms of how it feels about the client's perceptions of, and actions toward it. Both should be encouraged to identify what they need from each other to be more connected. If women have difficulty with the verbal modality, they can be directed to draw or paint the feelings stored in this part of their body. They may find it useful to select a metaphor that represents their feelings toward this disowned body part. Movement may also be used as a form of expression in facilitating this exploration. This exercise can be extended over time to include other disowned body parts, thereby facilitating greater bodily acceptance and integration.

This exercise can be particularly powerful for women who have experienced a sense of bodily betrayal through illness or disability. For example, through psychodrama, a woman I worked with several years after a hysterectomy was able to give her lost uterus a voice. In so doing, she was able to express the depth and extent of her feelings of anger and loss over what for her was a very defining and significant aspect of her female identity. Through this session, she was able to identify the meaning of her uterus to her. She perceived this organ as "the center of [her] creativity . . . where [she] created the most beautiful creation in [her] life, [her] daughters." Through this process, she was able to begin to heal from the loss of her "creative center" and came to see herself as whole again. In her words, "I mean whether or not that organ is there, that's still my creative center, my spiritual center. I'm still a woman, and I still have a uterus, if only symbolically." This type of exercise was also very facilitative in working through the grief and loss experienced by an infertile woman. This woman felt that her body had betrayed her in not allowing her to bear children. Another client who had experienced disfiguring facial lacerations following an automobile accident was able to come to terms with her appearance by giving this part of her body a voice through the use of clay.

CONCLUSION

The possibilities in adapting these exercises are virtually limitless. Counselors need only recognize the importance of helping women to live comfortably and more fully in their bodies. This is critical to experiencing the full range of women's sensory and erotic potential. It is fundamental to women's embodied sexuality.

The goal is not to encourage women to reject any and all efforts to change or alter their appearance. Seid (1994) suggests that a complete rejection of our normal human impulses toward self-beautification and bodily adornment would only serve to reinforce the "treacherous polarities that dominate our thinking" (p. 13). Rather, "we must restore a humanistic vision in which self-improvement means cultivating the mind and enlarging the soul; developing generosity, humor, dignity, and humility; living more graciously with biology, aging, and death; living with our limitations" (p. 15). Only then will women be free to really celebrate beauty and "encourage the imagination and play involved in bedecking ourselves and molding our own images" (p. 13). These sentiments are eloquently stated by Adrienne Rich (1976):

> The repossession by women of our bodies will bring far more essential change to human society than the seizing of the means of production by workers. . . . We need to imagine a world in which every woman is the presiding genius of her own body. In such a world, women will truly create new life, bringing forth not only children (if and as we choose), but the visions and the thinking necessary to sustain, console and alter human existence—a new relationship to the universe. Sexuality, politics, intelligence, position, motherhood, work, community, intimacy will develop new meanings; thinking itself will be transformed. This is where we have to begin. (p. 292)

10

FANNING THE FLAMES OF DESIRE

To love women
is holy and holy is the free love of men
and precious to live taking whichever comes
and precious to live unmated as a peachtree.
—MARGE PIERCY,
"The Sabbath of Mutual Respect"

in celebration of the woman I am
and of the soul of the woman I am
and of the central creature and its delight
I sing for you. I dare to live.
—ANNE SEXTON,
"In Celebration of My Uterus"

I've learnt that it's the journey into sleep that matters;
the lovemaking part is easy, but you can't sleep with
everyone. We sleep upside down in the end. When did
we move to breathe deeply into each other's faces,
mouths, eyes . . . some time deep in the heart of sleep
. . . I don't know. We wake up early and together,
discovering that we are holding hands.
—RAMABAI ESPINET, "Erotic Fragments"

After 20 years of intense physical change and growth, and with the groundwork for their adult identities well in place, young adults ostensibly turn their attention toward creating a space for themselves in the world. They further define and distinguish themselves in terms of their commitments to particular roles and relationships. They begin to create a lifestyle that reflects their unique needs and desires (Stevens-Long & Commons, 1992). For the current generation of young women, it is a time when they are freer to explore the various dimensions of their sexuality. It is a time when they can begin more fully to connect with their erotic and sensual selves.

The last several decades have certainly been characterized by considerable hype about women's capacity for unbridled sexual pleasure in the form of multiple partners and multiple orgasms (e.g., the "G"[rafenberg] spot, clitoral orgasms, etc.). The realities of AIDS aside (Lear, 1997), young women today supposedly have a newfound freedom to pursue their erotic fantasies and indulge their carnal desires without fear of pregnancy or reprisal (Denfeld, 1995; Wolf, 1997). And indeed, it would appear that women's patterns of sexual activity have undergone some rather dramatic changes in the last 50 years. Young women reportedly initiate intercourse at an earlier age, have more sexual partners, and participate in a broader range of sexual behaviors than women of previous cohorts (Wyatt et al., 1988a, 1988b).

However, despite these reported changes in behavior, and the promise of erotic pleasures previous unknown, young women today may not be freer to explore and express their sexuality than their sisters of previous generations (Lear, 1997; Ussher, 1989). To understand why this is so, it is necessary to examine more closely the dialectic between the body, the person, and society in the construction of women's sexual meanings and experiences. While we may as yet know little about the psychology of women's sexuality, we do know that language and culture play a significant role in promoting particular messages regarding women's sexual nature and expression. We also know that these messages are taken in to varying degrees and interpreted by women in understanding and making sense of their sexual needs and desires. They are significant in determining how these desires are expressed (Gagnon & Parker, 1995; Tiefer, 1995; Weeks, 1985, 1995). According to Weeks (1987) the things we perceive to be sexual are as much a product of our language and culture, as they are of nature.

And in looking outward at the context within which young women negotiate their sexuality and sexual expression, there can be little debate about the fact that the dominant model of sexuality promoted in North American culture may be problematic. This model is taught through the media, and "even in the present, supposedly enlightened, sexual climate, it is passed on from parents, peers, and teachers. . . . It is so pervasive that most people are not usually aware they are being taught this information; they believe it is *natural* or *just the way it is*" (Golden, 1988, p. 79). An overview of the prevalent model of sex is presented.

HE SHOOTS, HE SCORES: THE MALE MODEL OF SEXUAL EXPRESSION

At the center of our dominant model of sexual expression is the penis, a "magical instrument of infinite powers" (Zilbergeld, 1993, p. 42). Like the

Duracel battery rabbit, the penis is portrayed as always being charged and ready to fully satisfy the sensual and erotic needs of women (Morris, 1997). As for her part, the woman's role is

> to be instantly ready for intercourse when confronted with a *big enough* penis and be orgasmic merely because it is contained in her vagina. In addition, a vagina is supposed to be delighted to lend itself to the effort every time a penis needs to ejaculate [*the service center model of women's sexuality*]. If the owner of the vagina is not instantly orgasmic with vaginal containment of the penis, something is surely wrong with her. (Golden, 1988, p. 79)

The centrality and privilege of the penis in this model of sex is readily apparent. It has long been revered as *the* symbol of masculinity, fertility, and power. "The phallus stands not just for male desire, but all desire. . . . We have no female image or symbol to counterbalance the monopoly of the phallus in representing desire" (Benjamin, 1988, p. 88). From this perspective, then, to be considered "normal," women's sexual and erotic desire cannot exist outside of women's relationships with men.

Orgasms are also central in this model. Those genital spasms that occur at 0.8-second intervals are commonly promoted as *the* goal of sex. Genital contractions and the exchange of bodily fluids are the benchmarks of a successful sexual encounter, not the experience of communion with another, a joining of two souls or spirits, a moment of tender touch. And while the man's own orgasm is certainly important in this model, so, too, are the woman's. Orgasms are something that men are suppose to "give" to women, as much as proof of their own masculine sexual prowess as in service to the pleasure of their female partners. Orgasms are so important in this goal-oriented model of sex that many women admit to having "faked" the experience to protect the sensibilities of their male partners (Hite, 1981, 1987; Rubin, 1990). To do otherwise would be to risk inferring that the man's sexual equipment or performance was somehow inadequate or lacking.

The model is based on the assumption that somewhere deep inside every woman, a fierce erotic desire exists, waiting to be unlocked by the lovemaking talents of an erotically skilled man. Ironically, if women admit to not experiencing orgasm, however *skilled* their male partners may be, their *failure* to do so is often viewed as a reflection of the inadequacy of their bodies. It is a reflection of their lack of sexual responsiveness.

Underlying this prevalent model of sex are a host of dichotomous myths and assumptions about women's and men's sexual needs and natures. The myths outlined here continue to be regarded as essential "truths" about how men and women should conduct their sexual interactions, although they are not based on any objective fact.

Men are sexually aggressive—women are passive.
Men push for sex—women resist their efforts.
Men are skilled lovers—women must not be too skilled.
Men engage in sexual practice—women engage in restraint.
For men, sex and love are separate—for women, sex and love are inseparable.
Male sexual desire is relatively indiscriminate—female sexual desire is highly selective.
Men always want sex—women rarely want sex.
Men "need" sex—women "need" love.
Sexual exclusivity (monogamy) is difficult for men—for women, monogamy is "natural."
Men who love sex are normal—women who love sex are nymphomaniacs.
Men who force themselves on a woman "can't really help themselves"—women who give in "really want it."
Men never say "no" to sex—when women say "no," they really mean "yes."
Men give sex—women withhold sex.

The list is virtually endless and the dichotomies do not end with comparisons between the "basic" sexual natures of men and women. Women are also compared to other women in terms of their "sexual responsiveness." Women who are not interested "enough" (a word whose meaning is very context-specific) in sex are frigid. Women who enjoy sex "too much" are promiscuous "whores." Women who resist intercourse ("going all the way") are withholding "tight-asses" and "teases." Women who do not resist "enough" are "easy." Women who select sexual partners that dominate them are masochists. Women who prefer to dominate in their sexual relationships are "castrating bitches." And perhaps the ultimate irony is the commonly held assumption that although women do not want or need sex the way men do, a good "roll in the hay" is exactly what every woman needs. This is especially the case if she competes too aggressively or successfully in the male world, in which case, the assumption is that she "must have gotten there on her back." Even the words used to categorize women relative to sexual expression reflect this dichotomous thinking: hot–cold, tight–loose, frigid–easy, good–bad, virgin–whore, femme–dyke, normal–abnormal. The list goes on. (For an amusing and detailed review of the many myths that underlie our popularly held beliefs and assumptions regarding the sexual "nature" of women, the reader is referred to Chapter 6 of Carol Tavris's [1992] book, *The Mismeasure of Woman.*)

Based on this dominant model of sex, women are clearly disadvantaged in the sexual arena. These sexual myths are widely promoted in our culture (Wyatt & Riederle, 1994). They make it especially difficult for young adult women to experience a sense of sexual agency and entitlement. They impede women's ability to freely explore the range and possibilities of sexual and erotic potential within their lives. For example, Darling and Davidson (1987) conducted a study of the sexual feelings and behaviors of 212 never-married, coitally active, undergraduate students. They found that both men and women reported feelings of guilt associated with masturbation and intercourse. However, significantly more women than men reported feelings of guilt when engaged in sexual intercourse. For women, this was especially the case when they did not experience "emotional arousal" with their partners. The authors attribute this finding to the way in which "females have been socialized to regard the prerequisite of love as a necessity for the acceptability of sexual intercourse" (p. 267). Feelings of sexual guilt were also found to have a greater negative impact on the sexual satisfaction of the women in the study than the men. In 1993, these authors conducted a similar study of 805 adult women (mean age 33.6 years). They found that of the 88.5% of participants who reported engaging in masturbation, 64.7% of these women experienced masturbatory guilt. The origins of this guilt could be traced to negative, early socialization experiences. The authors concluded that "those women who reported guilt feelings associated with masturbation were . . . less likely to report sexual adjustment, physiological sexual satisfaction, and psychological sexual satisfaction" (Davidson & Darling, 1993, p. 289).

Hyde (1990) and others (e.g., Smith et al., 1996) also note persistent sex differences in the masturbatory experiences of women and men. These authors confirm that early messages and negative sanctions shape the behavior and sexual experiences of girls well into adulthood. In Kinsey et al.'s (1953) survey, only 58% of adult females reported "masturbating to orgasm at some time in their lives" (p. 143). They also reportedly engaged in this form of self-pleasuring much later than men. As noted earlier in this chapter, more women today report engaging in masturbation. However, despite the "sexual revolution" of the 1960s and the gains made by the women's movement toward sexual equality, for many women, this form of self-pleasuring still engenders feelings of guilt (Rubin, 1990). Tiefer (1996) advocates "affirmative genital education" to counter the "inhibiting insecurity" (p. 57) so many women appear to have about their bodies and their sexuality.

Sexual guilt and shame are often a particularly difficult legacy of childhood and adolescence for women who were indoctrinated into traditional patriarchal religions (Gil, 1990). In a study of sexual guilt and permissiveness in a sample of African American and white women, Wyatt and Dunn (1991) found that although African American women scored higher on sexual guilt measures than their white counterparts, religiosity was a stronger predictor of sexual guilt than ethnicity or socioeconomic status. Linda Hurcombe (1987) notes in her book, *Sex and God: Some Varieties of Women's Religious Experience*, how traditional religions are noteworthy in their complete absence of any "woman-defined God talk" (p. 2). She underscores the importance for women of envisaging other possibilities, of "chasing the old white man out of our heads" and engaging "in the journey towards a self-defined spirituality" (p. 3). Given the significant and often unacknowledged link between sexuality and spirituality, such a journey may well lead to a sexuality that is based less on guilt and shame for women and more on joy.

We turn now to an examination of the various ways in which the myths and assumptions that underlie this model are embedded in the messages young adult women receive about their sexuality and sexual expression from the media, sexologists, and intimate partners.

TOO HOT TO HANDLE: MEDIA PORTRAYALS OF SEX

The movies are filled with images of strong, macho men, who charge across the screen fighting villains, and young, beautiful women, who literally fall at their feet and collapse in a heap of orgasmic shudders at their very touch. In what Zilbergeld (1993) refers to as the "Fantasy Model of Sex," the media continue to portray men as always wanting sex and women as being ultimately unable to resist their charms. He goes on to underscore how these "fictional accounts of sex almost invariably depict male performance and female pleasure. He acts (rams, pounds, thrusts, bangs) and she feels ('unbearable pleasure,' 'overwhelming joy,' 'delirious ecstasy')" (p. 53).

The women in these scenes are no longer necessarily portrayed as the bubble-headed Marilyn Monroes of the past (*Married With Children* aside), who would have trouble running together a full sentence. Some are capable of organizing a successful corporate takeover (e.g., Melanie Griffith in *Working Girl*). Yet, however successful and competent these "new women are," when it comes to the sexual arena, they are shown as unable to resist the raw sexual magnetism of a "powerful" man. Male sexual power is still very much at the center of these images.

The women in current media accounts are almost always young women who are portrayed as being "seriously into sex." The messages promoted in most current popular fiction and visual media accounts of sex suggest that young women of the 1990s are "ready for action at a moment's notice. . . . Unless they're virgins, foreplay is not something they need much of. Orgasms, dozens of them, come quickly and easily to them" (Zilbergeld, p. 43). In a paper entitled "The Theory of Sexual Relativity: Female Reality/Male Myth," Gale Holtz Golden (1988) discusses this more current adaptation of women's role in the sexual drama: "After showing her boyfriend how to get rid of 'ring around the collar,' our 'new age' woman settled in front of the T.V. with her 'new age' boyfriend and grabbed the remote control out of his hand. She then turned off the T.V. and seductively demanded his attention (and his sexual favors, the commercial implies)" (p. 77).

Far from the bashful image of her sisters of previous decades, the "new age" woman is portrayed as knowing what she wants in bed and having few reservations about going after it. In fact, to read the captions on the cover of most "women's" magazines at the grocery checkout stand, one might actually conclude that young women today are all having a great time in bed. They appear to have no difficulty in asserting their erotic desires and in ensuring that their "sexual needs" are being met (Prusank, Duran, & DeLillo, 1993).

However, although the role of women may appear to have been transformed from one of sexual submission to sexual agency, in reality, the fundamental assumptions and characteristics of the model itself have not really changed much. Men, and the magical penis, still play a central role. Orgasms are still promoted as the goal. These largely decontextualized images of human interaction depict passion and lust, devoid of intimacy. Sex is portrayed as a commodity to be exchanged between men and women. It is something women can become skillful at and use when necessary to "keep their men." It is not an expression of something more intimate and tender (movies such as *Witness* being a notable exception). This may help explain the results of the study by Bielay and Herold (1995), mentioned in Chapter 6. In this study, *Cosmopolitan* was identified as the primary source of information on sexual topics for young university women. Next to seeking information on improving their sex lives, the topic of greatest interest to these women was learning "what *men* like/desire sexually" (p. 254).

In most forms of the popular media, women today are explicitly portrayed as having sexual needs. Women *appear* on the surface to be freer to pursue their own sexual pleasure on their own terms. In reality, however, media sex is actually a double-edged sword. The implicit message is that considerable *danger* lies in wait for the woman who dares to act too forcefully in serving her own sexual self-interests (Demi Moore's role in *Disclosure* is a good example of this). Physical and sexual violence are subthemes that always lurk beneath the main plot (Malamuth & Briere, 1986). They are there to ensure that women do not step too far out of their required sexual roles (e.g., *Looking for Mister Goodbar*), much less dare to remove men from the picture altogether. The pornography market strongly reflects this theme of female sexual submission (Dworkin, 1983).

Safety is promoted in the popular media as being found within the context of a monogamous heterosexual relationship. As McMahon (1990) notes in her description of the portrayal of the "*Cosmopolitan* Girl," women must be " 'sexy and wild' but 'also romantic and conservative,' a good/bad girl, sometimes promiscuous, yet still respectable" (p. 391). In other words, she must be *hot,* but not too hot to be handled by her man. These media representations of heterosexual relations "ensure that women see themselves to some extent through men's eyes" (Crawford, Kippax, & Waldby, 1994, p. 573) and act accordingly.

SEXOLOGISTS: THE PURVEYORS OF SCIENTIFIC "TRUTHS"

The media can always be criticized for creating "fictional" accounts of women's sexual desires and behavior. So what then are young adult women and we as mental health professionals to do if we really want to know about women's sexuality and sexual functioning? We may decide to turn to those experts who promote sexual "facts" based on scientific evidence—sexologists. After all, science, and, in this case, sex research, is suppose to be an objective, value-free endeavor. It is aimed at understanding the sexual development, motivations, and behaviors of women and men. Its goal is to determine how problems in sexual functioning may be rectified. And in turning to this scientific literature, what messages are promoted regarding women's sexual natures and "normal" sexual functioning?

The young woman who is looking for some confirmation of her sexual normality, and some way to understand her sexual feelings and experiences, will quickly learn from this literature that sex is about genitals and how they operate. The penis and vagina (and to a lesser degree, the clitoris) are the primary organs of focus in this literature. A review of the sex-therapy literature will uncover a preponderance of articles on how to have orgasms either through masturbation or coitus. It will detail the various ways that women's genitals fail to function "normally" in response to penile penetration (hypoactive sexual desire, vaginismus, nonorgasmia, dyspareunia, etc.). It will be filled with dozens of articles on "erectile failures."

With few exceptions (e.g., Barbach, 1975, 1984, 1988; Tiefer, 1995), the significance of coitus and orgasm is repeatedly underscored in the sex-therapy literature. There is also a noticeable dearth of attention to the sexual concerns of lesbian and bisexual women by sexologists (Matteson, 1996; McCormick, 1994). In effect, the prevalent model of sex, and many of the myths and assumptions that underlie this model, are reinforced. Some current literature proposes a more "integrated approach" to "the formulation and treatment of sexual disorders" (Rosen & Leiblum, 1995, p. 877). The intentions of these authors are laudable. However, even this work continues to reinforce the centrality of genital sexuality. Emphasis is placed on "the role of biomedical and organic factors" in remediating "sexual dysfunctions" (p. 885).

Several writers (e.g., Tiefer's work [1987, 1988, 1991, 1995, 1996] is particularly noteworthy) have soundly criticized the pathologizing, phallocentric emphasis of the discipline of sex therapy. Much of this work is based on biased and faulty assumptions regarding the sexual needs and desires of women (and men). It emphasizes the importance of biology in defining what is sexual and in circumscribing what is "normal." It pays little attention to the importance of nongenital affection and intimacy in creating satisfying sexual relationships. Women's sexual desires and behaviors are pathologized when these do not conform to societal expectations. These concerns have led Tiefer (1996) to suggest that what is presented in this literature as a "coital imperative" actually "represents a social imperative" (p. 60).

In her article entitled "Propping up the Phallocracy: A Feminist Critique of Sex Therapy and Research," Wendy Stock (1988) underscores the phallocentric assumptions that underlie much of the sex research that has been undertaken to date. She challenges therapists to maintain an "awareness of the power asymmetry within and outside relationships, and the effect of this on the sexual politics of relationships and on the individual psyche" (p. 39). Cairns (1990) concurs with these sentiments when she says, "Any approach to assisting men and women to experience sexual and emotional intimacy, that treats life in the bedroom as separate from life in the kitchen or the workplace, or that treats sexual behavior and emotional expressions as separable from one another, is doomed to perpetuate the problems it claims to address" (p. 7).

Indeed, this intersection between passion and power is inevitable when scientific and therapeutic "truths" are constructed within a social and political context of gender inequality (Goldner, 1987, 1991). As such, the discipline of sexology does not provide direction for a more expansive and affirming understanding of women's diverse sexualities. Rather, it replicates and reinforces the dominant model of sexuality discussed earlier. This literature leaves counselors ill-equipped to know how to assist women who are struggling to create a space for their sexual exploration and expression. Webster (1988) highlights this dilemma when she says,

> As a therapist, I find myself asking questions about the questions we ask. What is sexual "dysfunction"? Who decides? Based on what "norms"? When what is called "normal" sexual behavior/thoughts/feelings can be redefined at frequent intervals within one's lifespan, between generations, and within different cultures, how do we know if "we/they" are "normal"? Has confusion between the "sexual revolution" and the women's movement led women to confuse sexual conquest (their own and others') with a promise of "freedom," which somehow still eludes us? (p. 297)

These are very important questions. As mental health professionals, it is especially important to ask whose needs are really being served by the continued promotion of this model of sexual "adequacy" and functioning?

INTIMATE PARTNERS: MYTHS AND MISCOMMUNICATION

As young adult women attempt to negotiate their intimate and sexual relationships, it is this model, and the myths and assumptions that underlie this model, that guide their sexual interactions. It is this model that provides a way for them to make sense of their needs, desires, and behaviors. These myths pervade the sexual discourse and muddy the sexual waters. They convolute the communication between women and their partners. They can turn an avenue of potential pleasure and connection into a "hotbed" of miscommunication and dissatisfaction (Meuhlenhard, 1988).

The dominant sexual discourse appears to powerfully shape women's and men's sexual understandings (e.g., Crawford et al., 1994; Gilfoyle, Wilson, & Brown, 1993; Hollway, 1989; Ussher, 1994). This is reflected in the communications between women and men related to their heterosexual interactions (Muehlenhard, 1988). For example, based on her analysis of the conversations of women and men as they talk about sex, Hollway (1984, 1989) identifies three distinct discourses that appear to underlie women's and men's sexual communications: the have/hold discourse, the male sex-drive discourse, and the permissive discourse. The have/hold discourse emphasizes the acceptability of sexual expression for women, but only within the context of a socially sanctioned (and traditional) heterosexual relationship. This is consistent with traditional religious beliefs and doctrine. It is also apparent in the current "relational" theories of women's development (Jordan et al., 1991). The male sex-drive discourse reflects the belief that men have a natural, biologically based need for sex, whereas women are more driven by their drive to reproduce. This is consistent with sociobiological assumptions and is very prevalent in many media and literary portrayals of sex (Tavris, 1992). The permissive discourse, promotes sexuality as a natural component of human experience that is deserving of free expression. In this goal-oriented discourse sex is still equated with coitus and orgasm. It is consistent with the uncomplicated sexual pleasure ethos that was predominant during the 1960s and '70s (Marin, 1983; Rubin, 1990).

To this list, Gilfoyle et al. (1993) add the "pseudo-reciprocal gift discourse" in which women are perceived as "giving" themselves (their bodies, their virginity, etc.) to men. Men's explicit gift to women is sexual satisfaction in the form of orgasms. The implicit gift is their protection. This is consistent with cultural and religious beliefs regarding the importance of women saving their virginity for a worthy partner. It reflects the belief in male sexual prowess and the importance of orgasms as the goal of sexual interactions.

Women are positioned within these constructions as passive rather than active subjects (Muehlenhard, 1988; Muehlenhard & McCoy, 1991). Women act in response to male initiative rather than basing their actions on their own, self-defined needs and desires. Although many women attempt to negotiate and resist these limiting constructions, years of socialization are not easily erased. Deviation from what is considered "normal" sexual thoughts or behaviors often engenders feelings of guilt, shame, and confusion for women (Ussher, 1994). The "permissive discourse" and media representations of the lusty, multiply orgasmic female, who acts in the service of her own sexual self-interests, are currently popular (Tavris, 1992). Despite this fact, women are still reminded of the penalties that exist if they step too far over the line of acceptable sexual desire or behavior. Many lesbian women have lost custody of their children based on their sexual orientation (Gottfried & Gottfried, 1994). Sexual violence continues to be "excused on the basis of a woman appearing to be 'asking for it,' or being sexually provocative" (Ussher, 1994, p. 165). However "liberated" young women may appear to be in their sexual interactions, many experience feelings of guilt "in relation to acting out of desire, in relation to enjoyment, and in relation to desire itself" (p. 166).

Crawford et al. (1994) note how, in the absence of other acceptable constructions to make sense of their experiences, women and men turn to prevailing discourses. In particular, the "male sex-drive discourse is one which is [frequently] drawn upon in determining what takes place" (p. 571) in sexual liaisons and in making sense of these interactions. What constitutes a sexual experience? What is a "normal" level of sexual desire? Who needs sex more? Who should initiate sexual encounters? Are we having sex enough, too much? Are orgasms important? Is intercourse necessary? Is masturbation natural? Are sexual fantasies OK? The dominant model of sex informs the questions young women and their partners ask about their sexual desires and expression. This model, and its underlying assumptions, provides the basis for their answers, and for their subsequent self-evaluations.

We do not have alternate, more expansive constructions of sexual expression that affirm women's sexual agency and the diversity of their sexual feelings and desires. As such, women (and men) necessarily turn to the dominant model of sex to guide their behavior and to understand their sexual and erotic feelings. "The parts to be played by the actors in the scene are set and no negotiation is possible. Not only is there no negotiation, there is in a very important sense no possibility for negotiation" (Crawford et al., p. 579). In this way, current sexual myths continue to be perpetuated and the dominant model reinforced. While "different gendered, occasioned meanings may coexist . . . given the power differential" (p. 574) between women and men in our culture, in the sexual communications between individual women and men, male meanings are still privileged.

Unfortunately, the problem is not restricted to heterosexual interactions. Even in lesbian relationships, the absence of alternate discourses for guiding and understanding sexual feelings and interactions results in problems in communication for many women and the adoption of "traditional" male–female roles (i.e., butch–femme roles). Many writers (e.g., Golden, 1987; Loulan, 1987; Sang, 1991) have talked about the internalized homophobia that results from living in a culture where the only acceptable model of sexual expression and experiencing is a male-centered, heterosexist model. This model portrays erotic feelings and experiences between women as sick and deviant.

In a chapter entitled "Lesbianism: A Country That Has No Language," Valverde (1985) underscores the invisibility of lesbian erotic images and power within North American culture. As a consequence, many lesbian women experience difficulty in attempting to make sense of their sexual feelings and negotiate the expression of their erotic desires within the context of their intimate relationships. Loulan and Thomas (1990) note lesbians' fear of lesbian sex, and suggest that

> the coded and hidden language of our sexual archetypes has its roots in a silence about even our most common activities. There are few words that describe any part of our unique culture. Except for "lover," we cannot even find a word that truly describes our most intimate relationships. . . . The fact that we can't have even one word that fully explains this most important of our connections is remarkable. "Lover" hardly covers what a partner, soul mate, heart connection means to us. . . . "Lover" does not say what is really true about our relationships; it connotes a lack of substance. (p. 21)

In the absence of more inclusive language and models of sexual expression, bisexual women struggle as well to make sense of their sexual desires and to fulfill their needs for sexual intimacy without guilt and shame (Firestein, 1996; Fox, 1996). The development of an integrated sexual identity based on self-acceptance is especially challenging for this invisible minority (Rust, 1996).

SUMMARY: PROBLEMATIC MEANINGS

The model of sex discussed earlier is promoted in virtually every domain of life and through every medium of communication. It is the stuff girls and boys are raised on and, to varying degrees, come to believe in. The myths and misinformation that are embedded in this model are often accepted by women and their partners as implicit truths about how they should feel, what they should find erotic, and how they should express themselves sexually.

This model severely limits and circumscribes the wide range of sensations and activities that may be experienced by women as erotic and sexual. It also demands the involvement of men. In this way, it delegitimizes interactions between women and devalues a woman's erotic relationship with her own body (Tiefer, 1996). Wooley (1994) notes how "representations are objects created by subjects for other subjects." He suggests that these dominant representations of women's sexuality and sexual nature are man's "way of creating, defining, and empowering himself" (p. 46).

It is within this context that young women negotiate and make sense of their sexual and erotic desires, and the sensations of their bodies. There are no other socially sanctioned models available through which women (and men) can make sense of and talk about their sexuality and the many ways this is expressed throughout their lives (Gagnon & Parker, 1995; Morris, 1997; Tiefer, 1995; Zilbergeld, 1993). "Women have no discourses with which to speak about female sexuality and female desire" (Crawford et al., 1994, p. 574). At present, there is no acceptable vision of a woman "self-choosing, enjoying, directing and controlling her own pleasure" (Janeway, 1980, p. 9). This makes it difficult for most young women to develop and maintain positive sexual self-perceptions—to see themselves as the authors, rather than the subjects, of their own sexuality.

In light of the dichotomous myths and assumptions that underlie this model of sex, it should not be surprising that many young women experience conflict and confusion regarding their sexual desires and expression. For many women, experiences of lust and passion are laced with feelings of shame and guilt. Young women struggle to reconcile the contradictory messages of society regarding their purported sexual natures and the sexual behavior that is considered "normal" and "appropriate" (Darling & Davidson, 1987; Davidson & Darling, 1993; Wyatt & Dunn, 1991). As Plummer (1982) points out, there is continuity between the cultural meanings and the personal experience of sexuality. Where conflicts exist in the culture, they are inevitably mirrored in the person. Women are faced with messages and meanings that on the one hand promote sexuality as a powerful and pleasurable human drive, but on the other hand prohibit the free expression of it (sex as bad and sinful). This paradox plays itself out in women's inability to explore and abandon themselves (even momentarily) to the intensity of their eroticism. It makes it difficult for many women to become the initiators of sexual pleasure or diversity. It makes it difficult for them to step outside the dominant sexual script (in choosing to be celibate, in loving women, in having "casual" sex, etc.) without shame or guilt (Kitzinger, 1985; Wolf, 1997). It makes it difficult for young adult women to develop sexual self-perceptions based on a sense of efficacy and entitlement (Bartky, 1990).

Although this dominant model of sexual expression necessarily shapes sexual experiences and expectations, women do not passively and unquestioningly accept these socially constructed "truths." Despite the pervasive imposition of patriarchal sex and gender systems, women struggle to resist. They attempt to "develop new and more gratifying [sexual] definitions, identities, meanings, and freedoms" (Vance & Pollis, 1990, pp. 4–5). Some resist through celibacy, some through a refusal to participate in heterosexual interactions, and some through their insistence on negotiating shared meanings in their intimate interactions that are based on reciprocity, mutuality, and respect. On both an individual and interpersonal level, women and their partners have some latitude in the degree to which they accept or reject the dominant discourse. As indicated throughout this book, sexual meanings are negotiated and are therefore subject to modification.

CHALLENGE AND CHANGE: CREATING NEW MEANINGS

It is important to remember that "there is much in female sexuality that is truly unique . . . but inhibitions, stereotypes, and false premises must be disposed of before this uniqueness can be fully discerned" (Lewis, 1980, p. 36). To expect young women to experience "their bodies as ever-changing individualized sources of sensations and competencies" (Tiefer, 1996, p. 58) or to comfortably explore the boundaries of their erotic potential alone, and in their relationships with others, is to expect behavior devoid of context. As counselors, we need to attend to this context by helping to make women more aware of the sociocultural factors that generate distress and shame in their sexual experiences and self-conceptions. We need to alert them to the paradoxical images that currently represent our images of healthy female functioning and sexuality. One goal of this work is to assist each woman to "define the boundaries of herself" and to guide her as she learns

> to incorporate men's definitions, sexuality, and needs not as part of herself but as part of the context. She does not belong to them: the power concealing itself and lurking in the background must devote itself to itself, to its own aims, to its own manifestation. This involves recapturing the early ties with mother/woman/self and transforming them into a return to herself as a woman. (Kaschak, 1992, pp. 87–88)

Vance (1984) notes how "it is not enough to move women away from danger and oppression: it is necessary to move toward something—toward pleasure, agency, self-definition" (p. 24). Indeed, if we are to foster positive sexual self-perceptions and experiences, it is important to help young women construct more expansive and affirming visions of women's sexuality. We need to help young women expand their conceptions of sexual pleasure and ecstasy beyond a strictly genital focus to encompass a broad range of human experiences (Ogden, 1985, 1994). Attention needs to be paid to the emotional, cognitive, and spiritual aspects of women's sexual feelings and experiences, as well as the more physical dimensions.

It is important "to draw on women's energy, . . . on women's experience of pleasure in imagining the textures and contours" (Vance, 1984, p. 3) of a more woman-centered, as opposed to phallic centered, vision of sexuality and sexual pleasure. As Crawford et al. (1994) note,

> A discourse of sex as pleasure, separating pleasure from procreation, and acknowledging women as active, desiring and sexually assertive subjects,

> not necessarily centered around the erect penis, will challenge and confront established power structures. What is needed is a new mythology, one which speaks about mutual exploration, communication, discovery and pleasuring one another, where penetration is not an end unto itself, but one of many possibilities for erotic enjoyment in heterosexual relationships. (pp. 584–586)

We need to help women reject the emphasis in our current models of sex as achievement and women as recipients of sexual pleasure. Women need to take their place at the center of their own sexual dramas. They need encouragement to assume responsibility for determining and fulfilling their own erotic needs and potential. The importance of playfulness and fun in women's sexual and erotic experiences and sexual self-constructions also needs to be underscored.

According to Janeway (1980), "Our best chance of finding our way toward new paradigms of female sexuality would be to widen the range of personal connection from which we draw the values we use in assessing interpersonal relations, beyond the strictly and narrowly sexual" (p. 25). Because "women have no written tradition of sexual ecstasy, and no consistent language to describe it" (Ogden, 1985, p. 46), it is important to help young women find a voice and create language for their sexual feelings and experiences (Ogden, 1994). As counselors, we need to promote women's discovery of their own bodies as joyful sources of sensual and erotic pleasure, and assist them in exploring and identifying what is pleasurable to them, and where relevant, to help them find ways to communicate this to their partner(s).

It is important "to emphasize the rich diversity of personal meaning and experience" (Tiefer, 1987, p. 77) in our goals of counseling and in our choice of interventions. There are many activities that counselors can use to begin this process of exploration and expansion. To get past the layer of socially imposed feelings and meanings, and to access the subconscious and more creative processes, the use of expressive nonverbal techniques, as well as exercises that allow women to engage in an insight-oriented exploration while maintaining some safety and distance, are highly recommended. In particular, the use of life histories, journaling, and affective techniques such as imagery and metaphor may be very powerful tools in exploring past and current beliefs and meanings. These types of exercises underscore the power and validation that women can gain through externalizing their inner fears, thoughts, and desires (Capacchione, 1985). However, it is important to remember that discussion of sexual desire and behavior often elicits feelings of considerable vulnerability, fear, and shame for women. For some, this is associated with memories of pain and violation. The pacing and timing of this type of exploration are important. Clients also need to maintain control over this process.

Several clinicians (Boston Women's Health Book Collective, 1992;

Covington, 1991; Ogden, 1985, 1994) have noted the healing power for women of working in groups on issues related to sexuality. Other women can be an important source of validation and healing. Covington notes that

> when we share our sexual experiences with other women, something wonderful happens: what we previously thought of as individual pathology . . . gets put into a universally female context. We see that we are doing and feeling what most other women are raised to do and feel. We begin to see the limitations of the provisions that society offers women. We come to have compassion for ourselves. (p. 12)

Whenever possible, counselors are encouraged to employ a group format when undertaking this work. As always, care should be taken to ensure that a climate of safety, trust, and acceptance is fostered. The activities presented here are appropriate when young women present with general concerns related to their sexual self-perceptions, expectations, or feelings of guilt and shame.

Although the exercises in this chapter are devoted to work with women, attention may also need to be paid to the "intersubjective" realm of their experience. Couple work can be especially important in helping women and their partners negotiate more mutually satisfying sexual meanings and interactions based on broader and more inclusive conceptualizations of sexual intimacy, activity, and fulfillment. Examples of resources to facilitate this type of couple work that avoid the tendency to pathologize include Barbach's *For Each Other: Sharing Sexual Intimacy* (1984) and *Erotic Interludes* (1988), Schnarch's *Constructing the Sexual Crucible* (1991) and *Passionate Marriage: Sex, Love and Intimacy in Emotionally Committed Relationships* (1997), as well as more popular literature that expands the range of erotic possibilities (e.g., Crosbie's [1993] *The Girl Wants To*; Friday's [1975] *Forbidden Flowers*; Loulan & Thomas's [1990] *The Lesbian Erotic Dance: Butch, Femme, Androgyny, and Other Rhythms*).

Assessing the nature of young women's concerns related to their sexuality and sexual expression requires exploration on the following three levels: (1) the individual level (sexual self-esteem, identity, and pleasure); (2) the relational, intersubjective level (significant others); and (3) the level of the larger social context. Certainly, these areas are not discrete. Each interacts with, and reciprocally influences, the others in contributing to the sexual self perceptions and experiences of young women. These areas are addressed in the following exercises.

In the Beginning: Exploring Past Messages

The experiences and messages of childhood and adolescence, both positive and negative, are an important focus of exploration in understanding the current sexual self-perceptions and experiences of young women (Tiefer, 1996). However liberated adult women may be in their beliefs about women's sexual entitlement, for many, the messages and experiences of childhood and adolescence continue to creep into their consciousness, influencing their sexual interactions and their perceptions of themselves based on their erotic feelings and desires. It is often these childhood admonishments that result in the inability of women to freely abandon themselves in the moment, that result in assuming a critical-observer posture when engaged in sexual activities (including self-pleasuring) (Frederickson & Roberts, 1997; Ussher, 1989), and that engender feelings of sexual shame, guilt, and inadequacy (Kitzinger, 1985). It is necessary then, to assess the prevalence and power of these early messages in impairing adult women's abilities to freely explore and spontaneously express their sexuality in the ways that are most satisfying to them.

As noted in previous chapters, there are many ways to conduct this type of historical review. Lifelines, collages, photo albums, guided fantasy, and guided autobiography are only a few of the possible techniques. For example, individually or within a group, women can be asked to create a collage of all the messages they can remember receiving about sex and women's sexuality while they were growing up. The activity can be structured in such a way that the positive messages are placed on one side of the paper, and the negative messages are placed on the other. This usually results in a rather dramatic pictorial representation of the tremendous dearth of positive, woman-affirming messages throughout most women's early lives. In processing their collages, participants can be encouraged to identify the primary sources of these messages (including parents, teachers, priests and ministers, friends, magazines, television, etc.). They can also rank these sources in terms of those that had the most negative impact on their past and current sexual self-perceptions and behaviors. As well as ranking these regulators of their sexuality, it is important for women to rank the liberators as well. These include the significant others whose messages help to affirm their sexual self-perceptions, and reinforce a sense of their sexual entitlement.

Because this type of exercise requires the use of current magazines, collages serve the additional purpose of helping women become more aware of the way in which women's sexuality is portrayed in the media, thereby moving their exploration to the broader social level. To this end, the exploration can be expanded to include other media forms (i.e., television, movies, books, videos). Women can be assigned the task of bringing in examples of these dominant portrayals of sex and women's sexuality.

A particularly humorous way to examine the portrayals of women's sexuality in books, magazines, and popular media is to ask women to undertake a type of discourse analysis. They can pretend they are beings from another planet who are interested in learning about how women and men on earth conduct their sexual interactions. Specific reading material can be recommended from some of the more popular fiction writers (e.g., Judith Krantz, Danielle Steele, Harold Robbins, John Grisham). Or women can make their own selection of books, articles, movies, and so on. It is also useful to include self-help books (e.g., Gray's [1997] *Mars and Venus in the Bedroom: A Guide to Lasting Romance and Passion;* Norwood's [1997] *Women Who Love Too Much: When You Keep Wishing and Hoping He'll Change)* in this type of analysis. These books tend to reinforce the dominant sexual paradigm and perpetuate many of the popular myths and assumptions regarding the sexual needs and natures of women and men. Questions that are useful in guiding this type of analysis include the following: What are the themes, beliefs, and values being promoted and reinforced? Who is the active agent? Who is the respondent? What is the goal? Do they both have the same goal? What are the rules the players are following in these interactions? Whose needs are being met? Who has the power and how is it used? Verbally, or in writing, women can be asked to report what is being communicated about women's sexual and erotic pleasures and desires, and how these are expressed and satisfied. In processing, counselors are provided with an opportunity to debunk many of the myths that are promoted in our society as "sexual truths." This is an opportunity to provide concrete information regarding what is actually known about the ways in which women's sexuality is lived and expressed.

Women may also need assistance to explore how past and current sexual messages and meanings are still operative in their lives. It can be important to begin the process of attempting to determine which rules are "old baggage," and which are still congruent with women's current beliefs and values. Any number of values clarification exercises can be useful in identifying women's sexual beliefs and values (e.g., use of vignettes depicting various sexual scenarios, responding to a list of sexual belief statements, etc.). Women should be encouraged to consider whose "voice" is behind each of these belief–values statements. For example, on her list, one woman had the following statement: "Sex is dirty." She said that "at one level" she did not really believe this to be true. In her own life she had "occasionally" had sexual encounters that were "incredibly moving and almost spiritual." She even recalled a few that were "terrific fun." But despite what she knew in her head and believed in her heart, the "Sex is dirty" refrain continued to ring in her ears. Deeper down, it was internalized to mean "I am dirty." I asked her to close her eyes, relax, and play the refrain over and over again in her head. She was to "allow the voice behind the refrain to emerge." Eventually, this woman was able to identify the source of this message as the nuns from her Catholic school education. In the future, whenever the "Sex is dirty" refrain rang in her ears, she was able to experience the words not as her own, but as belonging to others. This diminished their power in eliciting feelings of shame and guilt related to her sexual self-perceptions and behaviors.

Writing an "as if" autobiography is another potent way to help women begin to understand the extent of the baggage that they may be carrying into adulthood. This can be especially useful in helping women gain some insight into the differences in the sexual socialization of men and women. In this autobiography, women are asked to recount their sexual development and experiences throughout childhood and adolescence "as if" they had been born a boy rather than a girl (*Note.* I often use an expanded version of this exercise with female and male graduate students as a very powerful mechanism to begin their understanding of the tremendous impact of gender-role socialization in shaping and circumscribing all of the experiences and choices available to them throughout their lives.) In completing and discussing this exercise, women are usually able to see how tremendously different the sexual socialization is for boys versus girls. The differences in the male sexual script versus the female sexual script become very apparent through the completion of this activity. Sometimes, for the first time in their lives, women are able briefly to capture a sense of what it might be like to have *their* needs and desires at the center of their sexual considerations and constructions.

Sex and Sexuality: Definitions and Meanings

Another important component of this work involves exploring how women define sex and what it means in their lives and experiences of self. An easy way to begin this process is to use a simple word-association exercise. For example, individually or within a group setting, women can be asked to spontaneously generate as many words as possible that come to mind in response to the word "sex." Frequently, the words generated involve both the behavioral components of the activity of "having sex" with another person (e.g., breast stimulation, kissing, genital manipulation, intercourse, orgasm). As well, some words relate to women's affective reactions to these behaviors (e.g., pleasure, fun, scary, great, pain, stimulating). Responses to the word "sexuality" and "sensuality," however, are usually more varied. They often include a wider range of affective, attitudinal, behavioral, and sometimes spiritual components. These words tend to reflect the sense of sexuality as being an energy, way of being, or set of attitudes unique to each individual (similar to Anna Freud's contention that sex is something you do, and sexuality is something you are). More frequently, these associations are positive and powerful (e.g., "energy," "vitality," "passion," "flame," "god," "goddess"). Subsequent discussion and processing of these two different lists of words is often quite beneficial in helping women to see how much of the dominant model of sex informs their own thinking about sex and sexuality. This can be a springboard to a discussion of more expansive ways to define women's sexuality and the avenues to sexual expressions. This exercise can also provide useful information about women's past sexual interactions and their responses to these.

Counselors can also encourage women to explore the ways they have characteristically expressed their sexuality and the purposes/meanings that particular forms of sexual behavior and expression serve (and have served) them in their lives. This can be accomplished in a number of ways. One involves a historical review of women's previous sexual encounters and intimate relationships through the use of a lifeline or through guided autobiography. This activity usually begins with a deep breathing or deep-muscle relaxation exercise, followed by guided imagery in which women are asked to be observers of their own lives. They should begin with their earliest recollection of when they began to engage in sexual play and interactions in childhood, and continue throughout adolescence to the present time. This includes their first awareness of themselves as sexual, their first attempts at masturbation, the first time they remember responding to visual erotic stimulation, their first orgasm, their first experience of intercourse, and so on. They should be asked to remain aware of the context within which these experiences took place. They should also be sensitive to the thoughts and feelings that accompanied these experiences. When the guided imagery has been completed, women should be asked to engage in a guided autobiographical recounting of these significant experiences, or they may plot these experiences on a lifeline, with the horizontal axis representing age (birth through to the present) and the vertical axis representing intensity of feeling. Depending on the goals of the intervention, an adaptation of this exercise would involve the vertical axis representing the intensity of a particular emotion or experience, such as shame or guilt associated with the sexual events in question. Next to each item plotted on the line, women can list the accompanying thoughts and emotions, or they can simply indicate whether each experience was affirming (+) or invalidating (–) of their sexual self-esteem. In the case of group work, women should then be encouraged to share their lifeline with another woman in the group. When doing individual work, the woman can be guided to explore more fully the interactions that she experienced as disempowering, as well as those that helped affirm her sense of sexual agency. Particular attention should be paid to the relational and contextual factors associated with each.

A similar exercise can also be used to help women examine their past sexual and intimate relationships, the ways they expressed themselves sexually within these interactions, and the feelings that were associated with these experiences. Women should be asked to write a narrative account of their sexual relationships/encounters. They should attend to the various dimensions of their experiences, in terms of the way they expressed themselves sexually, the relational dynamics, the contextual circumstances, and the thoughts and feelings that accompanied each relationship. They should be encouraged to explore the types of relationships they have engaged in, the ways they have expressed their sexuality differently in each, and the purposes that sex served in these relationships. It is also important to explore the times when they felt validated and empowered in these sexual encounters, and the times these experiences engendered feelings of pain, shame, guilt, inadequacy, and so on. Women should attempt to indicate their "best" and "worst" sexual encounter. They should explore the individual, interpersonal, and contextual factors that contributed to making these experiences positive or negative (the level of intimacy, the nature of the relationship, the sex of the partner, the contextual circumstances, etc.). For example, one client I worked with indicated that her "best" sexual encounter from the standpoint of "pure pleasure" was one in which she spent a night of unbridled lust and passion with a man she had just met, and whom she has not seen since. This same client also spoke of a long-term relationship with a woman, in which their physical intimacy was "almost something holy." She reflected on how, when she was nestled in the arms of her lover, she felt "a peace and contentment" beyond anything she had ever experienced before. The two situations appeared to be quite different on the surface. However, with further exploration, this client was able to identify the fact that in both circumstances, she experienced acceptance, validation, and respect from these partners that allowed her to freely express herself within these relationships. A review of their narratives allows women to identify particular patterns in their sexual relationships. It can help them to see and understand the purposes that sex has served in their lives. They become more cognizant of the personal, relational, and contextual circumstances that are required if they are to experience a sense of sexual agency in their intimate interactions.

In completing this exercise, another client noted how her ability to experience sexual pleasure and empowerment was clearly contingent upon her ability to connect with her lover(s) "with her head and heart as well as [her] body." This exercise can provide a good vehicle for helping women to explore how they define intimacy, and what the role of sex, and intimacy, is in their lives and relationships.

When working with young women, it is also important to help them move past restrictive and confining notions of what constitutes "appropriate" sexual feelings, experiences, and behaviors. This involves expanding their awareness of the many positive ways in which their sexual vitality and energy are, or may be, manifested in their lives. Women may well come into individual or group counseling based on a belief that their sexuality or sexual functioning is somehow flawed or dysfunctional. However, it is important to remember that the emphasis in this type of work is not on dysfunction. Rather, the focus is on helping women to extricate themselves from the oppressive *shoulds* and *should nots* that are a part of our dominant sexual scripts. It is to facilitate an exploration of different ways of conceiving of the fabric of their own sexuality. It is about expanding the ways their sexuality may be comfortably expressed in their lives and relationships. The assumption is that the client who claims she is nonorgasmic, or who has accepted the label of "frigid" or "promiscuous," does not need help to "cure" her of these dysfunctions (in the traditional sense of sex therapy). She needs support and affirmation of what her sexuality *is* and *can be,* not of what it *is not.* The following exercises may help in this process.

Who Am I?: Redefining the Sexual Self

As counselors, we can help women redefine their sexual selves. We can help broaden their perspectives of the many ways their sexuality can be lived and experienced in their lives. Of the various affective/experiential techniques available to accomplish this, the use of art and metaphor can be especially powerful in helping women explore their current and desired sexual selves. For example, counselors can begin with a relaxation exercise and a guided imagery. Women are asked to attempt to visualize their sexual core. They are encourage to try to connect with their sexual energy (see Chapter 6, section entitled "Embodied Sexuality"). Following this, women can use clay or finger paints (linking to the tactile/sensory realm), to sculpt or paint their sexuality. They should be encouraged to allow the sexual energy that they were able to get in touch with during the guided imagery to infuse their artwork. Again, this activity is very powerful when undertaken in a group format, where participants can feed off of the energy of each other. They can inject humor and play in their "work" (reinforcing the importance of fun and playfulness in women's sexual expressions). The task of constructing this image of their sexuality can be quite powerful. The subsequent processing and sharing of these pieces of artwork with the other women in the group (examining and discussing colors and contours, etc.) can be both enlightening and empowering. Metaphors can also be used, in addition to, or in the place of, artwork. For example, women can be encouraged to select an animal guide that serves as a metaphor for their sexual selves. They can be asked explore the meaning of this metaphor in their lives and sexual self-constructions.

Guided imagery exercises, such as the one discussed earlier, can be used in a variety of ways to help women expand the boundaries of their sexuality. Movement and body work are also excellent mechanisms to access subconscious processes. They can assist women in identifying the various places in their bodies where their sexuality is "located." These affective techniques can facilitate more in-depth exploration of the feelings associated with these various body parts. Life review and narratives are also effective in helping women to explore the various ways they express their sexuality, outside of the physical act of "having sex." They can be used to examine the particular contexts within which women feel very sexual and erotic. For example, in response to a question about how she expresses her sexuality outside of the physical act of "having sex," one client disclosed that she frequently does her housework in her underwear. She recounted how sensual and erotic she finds this experience (not to mention the fact that it takes some of the boredom out of cleaning). Another talked about feeling most sensual when she chooses not to wear underwear. Although she is celibate by choice, and no one is aware of her state of partial undress, she feels "powerful and in control of her sexuality" when she "chooses" to express it in this way.

Another powerful technique to explore the different aspects and dimensions of the sexual self is called "The Sexual Self Box." This exercise involves asking women to bring in a box (a large shoebox is often appropriate), which they then decorate and fill with a number of different items/objects that represent the many aspects of their "sexual selves." Women are encouraged to decorate the outside of the box with images, colors and, words that reflect the positive and affirming aspects of their sexuality. They are to line the inside of the box with the messages they received from significant people throughout their lives regarding their sexuality and sexual expression. The objects contained inside the box should be personal representations of their sexual secrets, difficulties, messages from significant others, self-messages, treasured aspects of their sexual selves, creative aspects of their sexual selves, and their sexual losses, hopes, and expectations. Within this box, women may choose to enclose a smaller box containing representations of the "darker side" of their sexuality. The objects and images contained in this smaller box often reflect experiences of sexual pain, trauma, shame, guilt, and isolation. The task of constructing these sexual self boxes can generate considerable insight. The act of sharing the box and its contents with others (e.g., the counselor, other members of the group, partners, and, in some cases, mothers) can be very healing and liberating.

In completing some of these exercises, it may become apparent to women that they are still carrying a fair bit of emotional baggage from the lessons they learned in their families related to women's sexuality and how it *should* be expressed. This baggage may make it difficult for them to act on their sexual impulses and desires. They may find it hard to experience sexual pleasure without guilt. If these early messages are to lose some of their power, it is important for women to confront the significant others from whom they learned these lessons. This confrontation can be undertaken directly, or it can occur through more indirect avenues such as letter writing, or the use of a two-chair or guided imagery. For example, one client reflected on the fact that in her family of origin, sexuality was "never talked about." There were no demonstrations of touch or physical affection between her parents. The discussion or expression of sexuality was never overtly reproached per se. However, the implicit message she received in her family was that sex was somehow dirty and shameful. It was something not to be talked about, much less expressed publicly. As an adult, this woman felt she had a "good relationship with her mother." As such, she decided to take the risk of "interviewing" her mother about her life. The interview included asking her mother about the messages she received within her own family of origin regarding sexuality and relationships. As the dialogue between mother and daughter progressed, they were both able to talk more freely about their experiences of fear, anxiety, and pleasure. They both came to realize how, in many respects, they had walked parallel paths in their lives as women. This experience not only helped the client feel more comfortable about her own sexuality, but it also deepened her understanding of, and relationship with, her mother.

Psychodrama can also be a very powerful mechanism for women to work through and come to terms with particularly traumatic experiences that damaged their sexual selves. It can help reduce the power of messages that served to impair their ability to express their sexuality in the ways that are congruent with their sexual identities and desires. For example, in a group setting, a 32-year-old woman, who had been unable to acknowledge her lesbianism to herself and to her family members, was able to construct a psychodrama. In this psychodrama, the other group members played the roles of her parents, her grandmother (who had lived with the family during the woman's childhood, and who was a powerful figure in the family constellation), and her two siblings (both of whom had followed a more traditional path of marriage and children). With other group members giving voice to the various players during the psychodrama, the client was able to find her own "voice" and "speak" her truth to the others in her family. Through enacting the dialogue between these significant and important people in her life, while others in the group served as nonjudgmental and supportive witnesses to her struggle, she was able to achieve what she termed a "victory of the self." Participating in a psychodrama was also very healing for another woman in the group, who carried the "shame" of having been a prostitute during her adolescence. This impaired her ability to trust and be intimate in her adult relationships. Through the psychodrama, she was able to understand more about why she still seemed to choose sexual partners who were controlling and abusive (men whom she referred to as "the devil you know"). She came to appreciate the positive aspects of her previous experiences and was able to consider how these might inform her present sexual self-perceptions and expression.

Nourishing the Sexual Self

Helping young women to give themselves permission to enjoy and nourish the sexual and erotic aspects of the self is an important part of this work. Such nourishment includes attention to their bodies, minds, spirits, and souls. This work is based on the contention that women's sexuality exists as a life force, whether or not it is freely expressed, and whether or not it is validated by others. It involves acknowledging the autonomy of women's sexuality and normalizing celibacy. It involves encouraging women to assume responsibility for their own sexual needs and pleasures, irrespective of their relational status. In Loulan's (1987) words, this component of the process is about encouraging women to have "a love affair" with themselves.

For so many women, years of sexually oppressive messages leave them unable to connect with that part of the self that is their sexual vitality and energy. Inner-child work can be a very potent way for women to begin to reconnect with this part of the self. In her book *Revolution from Within: A Book of Self-Esteem,* Gloria Steinem (1992) underscores the importance of "entering inner space" and reconnecting with the "inner child." She provides several examples of how women might do this work (pp. 326–332). More specific to sexuality, in a workshop she gave in Long Beach, California, Gail Walker (1992) described a guided fantasy. In this fantasy, women are asked to imagine meeting and saying "hello" to their neglected childhood "sexual selves." They are asked to try to connect with the part of themselves that once felt freedom in their bodies, and that moved through the world with a sense of spontaneity, curiosity, and joy. Once they have found this child, they are directed to ask her what it has been like for her all this time; whether she has felt invited into their lives, and if so, at what times? They are to ask when she has felt most alive over the past years, and what things or experiences make her feel joy, pleasure, and pain. After they have asked these and other questions they are curious about, the child and the adult woman are to give each other a gift. It is to be something that represents their connection to each other, and something that will serve as a queue to remind them of the existence of each other. They are directed to make arrangements with the child to connect again, and are instructed to ask the child to give them a note that they can take with them into their adult lives (often this is the gift of self-acceptance, spontaneity, or playfulness). This note should contain something the child has not told them today, or something she would like them to remember. In processing this fantasy, women are encouraged to reflect on their visit with the child and share the message passed on to them by the childhood representative of their sexual selves. They are encouraged to contemplate the ways they might continue to reconnect with their earlier sexual selves and to consider how the child's desire for expression might be realized in their adult lives.

Women can also be encouraged through sensate focus exercises, massage, self-touch, fantasy, erotica, and other forms of stimulation, to explore their embodied sexuality (see Barbach, 1975, 1988; Freeman, 1982; Kaplan, 1981; Kitzinger, 1985). Through these and other activities, they can begin to define their own sexual energy, rhythms, and pulses. They can explore the boundaries of their erotic desires (see Loulan & Thomas, 1990, pp. 139–184, for a discussion of ways lesbian women can explore their sexual passions and rhythms). Women should be encouraged to move past a genital focus and to explore a broad range of sensory experiences that they find sensual or erotic (particular foods, clothing, music, bubble baths, etc.). Journaling is another vehicle by which women can explore their sexual and erotic interests and desires (see Barbach, 1975, 1984).

Fantasy is also an important component of sexuality for many women. It can be an avenue of tremendous (and safe) erotic pleasure and a potentially valuable source of knowledge regarding what women find sexually stimulating (Bennett & Rosario, 1995). Exploration of women's fantasies should include an examination of the fantasies that women have had in the past. It should include their current fantasies. And it should include the situations and circumstances that they could *imagine* finding sexually stimulating, if they were free to explore and express their sexuality in any way that they found exciting, without restraint or fear of reprisals. Again, for many women, context plays a critical role in their sexual stimulation and comfort. Their sexual fantasies often involve particular partners, body parts, clothing, and activities. They also frequently include certain places that generate feelings of sexual excitement and pleasure. During the exploration process, women should be encouraged to attend to all of the details of their fantasies. They should be encouraged to use these to learn more about what "turns them on," and what does not. For example, in exploring her past and current sexual relationships, one woman realized that as she came close to a climax, she usually allowed herself to fantasize that she was making love with a woman rather than with a man. As she explored the themes of her fantasies, she was able to acknowledge that she found men's bodies sexually stimulating and enjoyed heterosexual interactions. However, orgasm represented surrender to her, and she did not feel "safe" surrendering herself to a man. Eventually, she was able to reframe the experience of orgasm as surrender to her erotic desires, rather than as "surrender to male power." For her, this was an important step in the process of honoring her own body and her sexuality. She was also able to acknowledge the eroticism of women's bodies and her desires to explore this further in her future sexual relationships. Having women write a story of their "ideal sexual fantasy" can serve the purpose of normalizing and reinforcing the importance and value of fantasy in the experience of women's sexuality. It can also provide a "safe" and "private" vehicle through which women can explore the potential depths and contours of their erotic possibilities.

Finally, an important part of nourishing the sexual self involves helping women to reincorporate laughter and play into their sexual experiences and intimate relationships. As Estes (1992) so accurately points out,

> Laughter is a hidden side of women's sexuality; it is physical, elemental, passionate, vitalizing, and therefore arousing. It is a kind of sexuality that does not have a goal, as does genital arousal. It is a sexuality of joy, just for the moment, a true sensual love that flies free and lives and dies and

> lives again on its own energy. It is sacred because it is so healing. It is sensual for it awakens the body and the emotions. It is sexual because it is exciting and causes waves of pleasure. It is not one dimensional, for laughter is something one shares with oneself as well as with many others. It is a woman's wildest sexuality. (pp. 342–343)

Laughter is also one of the most powerful ways for women to bring playfulness, joy, and honesty into the sharing of bodies and sometimes of souls. At one level, shared laughter can be a most intimate act. It can expose the self in a way that can be more revealing than nakedness between partners.

> Laughter could do it, break down the ceremonial masculine–feminine barriers. I'd catch his eye, mid-laugh, and there would be an amused recognition of mutual humanness, of shared funny bones and flesh, no one on top, no one in charge. Ah, my giggling self said in tandem with his giggling self, so we aren't so different after all. (Fleming, 1994, p. 156).

CONCLUSION

These suggestions are only examples of the many ways that counselors can assist women in exploring their sexual beliefs, needs, and desires. They represent only some of the many ways women might begin to the expand their conceptions of what is possible in terms of their sexuality and sexual expression. What is most important in doing this type of work is providing a safe space within which all that is unique, rich, and vital about women's diverse sexualities can begin to emerge. The sacred and the sensual/sexual self live very near one another in the psyche,

> for they all are brought to attention through a sense of wonder, not from intellectualizing but through experiencing something through the physical pathways of the body, something that for the moment or forever, whether it is a kiss, a vision, a belly laugh, or whatever, changes us, shakes us out, takes us to a pinnacle, smooths out our lines, gives us a dance step, a whistle, a true burst of life. (Estes, 1992, p. 342)

In helping women to move past the rather limiting constructions of women's sexuality and sexual expression that are so prevalent in our society, and in facilitating a more expansive, woman-affirming vision of women's sexuality, we are helping to fan the embers that then become the flames of women's sexual desire. In so doing, we are better serving the needs of women and their partners.

IV

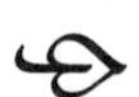

THE MIDDLE AND LATER YEARS

11

BIOLOGICAL AND PSYCHOLOGICAL DEVELOPMENT

BIOLOGICAL DEVELOPMENT DURING THE MIDDLE YEARS

When Hormones Stop Raging: Reproductive Changes

Prior to this century, the life expectancy of women was under 48 years, meaning that most women did not live long enough to experience the end of their reproductive cyclicity. Currently, however, the life expectancy of white women in North America is 80.9 years (Morokoff, 1988). For black women, it is an average of 6.5 years shorter (Unger & Crawford, 1992). Nevertheless, most midlife women can look forward to several postmenopausal decades. One might say that menopause has become a "normative" transition in the lives of adult women.

Distinctions are often made in the literature between *menopause* and the *climacteric*. The term "climacteric" is derived from the Greek words meaning "critical time" and "rung of the ladder." It is most commonly used to describe the biological changes that occur in all bodily tissues and systems for women and men during the 15- to 20-year period from middle to older age (mid-40s to mid-60s) (Delaney et al., 1988; Unger & Crawford, 1992; Weideger, 1978). Menopause, however, is a process specific to women. It is formally defined as the complete cessation of menses for a period of 1 year. The term "menopause" originates from the Greek words for "month" and "cessation" (Delaney et al., 1988). More euphemistically known as "the change of life" or "the change," menopause is the last phase of the menstrual cycle. This phase involves gradual, incremental decreases in the ovaries' production of estrogen and progesterone, resulting in the eventual cessation of menstruation. The process that leads up to menopause is referred to as the "perimenopausal transition." This transition begins almost imperceptibly with the onset of minor hormonal changes and frequently ranges from 10 to 15 years (Voda & Eliasson, 1983). Generally, menopause occurs between the ages of 45 and 55 years (Weideger, 1978). Approximately 8% of women experience a premature menopause that begins before the age of 40. The "typical age at menopause" for American women, however, is 51 (Golub, 1992, p. 213).

What do we really know about the biological changes that occur during the perimenopausal period leading up to menopause? Unfortunately, given the misconceptions that have guided much of the research in the area of women's reproductive health (Ehrenreich & English, 1978; Hubbard, 1990; Perrott & Condit, 1996), we may not know as much as we actually should. The menopausal research literature has come under considerable criticism in recent years. Problems have been noted in terms of definitional inconsistencies, sampling biases, and inadequate methodological procedures. Most notably, much of the available literature is "based on the assumption that menopause is a disease" (Glazer & Rozman, 1991, p. 237; Rostosky & Travis, 1996; Weideger, 1978). In particular, feminist researchers and scholars have indicted the medical profession for its use of the disease model of menopause as a mechanism to legitimize "sexism, under the guise of science" (McCrea, 1983, p. 117). They have called for cross-cultural investigations from a woman-centered perspective. In this way, we might begin to tease out the biological facts of the menopause experience from the societal messages that influence women's experiences of this transition (Voda & Eliasson, 1983; for an excellent review of the menopausal research reported in medical and psychological journals for the years 1984–1994, the reader is referred to Rostosky & Travis, 1996).

It is important to begin this discussion with the assumption that menopause is not a disease. Rather, it is an inherent component of the aging process that bears many physiological and emotional similarities to puberty. Both are times of hormone realignment and physical transition. Both are associated with a range of physical and emotional symptoms (Weideger, 1978). These symptoms vary considerably between women based on genetic predisposition, diet, ethnicity, and culture (Golub, 1992; Rostosky & Travis, 1996; Voda & Eliasson, 1983). Puberty involves incremental *increases* in the production of estrogen and the development of secondary sexual characteristics. Similarly, menopause involves a gradual *decrease* in the three types of estrogen in women's bodies: estrone, estradiol, and estriol (Morokoff, 1988). This is due to age-related changes in the functioning of the ovaries and endocrine system.

On average, this process begins for women in their late 30s, and is accompanied by very gradual changes in the length of the menstrual cycle and in menstrual flow. During this perimenopausal transition, blood estrogen levels decline to prepubertal baseline levels, where they stabilize and remain for the rest of a woman's life. This progressive reduction in estrogen production signals the inability of the ovaries to continue to release follicles (eggs). It marks the eventual end of a woman's fertility. The termination of ovulation usually precedes the cessation of menstruation. However, menstrual cycle changes generally become apparent approximately 7 years prior to a woman's last period. These changes vary from woman to woman. They may involve the shortening or lengthening of the cycle, and increased or decreased menstrual flow (Golub, 1992).

Other secondary symptoms that are characteristically associated with the "menopausal syndrome" include hot flashes, vaginal changes, urinary problems, night sweats, bone or joint pain, depression, irritability, nervousness, and sleep disturbance (Golub, 1992; Voda & Eliasson, 1983). Memory problems also are not uncommon (Leiblum, 1990). Menopause has been associated with bone decalcification, high cholesterol, high blood pressure, heart disease, and cancer. It is important to note, however, that the role of hormonal changes in the etiology of some of these problems is still not clear (Delaney et al., 1988; Morokoff, 1988). Some are more pronounced for women of particular races. For example, black women have a 1.5 times greater risk of dying of heart disease than white women. This appears to be due to a sharp decrease of high-density-lipoprotein cholesterol (the good cholesterol) among blacks after menopause (Barbach, 1993).

By far, the most frequently reported menopausal symptom is the hot flash. Approximately 60–89% of women in Western societies experience this vasomotor response during the perimenopause period (Flint & Samil, 1990; Golub, 1992; Voda & Eliasson, 1983). Hot flashes are characterized by a sudden, intense warming, usually beginning in the face and neck, and progressing down through the chest. This warming may or may not be accompanied by red blotches and sweating in the affected areas. Hot flashes range from mild to severe. They may be triggered by coffee, tea, alcohol, or the consumption of spicy foods (Golub, 1992). The frequency and intensity of hot flashes diminish over time. However, the feelings of dizziness, chills, or chest pains that accompany severe hot flashes can be quite disruptive and debilitating. For many women, hot flashes are associated with the occurrence of some combination of night sweats, nausea, headaches, and insomnia. The duration and intensity of these symptoms vary considerably between women (Morokoff, 1988). Some, but not all women, experience symptomatic relief of hot flashes and other menopausal discomforts with estrogen replacement therapy (Gannon, 1985; Golub, 1992; Kronenberg, 1990).

Changes in genitourinary function are also common during menopause. Some women report painful intercourse and stress incontinence (the leaking of small quantities of urine, particularly when running, coughing, or sneezing). This results from increased vaginal dryness and the thinning of the vagina and urethra due to estrogen reduction (Morokoff, 1988; Voda & Eliasson, 1983). The impact of these changes on the sexual responsiveness and comfort of women is discussed in detail later in this chapter.

The only other menopausal symptom that is clearly linked to the hormonal changes associated with menopause is osteoporosis. This involves a thinning of the bone density as a result of decreased estrogen. Painful joints, increased risk of fractures, and premature skeletal changes are commonly associated with reduced bone density. Osteoporosis is particularly common for fair-skinned, small-boned women. It is also linked to genetics. Those who have a family history of osteoporosis are more likely to develop this condition following menopause (Golub, 1992).

Some women also report mood swings during menopause. It is difficult, however, to ascertain the degree to which emotional fluctuations are precipitated by the hormonal changes versus the largely negative social and cultural expectations and messages associated with menopause. This may be further confounded by the many personal and relational challenges that characteristically occur for women during this "time of heightened reevaluation and reorientation" (health problems, family changes, responsibility for aging parents, etc.) (Klohnen, Vandewater, & Young, 1996). The fact that estrogen replacement therapy is no more effective than a placebo in curing the psychological symptoms associated with menopause suggests that external stresses may be far more significant than hormonal changes in contributing to the emotional responses of many women during this transition. Greater emotional distress is reported by women who experience an early menopause, and by those who are surgically thrust into menopause through hysterectomy (the removal of the uterus) and oophorectomy (the removal of the ovaries) (Golub, 1992; Leiblum, 1990; Morokoff, 1988). Approximately "30–40% of American women . . . undergo this operation." Most hysterectomies are "performed at midlife, between 40–45 years of age" (Leiblum, 1990, p. 500). According to Pokras and Hufnagel (1988), hysterectomy is the most frequently performed "elective" surgery in North America. An average of 650,000 hysterectomies are performed every year in the United States.

The onset of menopause and the length of the perimenopausal transition appear to be correlated with a number of individual variables and life events. For example, greater weight and height, being currently partnered, and having never been pregnant all have been associated with a later menopause. Conversely, an earlier menopause has been linked to heavy smoking, greater alcohol consumption, having had twins, and working outside the home. Golub (1992) also notes the possible role played by "lifelong nutrition, stress, illness, race, familial patterns, or geographical factors" (p. 215) in mediating or moderating the onset of menopause and its associated symptoms. Premenopausal health status also appears to be predictive of the experience of health-related distress during menopause. More menopause-related symptoms are reported by women with a history of prior health problems (Morokoff, 1988).

There is also some evidence to suggest that there are differences in women's perceptions and experiences of menopause, based on their socioeconomic and employment status, and their cultural background (Ehrenreich & English, 1978; Martin, 1987; Neugarten, Wood, Kraines, & Loomis, 1968; Gannon, 1985, 1994). For example, women who are employed outside the home tend to report fewer problems with menopause. It is also interesting to note that European and American women appear to have considerably more anxiety about the changes associated with menopause and the aging process than women from African and Eastern cultures. Based on her review of the research, Golub (1992) highlights the more positive perceptions and experiences of menopause for women from cultures that value and respect the contributions of older women. Unlike North America, in these cultures, the end of fertility frees women to move into positions of power and authority, and to achieve a status more closely resembling that of men. For example, few Japanese women report any problems with hot flashes during menopause. This fact may be related to the low-fat diets of these women, or to the fact that older, postmenopausal Japanese women are accorded positions of considerable status within their families. Research by Flint (1982) on high-caste women in India also indicates the relative absence of symptoms associated with menopause for these women, other than menstrual irregularity and changes. Research by Kronenberg (1990) further reinforces cultural and ethnic differences in the experience of menopause for women. This researcher found a *complete absence* of secondary symptoms at menopause for Mayan women in the Yucatan.

It is important to note that even among North American women, the literature indicates that only a minority of women experience menopausal symptoms severe enough to be disruptive to their everyday lives. Irrespective of their ethnicity or socioeconomic status, most women appear to find the reality of menopause to be considerably more positive than what they had anticipated (Golub, 1992; Unger & Crawford, 1992; Voda & Eliasson, 1983; Wilbur, Miller, & Montgomery, 1995). Roberts, Chambers, Blake, and Weber (1992) conducted a longitudinal study comparing the psychosocial adjustment of postmenopausal women on continuous hormone replacement therapy (HRT), women on cyclic HRT, and women taking only calcium supplements. No significant differences were observed among the symptoms of the women in these three groups. The results confirmed the continued well-being of the large majority of women. These authors noted that only 14% of women in the three groups were not adjusting well to menopause. Many of these women "had concerns about health care issues and difficulties in their sexual relationships. They experienced such psychological distress as anxiety, nervousness, anger, and body image difficulties" (p. 43).

Menopause is a universal phenomenon in the lives of adult women (whether naturally occurring or surgically induced). It is difficult to predict with any certainty, however, what constellation of secondary symptoms a particular woman will experience, if any, during this transition. Certainly, the research indicates that "women who suffer severely at menopause are, in general, those whose hormone supply has dramatically declined" (Weideger, 1978, p. 213). This may, in part, account for the greater symptomatic distress reported by women who experience a surgically induced menopause. There is also some evidence to indicate a relationship between negative menopausal attitudes and increased frequency of menopausal symptoms (Bareford, 1991). A relationship has been found between more negative attitudes toward menopause and higher levels of depression for both African American and white women (Wilbur et al., 1995). It is extremely difficult, then, to tease out the contribution of biological versus psychological or social factors in the responses of menopausal women. Certainly, some women appear to have a potential vulnerability toward a more difficult menopausal transition than others. However, "the meaning attached to each aspect of hormonal change, as well as the meaning attached to any symptoms which develop, is charged with the different values society attaches to each time of life" (Weideger, 1978, pp. 209–210). It would appear, then, that we need to look past the purely biological and physiological aspects of menopause to appreciate any woman's perceptions and experience of "the change" (Greer, 1991).

Fighting Gravity: Bodily Changes

There is a relative paucity of available information specifically related to the health and well-being of midlife women. This is in contrast to the amount of available literature addressing the reproductive health, body image, and sexual expression of women during adolescence and young adulthood. Leigh (1987) notes how, even in the feminist literature, there has "been hardly any discussion around the social construction of middle age as a distinct period of life." Little attention has been paid to "the way in which this affects attitudes and behavior towards middle-aged women, and the image we middle-aged women have of ourselves" (p. 22). Not surprisingly, the information that is available primarily focuses on the menopause.

This fact aside, we know that the midlife period for women is characterized by particular changes in metabolism and appearance (Stevens-Long & Commons, 1992). Some of these changes may be related to declining estrogen levels. Some are mediated by dietary, lifestyle, and hereditary factors. Others are simply a part of the process of living in an aging body. Certainly, for women, "it is difficult to differentiate between the body changes that are a result of aging and those attributable to menopause" (Golub, 1992, p. 227). This is particularly the case for changes in the elasticity of the skin, decreases in bone density (the bones of men and women become more brittle over time, but for women, this process appears to be exacerbated by the decreases in estrogen levels), and metabolic changes (which occur over time in women and men alike). In fact, most of the changes that characterize the normal aging process occur at a fairly steady rate throughout midlife for both women and men. "The changes in hair color and texture, the alterations in girth and visual acuity, the gradual decrease in energy level are incremental and barely noticeable" for most individuals (Cobb, 1988, pp. 156–157).

It is interesting to note that a redistribution of fatty tissues occurs for both sexes. This results in increased body weight and changes in girth measurements, beginning in the mid-20s through the 50s, and declining thereafter. Weight gain is particularly rapid for women, who "on the average gain almost ten pounds between thirty-five and forty-five and two more between forty-five and fifty-five." This extra fat appears to serve an important function in "the conversion of androgens into estrogen" after menopause (Boston Women's Health Book Collective, 1992, p. 538). Additional weight gain is also commonly reported by women who are prescribed HRT (Barbach, 1993).

For both men and women, there are other changes in physical appearance that characteristically occur during middle age. "The extremities and the face lose subcutaneous fat, and the excess appears in the trunk of the body." Men become more "apple-shaped" in terms of a "tire around the middle." Women become more "pear-shaped" with their weight being "less harmoniously distributed . . . on the hips and stomach areas" (Stevens-Long & Commons, 1992, p. 267). "The lips, breasts, eyelids, and often the lower portion of the face seem to shrink, whereas the nose, ears, and middle of the body seem to grow" (p. 266). Cross-linking of collagen and elastin protein molecules results in the skin becoming less elastic. Hair begins to thin, stiffen, and turn grey. "The weight of the bones begins to decline, at about 6 to 8 percent per decade" after the age of 30. "Age or liver spots proliferate and accumulate, especially on the hands" (p. 267). Changes in the immune system are responsible for "dramatic increases in the incidence of chronic and life-threatening disease during middle age" (p. 266). The most notable of these is cardiovascular disease, which "accounts for 40 percent of all premature deaths in this age group" (p. 269).

However, as discussed earlier, the social meanings of these changes, and the biological process these changes are attributed to, are different for women and men. For men, hair loss, age spots, and an expanded midriff are usually attributed to the normal process of aging. In some cases, these changes are even viewed as being indicative of a successful life (e.g., in response to comments regarding his "spare tire," it is not uncommon for a middle-aged man to say, "At least it's paid for"). These same changes in appearance and bodily functioning for women, however, are most often attributed to hormonal shifts associated with menopause—a process that has vastly different social meanings (Cobb, 1988). Based on these different meanings, midlife women and men necessarily understand and respond to the aging process differently.

The Short End of the Stick: Sexual Changes

Our knowledge about the effect of physiological changes on the sexual responsiveness and experience of midlife women is also quite limited. Greer (1991) notes that "most discussions of the sexuality of the fifty-year-old woman have concerned themselves exclusively with the category 'married woman, husband present' " (p. 280). This categorization clearly does not apply to a large number of midlife women who are not partnered (Anderson & Stewart, 1994) or are partnered with a woman (Sang, Warshow, & Smith, 1991). Also, most of the available research and literature is based on white, middle-class women who have sought assistance for their menopausal and sexual concerns. We know relatively little about the sexual satisfaction and expression of women who do not experience their menopausal changes as sexually problematic. Our current knowledge is also limited regarding the role of race, ethnicity, class, or sexual orientation in shaping the sexual experiences of women during midlife (Cole, 1988; Gannon, 1994; Morokoff, 1988).

With this caveat in mind, a number of changes have commonly been reported in terms of the sexual functioning and responsiveness of women during and following menopause. Cole (1988) conducted hour-long, semistructured intake interviews with 100 women attending the Yale University Menopause Program. She reports that "85 of the 100 women experienced one or more sexual problems that either began, or were exacerbated, at menopause" (pp. 159–160). These included vaginal dryness, loss of desire, loss of clitoral sensation, fewer orgasms, and decreased sexual frequency. Golub (1992) reports a similar decrease in sexual activity for 80 postmenopausal women attending a menopause clinic. Almost half of these women reported having intercourse only once a month or less. Sixty-eight percent reported having sexual problems, which included "decreased desire (77%), vaginal dryness (58%), painful intercourse (39%), decreased clitoral sensitivity (36%), decreased orgasmic intensity (35%), and decreased orgasmic frequency (29%)" (p. 230).

The literature on each of these changes is explored here. It is important to note, however, that many factors can contribute to the sexual concerns reported by midlife women. These include, but are not limited to, personal interest, difficulty in finding a suitable partner, lack of privacy in living arrangements, and having had a hysterectomy (Golub, 1992; Hallstrom & Samuelson, 1990; Hunter, 1990; Kitzinger, 1985; Leiblum, 1990). In her review of the literature on sexuality and menopause, Gannon (1994) suggests that there is "little or no predictable change in sexuality as a consequence of or coincident with menopause" (p. 104). Rather, the evidence for reduced sexual activity in postmenopausal women appears to be more highly correlated with factors "other than menopausal status, most notably the availability of a partner, insufficient emotional support from spouse, alcoholism in spouse and psychological problems" (p. 104).

Vaginal Changes

According to Barbach (1993), the vagina is "rich with estrogen receptors" (p. 112). A regular and ample supply of estrogen to these tissues helps to keep "the vaginal lining plump, lubricated, and pain free" (p. 114). Declining levels of circulating estrogens during the menopause are implicated in the thinning and decreased elasticity of the vaginal lining over time. These produce a shortening of the "vaginal barrel" (referred to in the medical literature as "vaginal atrophy") and result in reduced vaginal lubrication (Leiblum, 1990). Diminished vasocongestion of the genital tissues during sexual arousal, a decrease in the elasticity of the vaginal tissue, and the loss of subcutaneous fat in the vulva increase the time required for menopausal women to lubricate when sexually aroused. Although "the premenopausal woman takes from 6 to 20 seconds to lubricate when aroused . . . the menopausal woman takes 1 to 3 minutes" (Golub, 1992, p. 229). For some heterosexual women, these genital changes result in complaints of reduced clitoral sensitivity, painful intercourse, and decreased orgasmic intensity and frequency (Leiblum, 1990).

Vaginal changes are reported as problematic by 40–60% of women (Barbach, 1993; Cole, 1988, Golub, 1992; Leiblum, 1990). These women commonly experience painful intercourse and greater urinary urgency following coitus. Cole (1988) reports menopausal and postmenopausal women comparing their vaginas to "the Sahara desert," "white parchment," "fragments of cut glass," and "sand paper" (p. 162). She quotes a 47-year-old woman, who said, "My vagina's been dry for the last six months to a year. There's pain now, with intercourse. I just seem to be so sensitive" (p. 161). In the sex-therapy nomenclature, this is commonly referred to as "dyspareunia" (Leiblum, 1990, p. 496). It is not uncommon for menopausal women to experience

> painful insertion of the penis with intercourse (related to vaginal dryness); a burning sensation after ejaculation (also related to vaginal dryness—with no or little lubrication to neutralize the alkaline ejaculate); and pain from a vaginal infection (related to the increased susceptibility of women at menopause to vaginitis and cystitis). (Cole, 1988, p. 162)

Some women find inserting a tampon painful. Vaginal dryness is a common complaint of lesbian as well as heterosexual women (Cole & Rothblum, 1991).

Women who have had a hysterectomy often find intercourse particularly painful, "especially with deep penetration." This appears to be "due to tightening and shortening of the innermost part of the vaginal barrel, as well as problems with slackening of tone in the muscles of the pelvic floor which may change the sensation and intensity of orgasm as well as their ability to achieve orgasm" (Kitzinger, 1985, p. 304). Problems with vaginal dryness may also be exacerbated by the use of particular medications, including antihistamines, which dry out the mucous membranes.

Vaginal lubricants and estrogen creams, tablets, or suppositories, and in some cases estrogen replacement therapy, are the remedies most frequently prescribed to reduce vaginal discomfort and inflammation (Cole, 1988; Leiblum, 1990; Morokoff, 1988). Many women find relief of these symptoms from a combination of estrogen and androgen HRT administered through vaginal creams or subcutaneously (Morokoff, 1988; Leiblum, 1990). Some herbal remedies, such as chasteberry, are also reportedly useful in mitigating against vaginal dryness and infection (Barbach, 1993; Greenwood, 1992; Weed, 1992). In her book *The Pause*, sex therapist Lonnie Barbach (1993) recommends the following recipe to maintain vaginal "health" and avoid "vaginal atrophy": "It is in the best interest of your vagina, and possibly your psyche, to continue masturbating. . . . regular masturbation after menopause keeps the vagina healthy, . . . helps maintain the lubrication process, and masturbating with something inside the vagina like a dildo or cucumber keeps the vaginal walls stretched" (p. 120).

However, Kitzinger (1985) rightfully cautions us on the risks and dangers inherent in prescribing sex, especially genital sex and orgasm, as a therapy. She eschews the promotion of any kind of "sexual performance as a kind of health insurance" and warns that "any dogma about how we should feel and express ourselves through our bodies can degrade sex" (p. 241).

Orgasmic Responsiveness

There is some evidence to suggests that as women age, the duration of orgasm and the number of uterine and vaginal contractions are reduced (Gannon, 1994). Although most women retain the ability to be multiply orgasmic, many report changes in their orgasmic responsiveness. Notable changes include "taking longer to reach orgasm, reaching orgasm less frequently, or having less intense orgasms" (Barbach, 1993, p. 117; Kahn & Holt, 1987). Forty-one of the 100 midlife women followed by Cole (1988) reported changes in orgasmic responsiveness since menopause. Many experienced greater difficulty and less regularity in achieving orgasm. Comments such as "I had difficulty getting started," it takes "a long time to get hot," and orgasm takes "longer to get to" (p. 161) were common among these menopausal women, although they were by no means universal. In fact, some women in this study reported *enhanced* orgasmic responsivity following menopause. They attributed this change to having more time and energy for sex once their children left home, experiencing greater intimacy with their partners, and having a sense of freedom from the risk of pregnancy.

Changes in the genital tract and slackening of the pelvic floor muscles can reduce the intensity of orgasm. Changes in clitoral sensitivity and engorgement also make it more difficult for some women to achieve orgasm (Barbach, 1993; Leiblum, 1990). Decreased levels of estrogen can limit pelvic blood flow, thereby reducing the intensity of orgasm (Barbach, 1993). Again, this appears to be particularly true for women who have had a hysterectomy. "Many women who have lost uteruses and/or ovaries . . . report a complete absence of sexual arousal" because "the uterus itself may have important functions" in the experience of orgasm and sexual desire (Cobb, 1988, p. 62).

However, as always, the picture is likely more complex. These changes in sexual responsiveness and orgasmic capacity cannot be wholly attributable to menopause. As Masters and Johnson (cited in Morokoff, 1988) observed, "Sexual response in both older and younger women occurs across a number of systems and organs including the breasts, general muscle tension, clitoris, outer labia, inner labia, Bartholin's glands, and vagina" (p. 495). There are subtle changes in the sexual organs for *both* women and men as they age. Based upon their research, however, Masters and Johnson (1966) conclude that there is no time limit drawn by advancing years for female sexuality, and that women of any age are capable of having orgasms.

It is also important to note that in Kinsey et al.'s (1953) study, women under 60 reported no decline in the frequency of orgasm reached through activities that were not dependent on their male partners, such as masturbation. Similarly, Cole and Rothblum (1991) examined the sexual experiences of 41 postmenopausal lesbian women between the ages of 43 and 68 years. Although 20% of their respondents reported having fewer orgasms, 29% indicated an *increase* in sexual responsivity and *enhanced* orgasmic capacity. Notably, 100% of these women continued to be orgasmic after "the change." These findings suggest that reduced orgasmic responsiveness may be only minimally related to the aging process and the changes of menopause. Rather, decreased responsiveness may be specific to particular types of sexual activities, such as intercourse.

Barbach (1993) confirms that the changes encountered in sexual functioning and responsiveness during menopause seriously reduce sexual satisfaction for only about 20% of women. "For most women, however, these changes in orgasm are not significant and do not necessarily diminish sexual enjoyment. In fact, while women may experience less intense orgasms, they often describe them as gentler and sexier" (p. 117). In the words of one of the women in Cole's (1988) study, "What happens sexually is still very enjoyable. I can still achieve an orgasm, although it's now a *hill*, not a mountain" (p. 162).

Sexual Frequency and Desire

The literature related to declines in sexual frequency and desire is equally equivocal. Estimates of diminished sexual desire for women during and following menopause range from 35% (Barbach, 1993) to 77% (Golub, 1992). According to Barbach, about 35% of menopausal and perimenopausal women experience a reduction in sexual urgency and a decrease in sexual thoughts and fantasies. For most, this begins 1–2 years before their last menstrual cycle. She suggests that loss of desire may be gradual or sudden, transient or permanent. In Cole's (1988) study, loss of desire was reported by 66 of the 100 women who sought help for their menopausal complaints. In the words of one 47-year-old participant, "My desire's decreased, although a few months ago I went through a stage of wanting sex all the time. Nothing would satisfy me. It was kind of nice. A high sex drive makes me feel young and alive. But, overall, I feel like I'm losing it sexually" (p. 161).

Fifty-one of the women in Cole's study reported decreases in the frequency of sexual activity at menopause. Thirty-six reported periods of abstinence lasting sometimes for several years. Cole notes that "some women didn't mind the change," whereas others "minded terribly" (p. 164). For the 27% of lesbian women in Cole and Rothblum's (1991) study who reported decreases in the quality of their sexual experiences, lowered desire was cited as a factor.

Many women fear a loss of sexual desire and desirability during and following menopause (Barbach, 1993). However, a substantial portion of menopausal women report either no change, or an *increase* in their level of sexual interest and activity. For example, in their survey of the sexual functioning of 155 perimenopausal women, Cutler, Garcia, and McCoy (1987) reported little decline in sexual functioning and satisfaction for these women. In the Kinsey et al. (1953) sample of 127 postmenopausal women who had been sexually active prior to menopause, 39% reported no change in sexual activities and responses. Thirteen percent stated that their responses had increased. In the group of midlife women in their 50s and 60s, interviewed by Sheehy (1992), "most said they had negotiated the passage through menopause with a minimum of difficulty . . . [and] had enjoyed the best sex of their lives during and just after menopause, between the ages of forty-five and fifty-five" (p. 140). Sex also reportedly remained good for 62% of the 39 perimenopausal and 64 menopausal women studied by Leiblum and Swartzman (1986). Some of these women confirmed that their sexual interest and comfort increased following menopause. The literature also suggests that women with new partners often report increased sexual frequency and satisfaction (Gannon, 1994; Golub, 1992).

According to Ussher (1989), "The absence of fear of pregnancy, combined with a new sense of independence and power, can result in women feeling *more* sexual" (p. 129). Indeed, in her study of women's sexual behavior, Hite (1981) found that many midlife women reported "a liberating combination of experience, self-knowledge, and confidence, and an absence of pregnancy fears" (p. 509). For these women, this made sex *more* rather than less satisfying. Twenty-nine percent of the postmenopausal lesbians in Cole and Rothblum's study (1991) also indicated an increase in the quality of their sexual interactions. Overall, relatively little deterioration was reported by the 41 women in this study, leading the authors to conclude that "sex at menopause for lesbian women" seems to be "as good as or better than ever" (p. 193).

In attempting to understand these findings, researchers have suggested that changing levels of testosterone or androgens may be implicated. Commonly referred to as the "libido" hormone, some researchers blame lowered levels of "circulating gonadal hormones" (Leiblum, 1990, p. 499) for the decreases in sexual desire reported by some women during menopause. Some success has been documented in the use of estrogen–androgen replacement therapy in restoring sexual desire (Sherwin, 1988; Sherwin & Gelfand, 1987; Sherwin, Gelfand, & Brender, 1985). Others have argued that the natural decrease in estrogen levels experienced by women during menopause results in testosterone not having to "compete" per se with estrogen in the body. This might account for the *increases* in sexual desire reported by some women, and the sometimes total absence of sexual desire in women whose ovaries have been removed (see Gannon, 1994, Morokoff, 1988, and Sherwin & Gelfand, 1987, for a discussion of these changes). At this time, the jury is still out on the role of hormones in moderating sexual desire.

It remains difficult to account fully for the wide variation in the levels of sexual interest experienced by midlife women. Perhaps, as Tiefer (1996) suggests, some women may have more "sexual talent" and confidence based on their earlier life experiences. This may be "related in part to the ease with which a person adopts a sensual mode of being and feels spontaneous and at ease with bodies, movements, secretions, and intimate performances" (p. 62). The prevalence of other menopausal symptoms such as hot flashes, fatigue, and sleep disturbances may also play an important role in changes in sexual interest and desire for some midlife women. These symptoms can contribute to lower energy levels and a diminished sense of well-being during menopause (Cobb, 1988; Cole, 1988). Ill health and depression may also be implicated in diminished sexual desire (Barbach, 1993). Some menopausal women report periods when they are "extraordinarily sensitive to touch" (Cobb, 1988, p. 61), when "it hurts to be touched" (Cole, 1988, p. 162). During these times, any type of sexual contact borders on being physically painful. Barbach (1993) confirms that the loss of subcutaneous fat during menopause may "result in sensitivity or soreness of the clitoris in certain intercourse positions" (p. 120).

Other complaints that have been associated with reduced sexual desire and frequency include incontinence during sex, multiple role demands, lack of interest or sexual problems on the part of their male partners, lack of an appropriate partner, and concerns regarding their sexual attractiveness and desirability on the part of some women (Barbach, 1993; Cobb, 1988; Cole, 1988; Dowling, 1996; Gannon, 1985; Greer, 1991; Morokoff, 1988). It is noteworthy that of the women in the Kinsey et al. (Gannon, 1994) study who believed that their responses had decreased, the majority attributed this "essentially to their partners' declining interest in sex" (p. 103).

Previous sexual interest and responsiveness may also be an important indicator of midlife sexual interest and activity. Results of a survey of 967 women (Kahn & Holt, 1987) suggest that premenopausal levels of sexual activity and experience appear to predict postmenopausal sexual activity and satisfaction. Based on her survey results, Hite (1981) confirms that women's past sexual patterns of desire and behavior appear to be *the* best predictor of current and future patterns. For women who never, or rarely, enjoyed sex, menopause may be experienced as a relief from having to be sexually available and active (Barbach, 1993; Cole, 1988; Gannon, 1994). It is also important not to equate the loss of sexual urgency or frequency commonly reported by menopausal women with a loss of sexual desire. Although sex may not be experienced as frenetic or frantic, as it was in the past, it does not mean that midlife sex is not as desirable or satisfying. Sex may be experienced differently by women at midlife for a host of reasons, but different does not necessarily mean less satisfying than the way it was before.

Finally, Greer (1991) rightfully points out that to determine how many women experience a decline in sexual interest or responsiveness during menopause, it is first necessary to establish how much sexual pleasure they expect to get. "A woman who has never had any pleasure cannot very well experience a decline in it during the menopause" (p. 281). Kaplan's comments in 1974 (cited in Ussher, 1989) may best capture our present state of knowledge regarding the issue of sexual desire for the midlife woman: "Whilst some women report a decrease in sexual desire, many women actually feel an increase in erotic appetite during the menopausal years. Again, the fate of libido seems to depend on a constellation of factors which occur during this period, including physiological changes, sexual opportunity and diminution of inhibition" (p. 129).

Accordingly, "it is crucial not to presume that all menopausal women are the same" (Cole, 1988, p. 165). Citing the words of sex researcher Alfred Kinsey, 35 years ago, Cole cautions counselors to remember that " 'there is nothing more characteristic of sexual response than the fact that it is not the same in any two individuals' " (p. 167).

PSYCHOLOGICAL DEVELOPMENT DURING THE MIDDLE YEARS

"The End of the Line": The Loss of Fertility

Just as myths abound in relation to the *physical* consequences of menopause, there appears to be far more fancy than fact to many of the commonly held beliefs regarding the *psychological* consequences of this transition. Various mental disorders have been attributed to the "shutting off" of estrogen during menopause, from moodiness and irritability on the one end of the continuum, to profound depression and even insanity at the other extreme. In a remnant of biological determinism, women are led to believe that the hormones that purportedly caused emotional instability when they were turned on at puberty (e.g., estrogen) are also implicated in the impairment of their mental processes when they start to decline during the menopause. As Rostosky and Travis (1996) note, based on their survey of medical and psychological science-based journal articles on menopause from 1984 through 1994, the assumption is that both the presence *and* absence of women's hormones make women potentially crazy.

And if hormonal upheaval is not enough, the psychiatric experts propose that the menopausal woman experiences considerable regret over the loss of her fertility and the waning of youth. Based on the assumption that fertility is women's *raison d'être,* the end of menstruation has been conceptualized as a "partial death." The menopausal woman has been portrayed as having reacher her "natural" end as reproductive "servant of the species" (Deutsch, 1945). Menopause also purportedly heralds the end of a woman's natural feminine beauty. In the words of psychoanalyst Helena Deutsch, "Everything she acquired during puberty is now lost piece by piece; with the lapse of reproductive service, her beauty vanishes, and usually the warm, vital flow of feminine emotional life as well" (p. 461). To further compound the problems of the midlife woman, her children often leave home during this stage in life. The menopausal woman faces the double whammy of an "empty nest" and the loss of her fertility. A severe and debilitating depression is portrayed as an inevitable consequence of these losses. Women who have not fulfilled their reproductive role are considered most at risk of psychological problems by some experts. Others suggest that women who are "excessively attached to their mothering role" are most vulnerable to emotional upheaval and depression. As Greer (1991) notes, "There is no group of women which has not been identified as courting disaster at menopause" (p. 106).

Given the popular portrayals of the angst of the menopausal woman, it should not be surprising that some women facing this transition fear that they will become emotionally disturbed. Some worry about "going crazy" and losing their minds during menopause (Golub, 1992, p. 226). The comments of women interviewed by Emily Martin (1987) regarding their experiences of menstruation and their perceptions and expectations of menopause are quite telling in this regard. Martin found that many older women felt very positive about not having to deal with periods or the fear of pregnancy any longer. Younger women in her study, however, still associated menopause with mental and emotional instability. One participant in her research reflected on how her "grandmother almost went insane. . . . She almost didn't make it through menopause at all." Another talked about how her mother "almost went berserk" during the change. Similar sentiments are reflected in the fears of a 30-year-old woman who, in an interview with Ussher (1989), lamented, "I look at every new wrinkle, every grey hair and think of the time when I won't be able to cope with anything: when I'll probably finally go mad. Isn't it true that women who are going through the change are out of their minds for most of the time?" (p. 109).

These fears, however pervasive, are not substantiated by the research literature. According to Golub (1992), "Psychiatric studies have shown that hospitalizations for depression and suicide do not occur more often at this time of life. No differences in depressive symptoms have been found between women of other age groups and women during the climacteric" (p. 217). Results of a large-scale study of 2,500 middle-aged women between the ages of 45 and 55 years confirm these findings (McKinlay & McKinlay, 1987). According to these researchers, the hormonal changes of women who are allowed to undergo a natural as opposed to a surgically induced menopause are not significantly related to depressive symptomatology.

Rather, there are many stressors typically associated with particular life events and losses that occur for women during the middle years (caretaking responsibilities for adolescent children and elderly parents; death of a parent; ill health of friends or family members, etc.). These may result in the onset of depression, or may exacerbate menopausal symptoms (Golub, 1992; Kaufert, 1982). As members of what has sometimes been referred to as the "sandwich generation," midlife women may experience what McGoldrick (1989) refers to as a "dependency squeeze." Midlife women are frequently assigned the responsibility for the emotional and physical "care of their husbands, their children, their parents, their husband's parents, and any other sick or dependent family members" (p. 202). Women who are not partnered are even more likely to assume responsibility for the caretaking of sick and aging parents. This role falls on the shoulders of the daughters in most families. Greer (1991) cites Barbara Evans's contention that the complaints of midlife women of tiredness, irritability, and sleeplessness may not necessarily be due to the menopause. Rather, "menopause coincides with a period of life when stresses and domestic problems mount, and cause problems which are unrelated to the menopause" (p. 160; see also Klohnen et al., 1996, for a discussion of factors associated with midlife adjustment in women). In fact, "there seems to be evidence that stressful life events are more likely to influence a woman's menopausal symptoms than the biological event of cessation of menstruation, or the impact of aging" (Ussher, 1989, p. 120). However, we live in a culture that portrays menopause as a life crisis and menopausal women as suffering from a particular "syndrome." Within such a context, women are "conditioned to report certain types of symptoms" to their doctors (p. 121). Women are socialized to attribute their midlife feelings and reactions to menopause and the aging process, rather than to other stressful life events.

So what *can* we say with any certainty about the psychological changes that occur for women, during the menopause? Research suggests that for a majority of women menopause presents relatively few psychological problems (Golub, 1992; Martin, 1987; McKinlay & McKinlay, 1987). The end of menstruation represents a significant marker in the lives of most women, those who have mothered and those who were unable or who chose not to do so (Apter, 1995; Baruch et al., 1983; Mercer et al., 1988). It appears to be the *symbolic* closure of this part of their lives that is most meaningful to women. Despite the psychosocial and symbolic significance of menopause, however, research clearly indicates that most women welcome the cessation of both menstruation and fertility (Datan, Antonovsky, & Maoz, 1981; Golub, 1992; Martin, 1987). Women in general are relieved to be done with periods and maternity, and very few report feelings of regret (McKinlay & McKinlay, 1987). In the words of one client,

> "I felt very positive about the end of my menstrual cycle. No more concerns about being late, no more hassles with tampons, no more wet surprises when I'm least expecting it. I have not grieved one moment, or felt bad that I no longer menstruate. I guess maybe I'm different from other women, but I'm relieved to be rid of it."

Older women in particular (over 45) appear to reject the contention that menopause means the loss of femininity and womanhood. Many, in fact, report feelings of considerable well-being during and following menopause (Apter, 1995; Golub, 1992; Martin, 1987).

Contrary to popular expectations, the end of fertility also does not appear to precipitate a crisis for women without children (Ireland, 1993; Lisle, 1996; Minuk, 1995). Research suggests that some voluntarily childless women report a sense of loss at a door being permanently closed to them once menstruation ends. As one client who chose to have a tubal ligation in her 20s to ensure her childlessness said, "When I had the surgery I didn't grieve at all about not being fertile anymore, until I went through menopause and realized that a significant part of my life was really over." Overall, however, most appear satisfied with their lives and have "no regrets" about choosing to forego motherhood. Page (1993) quotes the sentiments expressed by a voluntarily childless woman: "I feel joy. I never had children, and now the whole question is no longer an issue, so I feel more expansive about the future" (p. 96).

Also contrary to popular beliefs, the majority of women do not appear to be emotionally devastated when their children leave "the nest." Rather, most actually *look forward* to having more time to engage in activities that nurture the self and other important relationships (Rubin, 1979; Unger & Crawford, 1992). These sentiments are captured in the words of one postmenopausal woman whose children had recently left home:

> I spent a large part of my early adult life on logistics—just getting from point A to point B with three young children and no money. Now, with no responsibilities with three functioning children who are off on their own, it's a liberation that is difficult to explain. . . . It's emotional, physical, financial—total. (Sheehy, 1992, p. 136)

Perhaps most importantly from the standpoint of counseling is the fact that, for many women, menopause serves as a signal event. It is a type of "wake-up call" to women regarding their mortality, or what Delaney et al. (1988) refer to as a time of "rebirth." What begins as an experience of bodily changes may actually precipitate a type of "stock taking" in women's lives, "of spiritual as well as physical change" (Greer, 1991, p. 5). This may lead women to assess the course their lives have taken thus far and to reevaluate the direction they wish their lives to take in the years remaining (Apter, 1996). Martin (1987) cites the case of a woman who experienced menopause as a milestone event that led her to assess her life and relationship. In her desire to reach for greater happiness, she chose to leave a stale and unsatisfying marriage. Terri Apter's book on the experiences of midlife women is also filled with examples of how women revision their lives and acquire self-determination and self-definition during this life stage.

Whatever their earlier feelings and fears, as women actually progress through menopause, their attitudes appear to become far more favorable (Datan, Antonovsky, & Maoz, 1981; Golub, 1992; Morokoff, 1988). This suggests that, contrary to popular stereotypes and beliefs, the gains associated with menopause and the midlife transition may indeed be greater for many women than the purported losses. In fact, many postmenopausal women report feeling better, more confident, calmer, and freer than they did before menopause (Apter, 1996; Neugarten et al., 1968). Many experience menopause not as loss, but "as a release of new energy and potentiality" (Martin, 1987, p. 177; Page, 1993). In response to the question "How did you feel after you finished menopause?", one of Martin's participants said, "It was just like somebody injected me with strength and energy and enthusiasm" (p. 177).

Diminishing Returns?: Body Image

It is also important to ask how middle-aged women respond to the changes that their bodies undergo in the aging process. According to the medical literature, women appear to have considerable difficulty coping with their changing bodies. Depression is reported as the most prevalent response to women's diminishing physical resources during midlife (Gannon, 1994). For example, in 1979, Kistner (cited in Voda & Eliasson, 1993), a well-known gynecologist, wrote that during the premenopausal decade from 40 to 50 years of age, women are preoccupied with the "deterioration of [their] feminine physical attributes." Particularly distasteful signs of aging apparently include "flabby skin, sagging breasts, increased skin pigmentation of the hand, chest or face, and flabby musculature" (p. 142). Even the tremendously bright and accomplished Simone De Beauvoir (cited in Greer, 1991) appeared to be tormented by a profound fear of aging and the waning of her physical beauty: "I loathe my appearance now: the eyebrows slipping down toward the eyes, the bags underneath, the excessive fullness of the cheeks, and that air of sadness around the mouth that wrinkles always bring. . . . When I look, I see my face as it was, attacked by the pox of time for which there is no cure" (p. 247).

According to Stevens-Long and Commons (1992), "Middle-aged women see themselves as less attractive than do any other age group" (p. 267). White, heterosexual women, in particular, appear to be more influenced by cultural pressures to be thin and to retain a youthful appearance, than black or lesbian women (Rothblum, 1994; Sang et al., 1991; Unger & Crawford, 1992). For example, Sang (1991) quotes one of the midlife lesbian women in her study as saying,

> One, if not *the* greatest blessing about being middle-aged dykes is that while heterosexual women are frantically chasing the rainbow of "lost youth" and are frightened by their loss of "beauty" and "sex appeal"—we old dykes are daily growing more comfortable and *accepting* of our aging faces and bodies and are therefore able to see beneath the superficial to the glowing beauty of a mellow soul. (p. 208)

However, even Sang noted how, for most of the 110 midlife lesbians in her study, becoming comfortable with the changes of age was not automatic. Rather, it involved a conscious process of rejecting the cultural messages that blame women for their *failures* to retain the appearance of youth. It involved a *gradual* process of coming to a place of self-acceptance.

Certainly, it is necessary for all women to adapt to the changes brought about by gravity, exposure to the sun, the physical wear and tear of pregnancy and childbirth, the demands of over 40 years of living, metabolic slowing, and diminished supplies of estrogen. As Cobb (1988) suggests, "There is always a time lag when there is a physical change: the self-image . . . and the real image . . . may not jibe and it takes time for these two images to match. This is true for those who lose a limb, those who lose weight, and those who gain it. It takes time to get used to the new shape" (p. 159).

In particular, "one of the most common complaints" of midlife women is their difficulty in controlling their weight. "Women talk about how it is harder to take off weight and easier to put it on" (Barbach, 1993, p. 97). They lament about their struggles to reconcile their ideal body images with the realities of their changing midlife bodies. The following words echo the sentiments of many women: "Around two years ago, when I was forty-six, my whole body started changing. I felt thicker in the waist. I'm working harder to keep ahead of weight gain, but the returns are diminishing. It's a real battle. Sometimes I can take off a few pounds, but the weight returns so rapidly" (Barbach, 1993, p. 97).

Just as the adolescent girl struggles to integrate her developing body into her self-structure (Cash, 1990), and the pregnant woman learns to psychologically accommodate the tenancy of another being within her body (Bergum, 1989), the midlife woman is faced with the psychological work of coming to terms with her changing body. She must deal with and make sense of all that these changes represent, literally and symbolically, in terms of her sense of herself as a woman and a worthwhile person. The words of one client characterize this process:

> "Working past the issues of aging is really tough. You come out at the other end and it's a different ball game; generally, you're fine. I think what happens is you get so far removed from the cultural ideal that you just say, well, to hell with it. It doesn't make any difference now. In other words, you're free—freed up to be who you are. But in the meantime, you go through anywhere from 2 to 10 years where you're doing all this struggling to get past that Madison Avenue image out there."

In her interviews with women between the ages of 40 and 54, Apter (1996) noted how, as they came to value their own visions, these women were "less daunted by negative views of others, and quicker to register others' positive views" (p. 74). "As women come to a road forked by liberation on the one hand, and the terror of meaninglessness on the other, they free themselves from the tyranny of that critical, overbearing reflection. As they are thus freed, they embrace their own vision" (p. 56). It is a testament to their strength of characters that most middle-aged women are able to work through the contradictions inherent in societies' messages regarding the acceptable standards of feminine beauty. It is to their credit that most are able to redefine and embrace a more generous, realistic, and accepting vision of what it means to be an attractive, middle-aged woman.

Sexual Self-Esteem

Similar to the medical community, psychological theorists have focused on the role of hormones in shaping the sexual identity and sexual expression of the midlife woman. Freud (1948) contended that menopause could elicit a reexperiencing of the "castration complex," thereby reawakening a woman's lifelong sense of inferiority. Ellis (1942) theorized that wild hormonal swings were experienced by women during menopause, resulting in the unleashing of an "overwhelming" sexual aggressiveness. He warned that younger men were the most likely targets of the midlife woman's uncontrollable, lustful desires. Helena Deutsch (cited in Greer, 1991) referred to the cessation of menses as "woman's last traumatic experience as a sexual being" (p. 241). According to McCormick (1994) and others (e.g., Apter, 1996; Greer, 1991; Kaschak, 1992; Rubin, 1979), a psychological theory has yet to be proposed that affirms the middle years as a time of potential growth and opportunity for women, personally and sexually.

Certainly, many social and biological transition occur in women's lives that affect their sense of themselves as sexually desirable and vital (Unger & Crawford, 1992). Hormonal changes, role changes, changes in physical appearance and health, and relationship changes may present challenges to the midlife woman's sexual self-esteem and identity. As Barbach (1993) notes, psychological factors play a significant role in women's experience of their sexuality. A woman's response to the changing circumstances of her life necessarily affects her psychological and sexual well-being. As well as dealing with changes in appearance and the experience of menopause, midlife women must also come to terms with the rather dramatic social changes in their sexual status and worth.

From the time women reach puberty and begin to show the signs of mature womanhood, women deal with being appraised and valued for the social symbols of their sexuality (breasts, appearance, fertility). Sex and sexuality are women's currency. To a degree, they are women's power. During midlife women experience a

> loss of a kind of power that occurs with the loss of youthful sexual attractiveness. Without even realizing it, many of us have received prompt or extra attentiveness from male clerks or salesmen throughout our lives, or perhaps we were readily assisted if the car broke down . . . simply because we were young and physically appealing. . . . With age comes invisibility. This means we may . . . no longer be able to trade our sex appeal for special favors. (Barbach, 1993, p. 96)

Bell (1989) also notes how, "as she approaches middle age" a woman "begins to notice a change in the way people treat her. Reflected in the growing indifference of others toward her looks, toward her sexuality, she can see and measure the decline of her worth" (p. 236). An experience when out with her teenage daughter brought this reality home to one woman: "I was walking down the street with my daughter the other day and a couple of men stopped and looked. Suddenly I became aware that they were looking at *her* and not me. It was a little hard on me. I felt proud of her, but at the same time, I felt bad about myself" (Barbach, 1993, p. 95). However high the costs of sexual objectification may have been for women during their youth, the sexual self must still find ways to accommodate the experience of sexual disqualification that occurs for women during midlife. The following quote from a 55-year-old attorney (cited in Cole, 1988) captures this struggle:

> It's not easy to see your chin get double and your waist get thick and see yourself as not sexually attractive. Things do happen to you that aren't nice. Sexually you don't feel the same way, there's no question about it. It takes longer to have an orgasm. Whether you want to put a lot of energy into it is the thing. You're tired; it takes longer. But it's not easy to relinquish your sexual self. (p. 163)

In fact, it would appear that not all midlife women do relinquish their sexual selves. Rather, with age and maturity comes increased confidence and a growing self-assurance. Many women report midlife as a time when they feel much more centered in, and connected with, their sexuality and sexual energy than they had felt earlier in their lives (Apter, 1996; Cole & Rothblum, 1991; Hite, 1981; Kitzinger, 1985; Loulan, 1987). Many report feeling more capable of giving and receiving sexual pleasure in their intimate lives.

The changes of the midlife decades may also result for some women in the growing realization of their lesbianism or bisexuality (McCarn & Fassinger, 1996; Weasel, 1996). For many, it is not until midlife that they begin to be aware of and acknowledge the strength of their erotic desires toward women. For example, in Sang's (1991) study of 100 midlife lesbians, almost half had been in heterosexual relationships at some point in their lives and had one or more children. Twenty-five percent reported experiencing their first erotic desires toward women at midlife. Kitzinger (1985) suggests that the identification or expression of lesbianism or bisexuality may be delayed or repressed by cultural attitudes and sanctions until late in life. Age, maturity, and circumstance seem to allow women the freedom to live more openly and to pursue other possibilities. In the words of one woman (cited in Porcino, 1983),

> I always suspected I was gay and spent many years trying to suppress those feelings and thoughts. Growing older gave me me. At last I'm able to do what I believe is right for me. Oh yes, society still said no loud and clear, but now I discovered that I am not alone, not the only one. . . . My life with my lover is the happiest, strongest love I know—just two beautiful people loving, living, growing, and sharing together. (p. 192)

There may indeed be freedom and contentment in coming to this self-awareness. However, the lesbian or bisexual midlife woman may still struggle with her own internalized homophobia as well as that of significant others in her life, and of society in general (Boston Lesbian Psychologies Collective, 1987; Hutchins & Ka'ahumanu, 1991). Coming out as a lesbian or bisexual woman and incorporating this reality into one's sexual self-structure is a complex and challenging task in a heterosexual world at any stage in life (Firestein, 1996; Golden, 1987; Penelope & Wolfe, 1990; Rust, 1996; Sang et al., 1991).

BIOLOGICAL DEVELOPMENT IN LATER LIFE: "YOU'RE AS YOUNG AS YOU FEEL"

As this century comes to a close, many women can expect to live well into their 70s and 80s (Unger & Crawford, 1992). The "elderly," or "elders" are generally defined as those 65 or older (Stevens-Long & Commons, 1992). The percentage of elders in the American population is larger now than at any time in history and is still increasing (Grambs, 1989), "from 4 percent, or 3 million in 1900, to 11 percent, or 125 million at present" (Dowling, 1996, p. 47). In setting their *Research Agenda for Psychosocial and Behavioral Factors in Women's Health* (1996) the Advisory Committee of the American Psychological Association noted that in 1990, 12.5% of the population of the United States was 65 or older. This figure continues to rise as the baby-boom generation ages. By the year 2030, there will be approximately 55 million persons over 65 years old. The majority will be women (Rotberg, 1987). Women outlive men by 3–8 years in every country in the world except India and Bangladesh (Grambs, 1989). Between the ages of 65 and 85, women outnumber men approximately three to two. For those over 85, there are five women for every two men (1992 U.S. Bureau of the Census, cited in Unger & Crawford, 1992). Women over 50 already form one of the largest groups in the population structure of the Western World. The threat of superbugs aside, there is every indication that older women today can look forward to very long and relatively healthy lives (Greer, 1991).

Not surprisingly, however, we know relatively little about the lives and sexuality of older women. Women have been

> largely invisible in . . . research on aging. Much research on older people has either used all-male samples or failed to analyze results by sex, so that possible differences between men and women are obscured. Moreover, biases based on stereotypes of women have affected researchers' choice of participants . . . result[ing] in research that has little validity for understanding the lives of today's aging women. (Unger & Crawford, 1992, p. 491)

The sparse literature that is available generally lumps together mid- and later life as one period in women's life span. Attention to the sexuality of midlife women is relatively absent in the literature, other than in books and articles focused specifically on menopause. The sexual needs, desires, and behaviors of postmenopausal women, and in particular, women over 65, are hardly a whisper in literature. It is as if, after menopause, women are destined to decades of living with only the memories of their sexual lives and selves as they once were.

Ageist attitudes are pervasive in North American culture. Nowhere is this more apparent than in our refusal to acknowledge the sexuality of the older woman. Gannon (1994) notes that in the 1,700 pages of the two reports by Kinsey and his associates, published in 1948 and 1953, respectively, only three pages were devoted to sexuality in older people. Almost 40 years later, the situation is not much better. Scientific research is still virtually nonexistent, other than surveys of the sexual attitudes and behaviors of small groups of seniors. What little information we do have must be interpreted carefully in light of cohort differences between the current generation of elders and those who have yet to reach this life stage. The women upon whom the current literature is based were born early in this century and grew up with different values and more restrictive norms. Nickerson (1992) notes how the present cohort of older women were raised during a time of tremendous sexual repression:

> Our generation was too often taught that sex was disgusting, nasty or bad. It was restricted by the Church, warned against by mothers and relegated to hushed, forbidden discussions. It's small wonder that we were often unable to understand our own sexuality even as hormones raced recklessly through our maturing bodies. . . . The pain and unhappiness of our suppressed sexuality still haunts many Age Mates in one way or another. (p. 217)

Cohort differences in sexual socialization make it difficult to predict the experiences of future generations of older women. These cohort differences must be kept in mind as we turn to a review of the limited, available literature.

Despite the prevalent myths and stereotypes of the asexual older woman, there is literature to suggest that women's sexual desires and expression do not cease to exist in later life. Masters and Johnson (1966), for example, indicated that 7 out of the 10 couples over the age of 60 in their study remained sexually active. Most reported progressive declines in their rate of intercourse and in the frequency and intensity of orgasm. However, their capacity to enjoy sexual contact did not deteriorate with advancing years. Good sex for the women over 70 was linked to good health and an interested and interesting partner.

Data gathered by Starr and Weiner (1981) on the sexual attitudes and activities of over 800 healthy U.S. seniors between the ages of 60 and 91 confirms the sexual interest and vitality of many older adults. The cohort of seniors in this study was born around the turn of the century.

Seventy-nine percent reported continued sexual activity, and 72% were satisfied with their current sex lives. Seventy-five to 80% believed that sex is good for one's health. Most indicated that sex was as good now, or even better, than when they were young. The vast majority also approved of widowed and unmarried older people having sex. Underscoring the multiple meanings of sexual intimacy, most felt that sex reaffirmed their identities and sense of aliveness. Sexual contact generated feelings of physical and emotional vitality. These seniors also enjoyed the enhanced intimacy and communication with their partners that having sexual contact provided.

Similar findings were reported in a study of 62 women and 40 men between the ages of 60 and 85, conducted by Adams and Turner (1985). These researchers looked at the changing patterns in respondents' sexual behavior from their 20s to the present. They found consistent declines in the reported frequency of sexual activity from young adulthood to old age. For women, however, the only significant sexual declines were in the reported frequency of intercourse. These findings support the "relative maintenance of *participation* in many sexual activities over time, especially among women" (p. 133). It is noteworthy that many of the women and men in this study remarked on the gradual improvement in their sex lives over time. They made reference to the "positive changes in sexuality that not only can, but sometimes do, occur in late middle age and beyond" (p. 138). Women of this particular cohort appreciated the release from the fear of pregnancy that occurred following menopause. They felt freer to enjoy their sexual encounters. Many women reported an increased sense of sexual agency and a greater desire to experiment and give sexual pleasure to their partners. They attributed this to the changes in traditional sexual scripts that have occurred over the past few decades, and to their exposure to feminism. The occurrence of masturbation among these women also increased significantly over time. This fact notwithstanding, 85% of women and 89% of men indicated a clear preference for interpersonal rather than solitary sexual activities.

The results of a more recent study by Bretschneider and McCoy (cited in Morokoff, 1988) shed some light on the sexual behavior of the group commonly referred to as the "old old," those 80 years of age and over. Popular myths and stereotypes would lead us to believe that people in this age group are too physically and psychologically frail even to think about sex. Some believe that to attempt intercourse at this delicate age would be to risk physical injury (e.g., "She might break a hip," "He might have a heart attack"). These researchers surveyed 202 healthy men and women between the ages of 80 and 102. Contrary to popular belief, most of these elders remained sexually active. Thirty percent of the women in the study said that they continued to engage in sexual intercourse. By far, the most commonly reported "sexual" activity for both women and men in this age group was touching and caressing (even though only 14% were currently married). It is also interesting to note that 75% of the men and 50% of the women reported that they often, or very often, fantasized or daydreamed about intimate relations.

Morokoff (1988) reviewed the literature on the sexual behavior and attitudes of the elderly. He notes that "a striking finding from this research is that while interest and activity decline on the average, a large percentage of older individuals maintain active sexual relationships, underscoring the fact that loss of sexuality is not inevitable" (p. 497). Certainly, women and men appear to be physically capable of giving and receiving sexual comfort and pleasure well into their later years (Boston Women's Health Book Collective, 1992; Kitzinger, 1985; Nickerson, 1992). However, certain physical changes and impaired health may preclude women from acting on their sexual desires, or may impede their sexual satisfaction.

Common physical changes that may noticeably affect the sexual comfort and self-esteem of older women include the loss of body hair, vaginal dryness, and urinary incontinence (Boston Women's Health Book Collective, 1992; Kitzinger, 1985). As they age, most women lose body hair, particularly those who are fair. Nickerson (1992) notes how "once-fluffy pubic hairs thin out to a semi-modest remnant. Underarm hair decreases. For a few, head hair thins. . . . Body secretions may also decrease—saliva, tears, vaginal fluids, even perspiration can be less copious than in younger years" (p. 79). The loss of body hair may leave the older woman feeling overly exposed and self-conscious, particularly if she is entering a new relationship. In the words of one older woman, "You end up feeling a little like a plucked chicken." Diminished vaginal secretions can result in painful intercourse for the older woman, as well an increased risk of vaginal infections. Some women may find vaginal lotions and jellies helpful. Others, particularly those in new relationships, may find their vaginal dryness to be reversible (Boston Women's Health Book Collective, 1992). Urinary incontinence, caused by a weakening of the muscles of the pelvic floor, is also very common among older women. This can be particularly embarrassing or problematic during intercourse or orgasm. However, the use of Kegel exercises (systematic contraction and relaxation of the abdominal and pelvic muscles), fluid-intake restriction, and complete emptying of the bladder prior to intercourse can help to remedy these concerns (Kitzinger, 1985).

Health concerns and a combination of prescribed medications can also interfere with, or reduce, the sexual responsiveness and desire of older women (Boston Women's Health Book Collective, 1992). Although women live longer, they have higher morbidity than men. Older women report more chronic, non-life-threatening impairments than men, and spend more years with chronic, debilitating diseases (American Psychological Association, 1996, p. 15). "Aging may bring physical disabilities that interfere with the way [women] express [themselves] sexually. Stiff joints, and aching back, difficulty in hearing and seeing, loss of taste and smell, may all mean that [women] need to adapt and experiment in lovemaking" (Kitzinger, 1985,

p. 247). Certain drugs (e.g., barbiturates, antidepressants, phenothiazines, diuretics, chemotherapy) and illness (e.g., lupus, chronic fatigue syndrome) can reduce sexual desire, decrease physical sensation, and diminish sexual functioning (Crenshaw & Goldberg, 1996).

Another very important factor to consider in any discussion of the sexuality and sexual behavior of older women is poverty.

> Today's older women are nearly twice as likely to be existing on incomes below the poverty level as same-age men, and Black and Hispanic women are worse off than White women. Overall, more than one elderly woman in six is poor. According to U.S. census data, 82% of elderly Black women are in "poor" or "near-poor" categories. (Unger & Crawford, 1992, p. 525)

The inadequate nutrition and poor living conditions that result from poverty can severely impair the health of elderly women. Poor health, in turn, can be a significant impediment to women's sexual functioning and satisfaction. Also, as Gannon (1994) points out, "The economic, social and medical problems of many of the elderly preclude a serious consideration of or interest in sex" (p. 120). Sexual pleasure may be very low on the priority list of women who cannot afford to feed themselves or their families. For some elderly women who are struggling to survive, "sexuality is simply irrelevant" (p. 121).

And yet Kitzinger (1985) underscores the fact that "for some women sex clearly improve(s) with age" (p. 243). Some report becoming orgasmic for the first time in their lives after the age of 65. It does indeed seem that "sex after sixty is much like any other activity—you get back what you put into it" (Nickerson, 1992, p. 207). As such, Nickerson offers the following advice to her female "age mates":

> Instead of writing your sexual obituary, be prepared for surprises, possibly even miracles. In this age of possibilities, new, compassionate relationships are free to develop based on love and understanding. . . . The fundamentals of "elder sex" are shared memories and warm familiarity. . . . Sexuality *is* always there. It may change in superficial ways, but for women, at least, this fundamental aspect of being human has the possibility of becoming more satisfying and more fulfilling as time goes by. Despite myths to the contrary, most women retain active interest in loving sex long past menopause. (p. 207)

PSYCHOLOGICAL DEVELOPMENT IN LATER LIFE: NOTHING VENTURED, NOTHING GAINED

Rotberg (1987) suggests that "the potential for sexual expression continues until the day we die" (p. 4). In later life, however, there are a number of changes, including "relationship and family transformations, . . . physical illness, normal aging and a continual resetting of priorities that could, and probably do, have an impact on a woman's sexuality" (Gannon, 1994, p. 119). Older women must psychologically accommodate the changes in their bodies that occur as they age. Many must learn to cope with, and adjust to, chronic health concerns (American Psychological Association, 1996). The loss of a breast, or leg, or hip, or receipt of a diagnosis of cancer can dramatically alter a woman's sense of herself as a woman, as a healthy person, and as a sexual being. All of these can affect a woman's interest in sex. They can significantly alter her ability to enjoy and express her sexuality.

Later life is also characterized by a number of personal and relational losses. These include but are not limited to the loss of energy, attractiveness, and health; the loss of valued roles; and the loss of partners, family members, and friends. There are many losses in later life that need to be accommodated, including "the experience of losing a valued part of the body, or that of losing a special, loved person—a sexual partner, a child or a parent" (Kitzinger, 1985, p. 281). Many older women are faced with the loss of their partner (Boston Women's Health Book Collective, 1992). The average widow lives 18 years after her husband's death (Unger & Crawford, 1992). Certainly, the loss of a partner is likely to limit the older woman's opportunities to express herself sexually with another. And research indicates that within months of a death of a partner, the survivor is likely to suffer a serious illness (Kitzinger, 1985).

Marked by periods of intense emotion, later life may be a time of great joy and accomplishment. It can also be marked by periods of pain and grief. "Any strong emotional state affects our feelings about sex, whether it is joy, depression, anxiety, anger—or grieving." Intense emotions and experiences can "change the way in which we experience sex and the meaning it has for us" (Kitzinger, 1985, p. 281). Kitzinger notes how "death and sex are intertwined. Death and the surrender of self in orgasm are inextricably bound up with each other" (p. 287). The experience of grief necessarily affects sex and how it is experienced. Grief is about bodies as well as minds. It involves a process with phases that affect a woman physically and emotionally in different ways at different points in the journey. For example, loss of libido is common when individuals are grieving or are depressed. Others may feel "almost driven to sex" in a striving for reassurance. In this way, sex may be a "determined affirmation of life" (p. 289; see Kitzinger, 1985, for an excellent discussion of the ways in which grief may affect women's sexual desires and functioning). Any older woman's ability to enjoy and express her sexuality will necessarily be influenced by the specific circumstances of her life.

Body image is another factor that to varying degrees will influence women's sexual comfort and expression in later life. We might assume that by the time women reach their sixth or seventh decades, they have worked through the body image struggles that plague most during their youth. We might expect that older women have come to a place of resignation, if not peace, with their appearance. For some, this appears to be the case. Wisdom supposedly comes with age, and with wisdom comes a greater acceptance of self—sags, wrinkles, and all. In later life, some women turn away from the brokers of beauty and youth and accept their bodies for what they are. In the words of one client,

> "I've given up trying to please everyone else. . . . Now I take care of myself, and my body, for me. It's interesting. . . . Whereas before I use to look at thin women and think they were beautiful, and lucky, I don't anymore—now I see them as frail. I walk and I do yoga to stay flexible, and I *appreciate* my body more now—for its strength and its good health. It's interesting how one's perspective changes with age."

Over time, some women learn to prize their bodies and make no apologies for carrying the marks (stretch marks, wrinkles, etc.) of a life well lived.

For many older women, however, letting go of the "illusion" of youth may not be an easy task. Rodeheaver and Stohs (1991) suggest that

> even women who can afford our culture's youth-preserving lotions, pills, surgeries, and exercise regimens over the course of their entire adult life cycles will, by old age, confront serious dissonances between subjective youthful body images and the reactions of others to their wrinkled, sagging, aged appearance. (p. 146)

In what these authors refer to as the "adaptive misperception of self" (p. 142), many older women appear to distort their perceptions of their appearance and body image in favor of maintaining a younger self-perception. In their interviews with women 65 and over, Rodeheaver and Stohs identified a recurring theme of "body dissociation" that occurs for women. This is a type of cognitive adaptation that women employ for a substantial period of the life cycle. It serves to "distance the self from the physical image the women confronted (in mirrors, store windows, or photographs) in favor of a subjective image of the physical self as more youthful" (p. 148). The women in this study appeared to be fully aware of their age and the changes that had occurred in their appearance over the years. Subjectively, however, they could not "relate" to the image in the mirror. They did not *feel* as old as they looked. Interestingly, rather than being a sign of psychological disturbance, the researchers found that subjective age was more highly correlated to the overall life satisfaction of these women. Their findings support the popular contention that you are "as young as you feel."

Indeed, research by Kaufman (cited in Rodeheaver & Stohs, 1991) suggests that most older people maintain a "continuity of self that is ageless regardless of the physical and social changes that accompany age" (pp. 147–148). Whether this continuity applies to the sexual self, however, is uncertain, in light of the almost complete invalidation of the sexuality of the elderly in North American society. Sexuality and sexual expression "deal with many facets of an individual's personality." These include but are "not limited to affection, companionship, intimacy and love. Love and belonging needs are timeless and ageless" (Rotberg, 1987, p. 4). Whether ill or in good health, partnered or living alone, women's needs and desires for companionship and intimacy do not end in later life. Women do not become asexual because they are old or unpartnered. Sexuality is a part of each woman's personhood until the day she dies, however she chooses to express this aspect of her self. As with other aspects of women's sexuality, however, the greatest barrier to this expression may well be the prevalent ageist attitudes that render the older woman undesirable and sexless.

In the chapters that follow, attention is paid to the sources of influence on the experiences of midlife women as they attempt to respond to menopause and the changes in body image and intimate expression that characterize this life stage. The final chapter addresses the experiences of women in later life.

12

WHEN BEING "HOT" TAKES ON NEW MEANING

Menopause

They tell her she is womb-man,
baby machine, mirror image, toy,
earth mother and penis-poor,
a dish of synthetic strawberry icecream
rapidly melting.
She grunts to a halt.
She must learn again to speak
starting with I
starting with We
starting as the infant does
with her own true hunger
and pleasure
and rage.
—MARGE PIERCY, "Unlearning to not speak"

it seems a pity to have a built-in rite of passage and to dodge it, evade it, and pretend nothing has changed. That is to dodge and evade one's womanhood, to pretend one's like a man. Men, once initiated, never get the second chance. They never change again. That's their loss, not ours. Why borrow poverty?
—URSULA LE GUIN, "The Space Crone"

= It is clear from the literature reviewed in Chapter 11 that most women find the physical experience of menopause to be far less problematic than they had expected it to be. Only a small percentage of women indicate that the cessation of menstruation and secondary menopausal symptoms are particularly disruptive or debilitating. In fact, some women report a sense

of renewed energy and creativity while going through "the change" (Barbach, 1993; Boston Women's Health Book Collective, 1992; Cobb, 1988; Golub, 1992). Psychologically speaking, like other transitions that occur throughout life, for most women, menopause is associated with both losses and gains. Each woman must incorporate these into her understanding of herself, as a woman, and as a sexual person.

The social and symbolic significance of menopause may be more important in understanding the experiences of menopausal women than the physical and psychological changes that occur when menstruation ends (Ahsen, 1996). Like menarche, the cessation of menstruation is both a physiological process and sociocultural event that is imbued with particular meaning and significance (Carolan, 1994). Within most cultures of the world, there is a powerful cultural link between fertility and femininity (Estok & O'Toole, 1991). As noted in Chapter 4, the onset of menstruation signals the beginning of fertility and marks the young girl's social passage into womanhood. It can be argued that the cessation of menstruation signals sterility, and by association, the symbolic end of womanhood. The importance of this connection is underscored by Paula Weideger (1978) in *Female Cycles.*

> Thirty or forty years pass in which recurrent cycles of hormone change have formed the substrata of woman's experience. During these years the litany is sung and repeated: you are your reproductive functions; you are the Madonna and the whore. Menopause occurs, and women will never again experience the monthly flow of blood or the monthly cycles of hormonal change. As soon as the bleeding ends, the menstrual taboo stops and the values attached to womanhood are no more. . . . Fertility and "dangerous" menstruation no longer form part of her being. Her body is no longer unclean, but it no longer serves its most "important" function—that of giving form to fertility. (p. 210)

Menopause marks the biological end of a woman's reproductive life. It is also an event imbued with social and symbolic meanings. These are communicated to women by medical practitioners, the media, and significant others in their lives. We turn now to a closer examination of some of these communications.

ALL "DRIED" UP: MEDICAL MESSAGES

Until recently, relatively little was actually known about menopause. However, this lack of scientific knowledge did not stop the medical profession from proffering opinions about this aspect of women's reproductive lives. Traditionally, the medical professionals viewed the process leading to the end of menstruation as pathological. It was believed to be associated with a range of symptoms including hot flashes, a "stiff and unyielding vagina," wrinkles, shrinking and sagging breasts, aching joints, palpitating organs, frequent urination, itchy skin, osteoporosis, irritability, depression, frigidity, absentmindedness, loss of memory, and insanity (Delaney et al., 1988; Ehrenreich & English, 1978; Martin, 1987). "Women entering menopause were viewed as diseased, hormone deficient, sexless, irritable, and depressed" (Golub, 1992, p. 215) human beings. The medical literature is full of terms such as "vaginal atrophy," "degenerative changes," "estrogen starvation," and "senile pelvic involution" (Kitzinger, 1985, p. 237) to describe this "death of the woman in the woman" (Ehrenreich & English, 1978, p. 111). These sentiments are captured in the words of David Ruben in 1969:

> As estrogen is shut off, a woman comes as close as she can to being a man. Increased facial hair, deepened voice, obesity, and decline of breasts and female genitalia all contribute to a masculine appearance. Not really a man but no longer a *functional* [emphasis added] woman, these individuals live in a world of intersex. Having outlived their ovaries, they have outlived their usefulness as human beings. (p. 287)

As recently as 1981, the World Health Organization defined menopause as an estrogen-*deficiency disease* caused by the "burning out" of the ovaries (Martin, 1987).

Greer (1991) and others (e.g., Dickson, 1990) underscore the "lamentable state of medical understanding" of women's reproductive functioning. This has resulted in the prescription of a range of experimental "palliatives" for women's menopausal and climacteric distress:

> They have let blood, prescribed violent purgatives, sent women to spas and mountain resorts, dosed them with bromide, mercury, sulfuric acid, belladonna and acetate of lead. Suspecting that the problems women encountered were directly caused by the cessation of ovarian function, they turned to glandular extracts, plant hormones, bits and pieces of the reproductive equipment of other species, dried corpus luteum from pigs, grilled ovaries from cows and sheep. (Greer, p. 161)

More recently, hormone replacement therapy has been promoted as the medical treatment of choice for menopausal symptoms (Sherwin, Gelfand, & Brender, 1985). This includes various combinations of estrogen and androgen replacement therapy. In the United States "between 1963 and 1973, sales of estrogen preparations quadrupled" and more than "half the post-menopausal female population was using Hormone Replacement Therapy" (Greer, 1991, p. 161). By 1975, over 26.7 million women were being prescribed hormone replacements. Estrogens were the fifth most frequently prescribed drug in the United States (McCrea, 1983). The risks associated with these exogenous hormone replacements reportedly include the increased incidence of uterine cancer, gallbladder disease, liver tumors, and blood clots (Glazer & Rozman, 1991; McCrea, 1983; Voda & Eliasson, 1983).

Advancement in the reproductive technologies may also further confound the issue of the medical management of menopause. With the aid of a powerful combination of hormones and the eggs of a younger woman, women are reported to be able to become pregnant well into their 40s and even into their 50s (Corea, 1985; Stanworth, 1987). The achievement of a pregnancy by a 63-year-old woman early in 1997 made headlines throughout the world. It served as a further testament to the possibilities available to women to extend the period of fertility well past the previous upper limit of age 40. If desired, women can also look forward to continuing to menstruate well into their 60s (Ehrenreich & English, 1978; Martin, 1987).

The theme of menopause as deficit and loss is still very prevalent in the medical literature. "Medical textbooks and research [still] tend to emphasize atrophic changes in the urogenital system, degenerative consequences associated with hormonal decline, and potential pathologic conditions associated with the menopause" (Choi, 1995, p. 58). Is it any wonder, then, that despite their often conflictual feelings about menstruation (Weideger, 1978), many women approach menopause with less than overwhelming enthusiasm? After all, who would want to rush into such a "rite-of-passage" when the destination of the journey is portrayed as one of physical and mental decline on the one hand, or the continuation of an artificially induced menstrual cycle on the other?

ALL "USED" UP: MEDIA MESSAGES

As noted in Chapter 11, the current middle-aged cohort is the largest in recorded history (Stevens-Long & Commons, 1992). Reflecting this demographic reality, media messages now abound regarding how a woman might best negotiate the menopausal "transition." Far from being a "taboo" subject, Ahsen (1996) underscores the increasing public emphasis on menopause. Only two articles, books, videos, and television shows focused on managing the menopause were logged by the Project for Automated Library Systems in 1986. Between 1993 and 1995, however, 349 titles were logged. There are now significantly more books and magazine articles directed at helping women to decide about the merits of hormone replacement therapy (as well as exercise and nutrition). There is no shortage of direction and advice on how women can best deal with uncomfortable menopausal symptoms.

Unfortunately, the emphasis in much of the available literature is on eliminating the symptoms of menopause and the signs of aging. For example, a recent ad for skin care products in *Psychology Today* magazine headlines

"Menopause, Daylight, and Your Skin: Why Your Skin May Be More Vulnerable Now (and What You Can Do About It)" (p. 3). The thrust of the ad is that menopause, and in particular, estrogen supplements may make women's skin "vulnerable to daylight damage." The company's special moisturizer is promoted to relieve the symptoms of "melasma" (which include freckles, blotchy spots, discolorations, premature lines, and wrinkles). The "self-help" and "health" sections of many bookstores are also filled with pocketbooks that emphasize ways women can unobtrusively manage (and hide) their menopausal symptoms and maintain their youthful appearance.

Fortunately, there are some recent books by women authors that attempt to present menopause as a natural transition (e.g., Germaine Greer's [1991] *The Change: Women, Age and Menopause*; Janine O'Leary Cobb's [1993] *Understanding Menopause: Answers and Advice for Women in the Prime of Life*; or Lonnie Barbach's [1993] *The Pause: Positive Approaches to Menopause*). These authors provide suggestions as to how women can maintain and enhance their health and well-being during menopause. However, a regular browsing through the shelves of many bookstores over the past 5 years suggests to me that these are not the types of menopause books carried or promoted by many retail outlets that routinely service the lay public.

Popular portrayals in the visual media also reinforce a stereotypical view of the menopausal woman as being on an "emotional roller coaster" (Barbach, 1993, p. 27). This unfortunate creature is "exhausted, irritable, unsexy, hard to live with, irrationally depressed, and unwillingly suffering a 'change' that marks the end of her active (re) productive life" (Lindemann, 1983, p. 103). In television shows and movies, women and their partners never actually sit down and discuss the realities of the climacteric changes that *both* experience as they age. Rather, there is an "inference" that the woman is going through "the change" or "that time of life," and that this is a difficult and tumultuous time for all concerned. And if having her hormones raging out of control is not enough to deal with, the midlife woman is also portrayed as grieving the departure of her children from the "nest" (irrespective of any other form of productive labor she may be engaged in). For example, in an episode of the television show *Picket Fences,* Joan, a family physician and once the town mayor, is portrayed as going through erratic fits of temper (throwing plates, screaming at her husband and children, dismissing the complaints of her elderly patients, etc.). As the story unfolds in stereotypical fashion, we learn that the onset of menopause, combined with the realization that her motherhood role is almost over (her youngest child is turning 13—the "empty nest") is responsible for this emotional upheaval and crisis in her identity as a woman and as a mother.

The power of the media in shaping women's expectations and experiences of menopause was underscored in a 1980 study by Kaufert (cited in Voda & Eliasson, 1983), of the help-seeking behavior of menopausal women between the ages of 40 and 60 years old. In this study, 83% of the respondents said they relied most heavily on popular books and magazine articles, rather than the advice of their physicians, for information and guidance on what to expect during menopause. They turned to these sources to learn how best to cope with menopausal symptoms. Twelve years later, similar results were reported by Mansfield, Theisen, and Boyer (1992). Of the 515 women between the ages of 35 and 55 years in this study, few women said that they had, or would, consult their health care providers for information about menopause. Rather, the majority relied on the "truths" contained within popular books, magazines, and television shows to help them prepare for, understand, and cope with their reactions to this transition.

It would be inaccurate to suggest that midlife women are passive recipients of the messages of the media. Many women manage to tease out some valuable information from the more balanced and informative books or articles that are available. However, it is difficult to completely disregard the overt and covert messages suggesting that menopause is associated with emotional instability and physical decline, that it is a "condition" that requires attention or intervention in terms of drugs, diet, and lifestyle changes.

SECRET SHAME: MESSAGES OF SIGNIFICANT OTHERS

Popular writer Gail Sheehy (1992) refers to menopause as *The Silent Passage*—a transition shrouded in secrecy. Greer (1991) says the menopausal woman "simply has to tough it out and pretend that nothing is happening" (p. 35). Women sometimes feel shame about experiencing this inevitable biological process. This is apparent in the euphemistic language women often use in reference to menopause (e.g., "change of life," "the change"). It is also reflected in the discomfort many women feel in discussing and sharing their menopausal expectations and experiences with significant others, including family members and friends (Roberts et al., 1992). For women to communicate openly with others in their lives about their menopause would be to acknowledge that they, too, now share the stigma of having reached this physiological and social crossroads.

Family members also internalize the largely negative social perceptions of menopause that have been discussed throughout this chapter. They are often guilty of communicating messages to menopausal women that reinforce the medical model of menopause as deficiency, and menopausal women as being held hostage to their diminishing hormones (Sheehy, 1992; Weideger, 1978). In most families, it is likely that menopause is not a regular topic of dinner conversation. However, inferences are nonetheless made within families attributing the behaviors and emotional reactions of midlife women to "the change." The hormonal fluctuations during menopause can serve as a catch-all explanation for any actions on the part of "women of a certain age" (Rubin, 1979) that are not considered desirable or acceptable by significant others. The comments of several of the young women in Martin's (1987) study reflect such perceptions: "Mom almost went berserk. I don't mean she really did, but it was hard." "Watching my mother go through that, I think that is why she is kind of whacko" (p. 174).

I, too, can recall chiding my mother (who had been propelled into a medical menopause in her mid-30s through an emergency hysterectomy) about it being time for her to visit her doctor to "get her shot" of estrogen. We each resorted to such diminutive comments whenever mom seemed a bit "out of sorts" or "bitchy," or whenever she was not being the ever-available, self-effacing, nurturant caretaker we had all come to expect her to be. The fact that she was raising three teenage daughters, working part-time nights in a neonatal nursery, and always living under the burden of insufficient money to "make ends meet" seemed lost on all of us, including my father, at the time. Rather, menopause was a much more acceptable rationale for her frustration and discontent.

Women's male partners may also not be a great source of support, acceptance, or understanding during menopause. Research confirms that men's attitudes toward menopause generally reflect the stereotypical cultural perceptions of this event as a major life "crisis" for women. For example, in a study of men and women's perceptions toward menopause, Bowles (1986) reported that the attitudes of the 180 middle-aged men toward menopause were significantly more negative than those of a group of 18- to 86-year-old women. Similar to the findings of other researchers (Golub, 1992; Martin, 1987; Neugarten, Wood, Kraines, & Loomis, 1968), the younger women in this study held much more negative perceptions of the menopausal transition than the older women who were experiencing menopause or were postmenopausal. The attitudes of the male respondents, however, were considerably even *more negative* than those of the *younger* women in the study.

Sheehy (1992) also cites the results of a 1991 Gallup poll commissioned by a company that manufactures estrogen-replacement patches. In this study, "one in four of the seven hundred women ages forty to sixty expressed concern about menopause, but two thirds of the middle-aged husbands were bothered about it" (p. 90). Specifically,

> two thirds of the husbands of premenopausal women expressed fears that their sex lives would be compromised by having a wife in menopause. A majority of the men married to women in the transition focused on the emotional impact on their wives, saying they manifested anxiety, irritability, and mood swings. Fewer than half the men took any notice of physical problems that underlay these emotional reactions . . . hot flashes, night sweats, and difficulty sleeping. (p. 91)

Interestingly, menopause was a convenient scapegoat/rationale for understanding and interpreting their wives' disagreeable behaviors. Many of these men were reluctant at best to admit openly that their wives were actually in menopause. To do so would have been to admit that they, too, were getting older.

So to whom, then, can midlife women turn to seek information and advice? With whom can women candidly and freely discuss their apprehensions, concerns, and experiences related to the menopausal transition, without fear of being shamed and judged? Ideally, we might expect that women might turn to their own mothers, or to other women as allies in this shared reality. Indeed, Choi (1995) suggests that

> mothers typically serve as the primary messengers of menopause for their daughters. Early views of menopause frequently emerge from women's recollections of their mothers' attitudes and responses surrounding this event. When mothers are pereceived to have gone through menopause without problems, daughters express that they are more ready to accept it as a natural life cycle event. (p. 56)

Unfortunately, however, many women indicate that they have little or no actual knowledge about their own mothers' menopausal experiences. Most are unaware of how their mothers negotiated the menopausal transition (Golub, 1992; Mansfield et al., 1992; Martin, 1987). Just as most women are reluctant to share the details of their sexual lives and activities with their mothers, menopause also appears to be a taboo subject between many mothers and daughters. The largely negative social meanings associated with menopause, and women's feelings of shame in undergoing this stigmatized process, often precludes such open communication between mothers and daughters, and between women and their peers (Greer, 1991; Page, 1993; Sheehy, 1992).

It would appear that just as many men hate to admit that their wives have reached this time in life, many women are reluctant to acknowledge that they are undergoing a process that is commonly associated with physical decline and emotional instability (Choi, 1995). Martin (1987) talks about the extensive attempts women in her study reported going to in order to "hide" their menopausal symptoms. She noted the "embarrassment" many felt when experiencing hot flashes. A rather striking example of this was relayed to me recently in a conversation with a 50-year-old colleague. She is currently undergoing the menopause transition and has been experiencing increasingly intense hot flashes and night sweats over the past 6 months. While having lunch recently with two of her close friends, both academically accomplished women who are in their late 40s, she disclosed that she was experiencing the symptoms of menopause. She asked if either of her friends had noticed any similar symptomatic changes, and inquired as to how they were handling them. She was quite "taken aback" by the responses of these well-educated and "enlightened" women. Both were quick to reply that they "absolutely were *not* going through *that* yet, thank God!" The focus of the conversation quickly returned to university politics. Ironically, this topic was obviously less emotionally loaded than menopause. My colleague reported feeling that she had somehow identified herself in this interaction as some kind of pariah from which her friends clearly wanted to dissociate themselves.

The women who participated in my research group on women's sexuality reported similar experiences (Daniluk, 1993). They talked about their comfort in sharing the intimate details of their personal and sexual lives with their women friends. Menopause, however, was a much more taboo subject. Consistent with the results of the study discussed by Mansfield et al. (1992) those who had experienced menopause said that they had learned about menopause through books and articles. None had openly discussed their experiences with other women. Those in the group that had yet to undergo menopause expressed similar discomfort in accessing information about "the change," either from their physicians or from other women.

It is important to note that while participating in this research group, the younger women and those just entering into this transition were able to express their fears and apprehensions, and ask questions about menopause, most for the first time. The postmenopausal women in the group served as resources in sharing what they had experienced and learned about menopause. The women asked questions about managing the common symptoms associated with menopause. They expressed concerns about the psychological and emotional instability that purportedly accompanies this transition. Of particular concern to the women was the issue of estrogen replacement therapy. Most were anxious to find a way to tease out accurate information and make an "informed choice" about the risks associated with estrogen replacement therapy versus the risk of suffering from osteoporosis. The women were also concerned about metabolic changes that might result in further weight gain, and were distressed to learn that weight gain is a common side effect of hormone replacement therapy. As one woman said,

> "I feel like I'm in such a double bind. On the one hand, if I'm too thin, the books I've read tell me that I'm going to be more prone to osteoporosis, but on the other hand, if I take estrogen replacement, I'll put on weight, and I'll increase my risk of uterine cancer. So what am I suppose to do? I can't win either way."

The importance of open communication between women, and within their families, regarding the menopausal transition was repeatedly underscored by the women in the group. However, the difficulty these and other women appear to experience in accessing information, discussing menopause, and sharing their experiences with others speaks to the profound stigma associated with this normative transition.

SUMMARY: PROBLEMATIC MEANINGS

It is "difficult to predict how any *one* woman will experience the menopausal transition" (Leiblum, 1990, p. 497). As with any developmental transition, this process is complex. It involves the specific biological realities of each woman's experience. These, in turn, are linked to family history. They may involve minimal or severe symptomatic distress (Golub, 1992; Kaufert, 1986; Rostosky & Travis, 1996; Voda & Eliasson, 1983). As the levels of estrogen slowly decline in their bodies, it is safe to assume that most women will experience at least some of the characteristic symptoms associated with this process, most commonly hot flashes and night sweats. For an estimated 20% of women, the symptoms will be severe and debilitating enough to require some type of medical intervention (Cobb, 1988; Flint & Samil, 1990; Golub, 1992; Voda & Eliasson, 1983).

The literature reviewed earlier suggests that the menopause is a process that, similar to other transitions in a woman's life, is not without its challenges. It occurs during a time of considerable change and growth in women's lives (Baruch, 1984; Gergen, 1990; La Sorsa & Fodor, 1990; Mercer et al., 1988). As such, the experience of menopause is confounded by a host of other significant developmental hurdles, role transitions, and changing life circumstances. As Dowling (1996) notes, the midlife period is a veritable "whirlwind of change, loss, and growth." It is a period marked by a sense of "urgency, a feeling of challenges to be hurdled, and maybe even drastic steps that need to be taken." It is a time when women are confronted with "the fact of aging, the possibility of illness, the onset of limitations . . . the gut-level acknowledgment of mortality—our parents', and our own" (pp. 10–11). It is often difficult, then, to know how much of what a woman experiences during midlife can be attributed to menopause, and how much to the other realities of her changing life. Clearly, they are all connected.

We do know, however, that for many women, the thought of entering menopause at best engenders feelings of ambivalence. More commonly, it is met with feelings of fear, trepidation, and sometimes dread (Gannon, 1994; Martin, 1987). It would appear that many women facing menopause perceive the losses associated with this unheralded "rite of passage" to be substantially greater than the gains. Menopause means far more to women than merely the end of menstruation (Choi, 1995). Negative expectations are particularly pronounced for younger women who have yet to experience the physical changes that signal the onset of menopause (Neugarten et al., 1968; Theisen, Mansfield, Voda, & Seery, cited in Golub, 1992). A menopause taboo appears to shape the perceptions of women, particularly young women. Many women equate the cessation of their monthly cyclicity with *endings*—the end of their womanhood, femininity, desirability, and in some cases, their sanity. These sentiments are understandable given the largely negative messages women receive in North American culture regarding menopause and the aging process (Choi, 1995).

How any woman experiences menopause involves each woman's particular constellation of psychological needs and disposition, the strength of her self-structure, and the degree to which her identity is based on her fertility (Barbach, 1993; Ireland, 1993; Lisle, 1996; Rubin, 1979). Being a social experience, menopause involves the specific economic, role, and relationship circumstances of each woman's life (Apter, 1995; McGoldrick, 1989). Adaptation to this transition will also be dependent upon the personal and symbolic meanings menopause holds for each woman. It will be contingent upon the degree to which she is able to reject the largely negative social meanings of menopause promoted in North American culture (i.e., loss of womanhood, youth, sexuality, fertility, usefulness, control, memory, sanity, health), and to construct more positive and affirming meanings.

CHALLENGE AND CHANGE: CREATING NEW MEANINGS

If women are to successfully negotiate this biological and social transition, it is necessary for them to look "outside their reproductive role" and find "meaning in life which is not restricted by biology" (Ussher, 1989, p. 132). There are many ways that mental health professionals can assist women in accessing information and resources, breaking the silence, coping with the changes, challenging cultural meanings, and creating new meanings related to menopause. "We need to listen carefully to what our clients at menopause are telling us about their . . . concerns. It is crucial to presume neither that they will sail through menopause nor that they will experience severe distress" (Cole, 1988, p. 167). It is important that we familiarize ourselves with the woman-positive physicians and medical services that are available within our communities, and assist women in accessing these services when necessary. Women may also benefit from information and education on menopause, including more holistic methods of managing this transition (see Appendix G).

It is important to help clients explore the personal and symbolic meanings they hold regarding menopause, and to help them work through and perhaps grieve the losses that are associated with this transition. We need to help normalize the menopausal transition and assist women in understanding their experiences and perceptions of menopause within the context of the other significant changes in their lives. Within the safety of the counseling relationship, and in the company of other women, we need to encourage women to explore and confront their fears, attitudes, and expectations regarding menopause, and help them separate the myths from the reality of this transition.

We also need to explore and challenge our own attitudes and assumptions about menopause. We too, are products of our socialization and cannot help but carry some of this baggage into our counseling. We need to

> publicize the fact that life does not end at forty, so that younger women do not approach these years with dread. We need to challenge the stereotypes which define women as useless when their reproductive function is ended. Ageist and sexist stereotypes . . . which reinforce the negative images of older women, must be continuously criticized and challenged. Positive images of older women, realistic and positive role models, must replace those which are currently available and which do so much damage. (Ussher, 1989, p. 132)

As with menstruation, childbirth, and infertility, we need to "take menopause out of the closet" (Page, 1993, p. 1) so-to-speak, by helping women to name and own their menopausal experiences without shame or apology (e.g., Goldsworthy, 1993; Sand, 1993; Taetzsch, 1995). Martin (1987) suggests that

> women are asked to do what is nearly impossible: keep secret a part of their selves that they cannot help but carry into the public realm and that they often wear blatantly on their faces. Resistance in the case of menopause . . . consists in the occasions when women publicly name their state, claiming its right to exist as part of themselves in the public realm. (p. 177)

We need to help women to challenge and resist negative cultural meanings and imperatives, and to create their own, more affirming meanings and rituals around the menopausal transition. In essence, we need to help women *reclaim* menopause.

> It is time for women to reclaim menstruation and menopause. Each day one of these cycles is part of our lives; yet we live with a male idea of how we ought to feel about them. We may clasp the earth mother to our breasts and proclaim the beauty of menopause and the marvel of menstruation, but this is no more necessary than hanging on to the witch who bears a curse. Somewhere between the goddess and the demon is the menstruating woman and after her the woman at menopause—living women with cycles of life not experienced by men, different and equal. (Weideger, 1978, p. 248)

The exercises and interventions that follow are examples of ways that mental health professionals may begin to meet these goals. These may be undertaken in individual counseling, although menopausal issues may be best addressed in groups. Several writers (e.g., Heilburn, 1988; Noble, 1990) have noted the power of women's stories and the importance of sharing these with other women. Indeed, Noble notes how women "need to hear the stories of other women . . . to appreciate the complexity and profundity of their own lives, to know that they are not alone, and to realize that their ability to face the pain and darkness in their lives is a heroic act evidencing strength, not weakness" (p. 17).

As with other uniquely female issues, within the safety of a group, women can begin to name their experiences and explore their fears. Groups can help reduce the shame and isolation that is so much a part of the menopause experience for women in our culture. They can help provide a positive setting within which women can reframe the menopause and their middle years in ways that are meaningful for them (Ussher, 1989, 1992b). Like the consciousness-raising groups of the 1970s, women's groups provide a rich forum in which participants can be the experts and authors of their own lives—sharing information and knowledge, and serving as role models for each other. As Choi (1995) notes, "As their own menopause grows closer, women begin to pay increasing attention to the responses and behavior or other women who are or have been menopausal. They may seek out older role models who cope with menopause and aging gracefully and healthfully" (p. 57).

In referring to her own midlife transition, Dowling (1996) underscores the importance of other women in her growth and development. "More and more, I turn to women for succor and guidance, for their special humor and down-to-earth willingness to look life in the eye" with "wit, wisdom, and inventiveness" (p. 12). The exercises discussed here are meant to assist women in "looking menopause in the eye." They are aimed at creating more affirming meanings and rituals to mark the significance of this transition in women's lives. Readers are also directed to Ahsen's (1996) paper for a detailed discussion and numerous examples of the use of imagery interventions when working with women's menopausal concerns. Books by Page (1993) and Cobb (1993) provide some excellent suggestions on coping with and working through the physical, social, and emotional responses of women to menopause. Some may also find the work of Drake (1992) and Noble (1990) useful in their work on this and other issues with midlife and older women. The focus of these writers is on guiding the female hero on her quest for healing and wholeness.

Exploring the Myths and Meanings of Menopause

Before we can begin to challenge the myths, stereotypes, and false expectations that women hold about menopausal changes, it is necessary to explore what myths they hold. There are many ways to do this. One that I have found useful is to have women brainstorm about their "worst fears" about the menopause. We can encourage women, individually or within a group, to identify all of the negative things that they have heard about what happens to women's bodies, minds, and sex lives during menopause. Initially, women laughingly begin with comments about "drying up," "getting fat and hairy," and "having hot flashes." As the exercise proceeds, however, they start to identify their deeper fears and concerns about "going crazy," "becoming frail," "getting osteoporosis," and becoming "old," "unattractive," and "sexually undesirable." The number of concerns and fears raised by women is often quite substantial. Sometimes they include a few dozen items. It is important to have women, either in pairs or in individual counseling, explore the common sources of these myths. They need to examine how they came to know about and believe these things about menopause. They need to identify the source of these messages (from family members, friends, magazines, the medical profession, etc.).

It is important to challenge any faulty attributions concerning the etiology of particular symptoms, such as depression or mood swings. We need to help women locate menopause within a larger social context, and to understand their menopausal experiences within the context of their own lives. Having completed this part of the exercise, counselors can then ask participants to brainstorm about the positive aspects of menopause. They can be asked to indicate the things that they have heard and experienced themselves, or that they anticipate. In stark contrast to the "negatives" list, the "positive side of menopause" list is generally significantly shorter and is often limited to "the end of periods," and "no more risk of pregnancy."

It is important to take this opportunity to educate women about the realities of the menopause and the frequency and intensity of common menopausal concerns such as hot flashes and night sweats. It may also be useful to provide information on the physical and social management of these symptoms should they occur. For example, the midlife women in Martin's (1987) study expressed tremendous embarrassment when they experienced hot flashes, particularly when these occurred in their work environments. As well as providing them with information on possible remedies for common menopausal symptoms, women can role-play ways that they might cope with social or work situations that they find especially uncomfortable. Also, as Kitzinger (1985) points out, hot flashes can be reframed as something quite attractive and distinctly female:

> A hot flush can look very attractive. . . . I like the rosy glow. . . . [It is] life-enhancing. Once you can think positively about a hot flush, the sensations experienced may change their quality too. Each flush is wave-like, rather like a contraction in labour, or like a wave of sexual feeling sweeping through the body. It is possible to go with it rather than against it or trying to pretend it is not happening. (p. 234)

This and other types of cognitive restructuring can be helpful in relabeling menopausal symptoms as another part of women's cyclicity (Ussher, 1989, 1992b).

In countering negative myths, women can be encouraged to generate more ideas on the positive aspects of menopause. They can be asked to consider and explore the ways that menopause might actually liberate, rather than constrain, women. In fact, a useful exercise is to ask women to seek out and talk to a family member or acquaintance whose menopause was at least a neutral, if not a positive, experience. This type of dialogue can help to counter the predominantly negative menopausal messages, and can provide a more optimistic role model for negotiating this transition. For example, one woman was quite affected by the way her mother spoke about having had hot flashes during her menopause. Rather than being irritating or problematic, she said that the hot flashes she experienced during the menopause were like "wonderful waves" that swept over her, leaving her feeling warm and peaceful.

It is also important to encourage women to explore the source of their fears and concerns related to menopause and their middle years. These fears often have their genesis in women's own families of origin, and in particular, in the menopausal experiences of the women in their families (mothers, grandmothers, aunts, etc.) (Martin, 1987). It can prove to be quite enlightening when women are asked to recall the messages they received in their families about menopause, from the women in their families (mothers, grandmothers, aunts, etc.), and also from the men (fathers, grandfathers, etc.). It is particularly useful for women to revisit their mothers' and even their grandmothers' menopausal experiences, and to examine their own perceptions of these (first through the eyes of the child or adolescent they were when this occurred, and then through the eyes of the adult woman they are now). Helping women to view and discuss their mothers' experience of menopause within the larger context of their mothers' lives is also important. When possible, it can be very facilitative for women to talk directly with their mothers (or the other significant older women in their lives) about their menopause experiences and the particular circumstances of their lives at that time.

It is also important to help menopausal women examine both the *social* meanings of menopause in our culture and their own *personal* meanings. The larger group setting is often an excellent venue for exploring the social meanings of menopause. Tools such as the creation of collages or the review of books or film clips can facilitate some very animated discussion about the way menopausal women are depicted in the media and treated by the medical profession. The virtual absence of menopausal women in the popular media, or their portrayal as comic and pathetic figures (Weideger, 1978) becomes readily apparent. It is also useful to ask women to discuss the meanings of menopause in their particular cultures and subcultures. Information about the menopausal beliefs and experiences of women in other cultures can help highlight how the meanings of menopause, the frequency of reported symptoms, and, subsequently, women's attitudes toward this experience vary considerably between cultures. In particular, women can begin to appreciate that although menopause is a biological event, there is no one pattern or profile to this experience. Rather, they learn that the experience of menopause is shaped significantly by the social and cultural context within which it occurs.

The *personal* meanings of menopause held by any woman are based on her past and present experiences, as well as on her future hopes and expectations and whether these will likely be fulfilled. For example, for a woman who wanted to have children but was unable to, menopause may signify the end of her hopes and dreams of becoming a mother. For a woman who watched her mother plunge into a deep midlife depression, menopause may be associated with incapacitation and despair. For a woman whose father left her midlife mother for a younger woman, thoughts of menopause may engender fear of being abandoned and discarded. And for a woman who watched her mother "come into her own" during her middle years and lead a vibrant and full life, menopause may be filled with promise and opportunity. Each woman's personal history combines with her present needs and future desires to create unique meanings of menopause. These meanings inevitably shape her experience of this transition. Counselors can play a very useful role by helping women explore these personal meanings. This can be done through art, metaphors, journaling, guided autobiography, or narrative review. When menopause is associated with losses and imbued with negative meanings, women should be assisted in grieving these losses. Rituals can be very helpful in letting go of past hopes, expectations, or self-perceptions. As with other life circumstances, experiences of loss can precipitate experiences of tremendous gain. Women should be encouraged to consider the ways that menopause may be a positive experience in their lives (e.g., it may serve as a benchmark event that is forcing them to revision themselves and their lives; it may help them achieve closure on issues related to childbearing).

Breaking the Silence

When an event as significant as menopause is shrouded in secrecy, as it is in North American culture, it can have even more power in oppressing and controlling women's lives. Greer (1991) refers to the pressure already brought to bear "upon the middle-aged woman to make herself inconspicuous" (p. 33). This pressure is particularly strong relative to menopause and the signs of aging. And with secrecy, there is always the undertone and inference of shame—of something being so disdainful that it cannot be spoken about openly (Karen, 1992). Indeed Barbach (1993) notes how

> it is only when hidden in secrecy that it becomes something to be feared.

> . . . Our culture needs education about menopause. . . . We also can create a new image, one that projects how *we* feel about ourselves during this stage of life rather than how others have chosen to view us. If we do it well, we will open the way for our younger sisters and daughters, just as we did with the women's movement in the late 1960's and 1970's. (p. 208)

In incremental steps, women can be assisted to begin to speak their truths about menopause and about the significance of this event in their lives. It is important to create safe and nonjudgmental forums within which women can openly share their fears and concerns about menopause (e.g., individual or couple counseling; women's menopause support groups). Within these settings, women can be encouraged to share their concerns and experiences, using woman-affirming language rather than the language of pathology. For example, women can be encouraged to replace the words menopausal "symptom(s)" with words such as menopausal "response" or "experience." In a fun and energizing exercise, women can be encouraged in fact to play with language, and to create their own menopause vocabulary and definitions. For example, Page (1993) refers to a short story in which author Margaret Atwood refers to menopause as "a time in which we pause to reconsider men." On a similar note, sex therapist Lonnie Barbach (1993) removed men entirely from the word menopause in titling her book *The Pause.* Emphasizing the hard-earned wisdom that comes with age and experience, one client redefined menopause as the "mental pause." Still another woman drew on the goddess literature in defining menopause as being in "the full moon" of her life cycle. Individually or within a group, women can be encouraged to rename and create new language to describe hot flashes, night sweats, even vaginal dryness—all common aspects of women's menopausal experiences.

Women should also be encouraged to talk to other women about their expectations and experiences of menopause. They can become spokeswomen for a more realistic and positive view of menopause. It is not necessary to deny the difficulties that some women experience in negotiating this transition to still promote midlife and menopause as a time of opportunities and possibilities rather than decline. Women can begin by identifying and seeking out one other woman with whom they feel comfortable talking about menopause. Step-by-step, over time, they can expand their circle to include other women and men in these discussions. And when in the company of others, women can be encouraged to talk about their menopausal experiences and reactions without shame. They can refuse to be co-conspirators in maintaining the menopause taboo. They can refuse to comply with having their feelings and behaviors attributed to their menopausal status.

Weathering the Storm

Estrogen levels begin to decline for most women in their early to mid-40s. This process continues until the cessation of their menses around the age of 51 (Golub, 1992). While the degree of discomfort varies from one woman to the next, most women can expect to experience some physical and psychological responses during this process. These are often relatively imperceptible and unobtrusive for several years. Generally, they become increasingly more noticeable during the final years of the menopause. For women whose menopause has been surgically induced, the symptoms are often more immediate and severe (Boston Women's Health Collective, 1992).

It is important to reframe menopause in positive and accepting terms and to "validate" this process as a normative part of women's reproductive lives. However, it is also critical that we do not dismiss women's legitimate discomfort and concerns. Some women experience up to 30 hot flashes per day. Some find that memory lapses impair their work performance. The lives of others are disrupted by the fatigue of continual sleep interruptions caused by night sweats. For these women, there is little comfort in being reassured that this is a "normal" part of being a woman. There is little relief in being encouraged to "tough it out" because "this too will pass." Rather, as several therapists and writers point out (e.g., Cobb, 1988; Cole, 1988; Kitzinger, 1985; Leiblum, 1990), we need to be aware of the common physical concerns of menopausal women. We also need to help women weather the storm by finding some symptomatic relief.

In some cases, this may mean providing information and referrals for medical intervention. As noted in Chapter 11, the current treatment of choice for women who do not have a family history of breast or reproductive cancer, or a history of high blood pressure and hypertension, is hormone-replacement therapy (HRT). Although women need to be apprised of the possible risks involved in HRT, it is important that counselors support women' choices if they turn to medical solutions to ease their discomfort. It is important to validate each woman's right to make the choices that are best for her. Women should not be made to feel that they have somehow "failed" either themselves or other women by choosing HRT (a parallel to this is the experience of many women who were unable to manage childbirth "naturally" and often felt tremendous residual guilt in having turned to drugs to ease their pain). In terms of education, it is also important when working with menopausal women to provide information in the form of handouts, pamphlets, and books (see Appendix G). Psychoeducation within a group format may include guest speakers who can teach women about various approaches to managing their menopause, such as herbal preparations (oil of primrose, don quay, chasteberry, etc.), nutritional suggestions (decreasing sugar and caffeine, increasing carbohydrates, etc.), exercise (yoga, walking, etc.), and so on. Information on osteoporosis is also an important part of women's menopausal preparations and decision making.

Endings and New Beginnings

Menopause marks an irrevocable change in the lives of women. Although that change heralds new beginnings, it also involves endings. Like all transitions, it involves losses as well as gains. Before we ask women to turn optimistically toward the future, it is often necessary to assist them in gaining closure on the past. Whatever their personal meanings of menopause, biologically, the end of menstruation marks the end of their fertility—literally and symbolically. It also marks the end of a woman's cyclicity. Irrespective of how a woman has come to feel about her periods, it is important to mark this ending. One way counselors may assist in this process is to ask women to write a narrative of their reproductive lives and to identify the predominant themes. They might begin with puberty and progress through their adult years until menopause, identifying their reproductive "accomplishments" and "joys" (e.g., regular cycles, sense of femininity and continuity with other women, pregnancy and childbirth) as well as their "pains" and "sorrows" (e.g., pregnancy loss, infertility, hysterectomy). For some, this might involve using a "lifeline" and writing a chronology of the significant events (or nonevents) in their reproductive lives. For others, it may take the form of a metaphorical story or journey. For example, the central theme in one client's story was one of "awe" and "wonder" at the experience of birthing her daughters (and symbolically herself). For another woman who had anticipated having children, but who never found a partner with whom she wanted to parent, the central theme of her story was "lost opportunity." For one voluntarily childless woman, the theme was one of "connection." Her story reflected her belief that her monthly cyclicity connected her in a fundamental way to other women and to the earth. For another woman, whose periods were always very problematic, the primary thread running through her story was of menstrual "tension" and "distress." Rather than writing narratives, some women may elect to paint pictures or write poems about their reproductive lives and experiences, or the passing of their cyclicity. Some might relate their stories through dance or music. Guided autobiography can also be an excellent vehicle for women to explore their reproductive milestones and the meanings of these in their lives. Using sensitizing questions to elicit autobiographical recollections, women can be assisted in identifying the salient themes related to their reproductive functioning, experiences, and histories (see Birren, 1987, and de Vries, Birren, & Deutchman, 1990, for examples of using and applying this technique). Whatever the modality women choose, this type of review often proves to be a powerful experience. Recounting this significant part of their female lives, complete with its joys and pains (and sharing this with other women if a group format is used), can be a very validating, and in some cases, healing process.

On an individual level, and based on their responses to the earlier exercise involving the personal meanings of menopause, women may find that the losses that they need to grieve are not reproductive losses. Rather, some may grieve the loss of youth. For women who have experienced illness, injury, or disability during midlife, their grief may be over the loss of their sense of themselves as they once were—healthy, vital, energetic, whole. For example, Bullard and Knight (1981) note how women with disabilities such as spinal cord injuries, or women who have had colostomies or mastectomies, need to grieve the loss of the self they once were. This is an important precursor to constructing and embracing a new sense of themselves as whole and vital.

Menopause may serve as a significant marker of the ending of life roles as well (e.g., for women who are now divorced and those whose adult children have moved on to their own lives). Menopause can mean many things to women. Each woman's unique history serves as the backdrop upon which her menopausal experience is painted. Helping women to acknowledge and grieve their actual and symbolic losses, as well as identifying and celebrating the gains, is an important part of the work of letting go and moving on at midlife (Barbach, 1993; Greer, 1991; Sheehy, 1992; Unger & Crawford, 1992).

Women should also be encouraged to create rituals to mark their passing into the next stage of their lives. In concluding her book *The Beauty Myth,* Wolf (1991) contends that "we need new and positive, rather than negative, celebrations to mark the female lifespan" (p. 279). In specific reference to menopause, Greer (1991) notes that although "there is no public rite of passage for the woman approaching the end of her reproductive years, there is evidence that women devise their own private ways of marking the irrevocability of the change" (p. 5). Mental health professionals can help menopausal women to construct rituals that acknowledge the personal significance of this part of their lives. For women who have experienced reproductive losses, this may involve facilitating closure (visiting the grave of a lost child; having the frozen embryos that have been kept in storage disposed of; writing a letter to an unborn child). Rituals such as these are often about making peace with oneself, with nature, with one's God. They can be powerful tools to help women move forward (Anton, 1992; Daniluk, 1991a).

For women who are delighted to be done with the "hassles and mess" of their periods, their ritual may be as simple as burning a box of "sanitary" pads or tampons. For women who relished their reproductive capacity, this may involve a ritual that helps them celebrate their creativity and its continuance in their lives in other forms (e.g., through their grandchildren, in their work). Women may wish to select a favored older woman to witness and participate in their ritual. Or they may share this passage with other women of a similar age who are important in their lives. They may mark this passage with a ceremonial dinner, a weekend retreat, or some other ritual that is personally meaningful to them. For example, my 40th birthday was marked by spending the weekend with my three closest childhood friends. Although our lives had gone in very different directions, we nonetheless had shared the most intimate details of our adolescent and young adult lives together. We all turned 40 the same year and came together from different corners of the country. We took up residence at a cottage on the beach, where we shared photos of our youth and stories of our parents and siblings. We laughed and cried as we recounted the adventures of our youth, and left at the end of the weekend feeling a sense of completeness and connection. Through this experience, each of us could better appreciate the continuity of our past and present lives. We plan to meet again to mark our 50th year. At that time, we will no doubt revisit the past and commiserate on the future, amid our sharing of remedies for hot flashes and vaginal dryness. The possibilities for marking the important phases of any woman's life are limited only by a client's own creativity.

Counselors might also note how the creation of a ritual can be very a significant way to conclude their individual work with a midlife client, or to end a menopause group. After sharing their fears and expectations together, and having borne witness to each other's pain and joy, a group ritual can be a powerful way to bring closure to this work (Page, 1993).

Taking Stock and Moving On

Menopause can also be a time of taking stock and making important decisions about what a woman wants her future to look like (Apter, 1996). It is a time of

> discarding the shell of the reproductive self—who came into being in adolescence—and coming out the other side to *coalescence*. (*Coalesce* means "to come together," "to unite"; *essence* denotes "action or process," a change state.) It is a time when all the wisdom a woman has gathered from fifty years of experience in living comes together. Once she is no longer confined to the culture's definition of woman as a primarily sexual object and breeder, a full unity of her feminine and masculine sides is possible. As she moves beyond gender definition, she gains new license to speak her mind and initiate action. (Sheehy, 1992, p. 135)

It can be an opportunity to redefine oneself. It can be a chance to "dig deep into one's character to discover what is most real, most enduring." It can be a chance to construct or affirm one's "life in a way that would give prominence to that deeper sense of self" (Dowling, 1996, p. 15). Based on her interviews with over 100 midlife women, Sheehy (1992) concludes that "how—or if—one *welcomes* postmenopause, and consciously prepares for the new freedom it offers, makes all the difference in reaping the benefits of the stages beyond" (p. 143). Menopause marks the end of an important part of each woman's life. Yet it can also be the "start of a new life . . . a stage of expansiveness or withdrawal. It [can] be a time of introversion or of worldly adventure" (Bateson, cited in Sheehy, 1992, p. 143).

> We have a second chance in postmenopause, unencumbered by the day-to-day caregiving and thousand and one details of feeling that most women put into the long parental emergency, to focus on the things we most love and to redirect our creativity in the most individual of ways. We must make an alliance with our changing bodies and negotiate with our vanity. No, we are never again going to be that girl of our idealized inner eye. The task now is to find a new future self in whom we can invest our trust and enthusiasm. (Sheehy, p. 136)

In some respects, the menopause for many women marks an opportunity to asses the past, reevaluate lost dreams, and make decisions about the future they want to create. Counselors can play an important role in facilitating this process by assisting women to "dig deep" into themselves at this crossroads in their lives. We can help them get in touch with who they are as women and as sexual persons, now that they are freer to act on their own needs and in their own self-interests. Individually or within a group, counselors can employ any number of affective exercises (e.g., life review, guided fantasy) to help women get in touch with the girls they were prior to their conscription into womanhood. Women can be assisted to reconnect with the abilities, hopes, and expectations that once filled their dreams and fueled their desires. They can be assisted in reevaluating the relevance and salience of their early motivations and dreams in light of their subsequent accomplishments and choices, and in consideration of their present life circumstances.

Some women may conclude this assessment with an overall sense of satisfaction and contentment with the choices they have made and the paths they have taken. They may feel no need to make significant changes in their lives. However, others may realize that they have lost touch with an important part of themselves. They may feel that the path they have forged has taken them too far afield from who they believed themselves to be, and what they hoped to accomplish in life. This realization may be met with shock and depression, or it may serve as a catalyst for change. Through this life review and assessment process, women may determine that to live more authentically and happily in the future, they must be true to themselves and make their own needs a priority (perhaps for the first time in their lives) (Dowling, 1996). For some, the awareness of "time running out" may create a sense of urgency—a "now or never" feeling. This may result in the instigation of significant life changes. As such, women may need for more in-depth work and ongoing support during this time of personal change and transition. Others may feel that it is "too late," and need help in realigning their goals and priorities, so that they are more realistic and attainable. For example, one very bright woman's early dreams of a career in the theater were subverted by an early pregnancy and subsequent marriage. She decided, at 52 years old, to take up acting, although she knew that this would not ensure her economic security in the years to come. However, 6 years later, at the age of 58, she has found a way to combine her love of acting with the necessity of earning a living. She puts her sewing skills to use in working as a costume designer, as well as acting in various local theater productions. In her words, "There isn't always a call for older women in the theater—but when there is, I'm there—and when I get a part, I just shine."

CONCLUSION

Sheehy (1992) suggests that "a great discovery of the fifties is the *courage to go against*—against conformist behavior and conventional wisdom" (p. 138), and against gender-role stereotypes. It seems appropriate to end this chapter on the menopause transition with a quote by one of the most prolific feminist writers. A passionate supporter of women's courage and entitlement to embrace their dreams and speak their own truths, Germaine Greer (1991) encourages menopausal women to

> let the Masters in Menopause congregate in luxury hotels all over the world to deliver and to hearken to papers on the latest astonishing discoveries about the decline of grip strength in menopause or the number of stromal cells in the fifty-year-old ovary, the woman herself is too busy to listen. She is climbing her own mountain, in search of her own horizon, after years of being absorbed in the struggles of others. The way is hard, and she stumbles many times, but for once no one is scrambling after her, begging her to turn back. The air grows thin, and she may often feel dizzy. Sometimes the weariness spreads from her aching bones to her heart and brain, but she knows that, when she has scrambled up this last sheer obstacle, she will see how to handle the rest of her long life. Some will climb swiftly, others will tack back and forth on the lower slopes, but few will give up. The truth is that fewer women come to grief at this obstacle than at any other in their tempestuous lives, though it is one of the stiffest challenges they ever face. Their behavior may baffle those who have unthinkingly exploited them all their lives before, but it is important not to explain, not to apologize. The climacteric marks the end of apologizing. The chrysalis of conditioning has once and for all to break and the female woman finally to emerge. (pp. 386–387)

13

THE FESTIVAL OF LIPID MIGRATION

Bodily Changes and Body Image

In this autumn of my being, parts of me
fly, like tossed and wintry-blasted leaves.
I don't regret their passing. I must work
to make a clean and crystal-perfect form.
I, alchemist, and I, philosopher's stone,
have sacrificed the fat, and froth, and fur
of youth, to walk through fire, leap in the dark,
swim inward rivers, pray at a wailing wall.
The wrinkles, sags, the graying hair are earned.
—HYACINTHE HILL, "Reaching toward Beauty"

Memorizing the seasons, I touch
things as if my fingers
will learn them
again; weary of explanations,
at midlife I am more comfortable
with the truth.

Outside, the mountain ash hangs
heavy with orange berries,
like overripe breasts they weight
the branches down; I feel
the tug, my flesh molding
itself to gravity; closer now
to the soil than ever
to the sky.
—SUSAN KATZ, "New Directions"

However healthy and vital the midlife woman may subjectively feel, the way she experiences and interprets the bodily changes inherent in the aging process must be understood within the context of our youth-oriented culture. While older men and women are both subjected to age discrimination, for women, ageism begins several decades earlier than for men (Ussher, 1989, 1992a, 1992b; Wolf, 1991). This appears to be particularly true in white cultures, where women are perceived as "over the hill" when they reach middle age (Banner, 1992). Referred to by Susan Sontag (1979) and others (e.g., Bell, 1989) as "the double standard of aging," North American society views the characteristic signs of aging much more harshly for middle-aged women than for men. Certainly,

> the prestige of youth afflicts everyone in this society to some degree. Men, too, are prone to periodic bouts of depression about aging . . . but men rarely panic about aging in the way that women often do. Getting older is less profoundly wounding for a man. . . . Society is much more permissive about aging in men. . . . Men are allowed to age, without penalty, in several ways that women are not. (p. 464)

The experience of aging represents the intersection of the biological and the social. The biological and physical changes associated with the climacteric and aging process are set against society's largely negative perceptions of the aging woman (Voda & Eliasson, 1983). As Sontag (1979) accurately points out, "Aging is much more a social judgment than a biological eventuality" (p. 466). Cultural values and beliefs about aging play a significant role in each woman's self-evaluations and perceptions of her aging body at midlife. For example, historian Lois Banner (1992) notes the differences in the perceptions of black culture toward midlife and older women. These women are viewed as active and forceful members of black society, irrespective of their size and the number of lines on their faces. This cultural acceptance lays the groundwork for much higher levels of self- and bodily acceptance among older black women.

It is from the vantage point of these socially held beliefs regarding the value of youth that women judge themselves. It is here that their meanings evolve. "Like sex, age has social meanings that transcend biology. Like gender, age is a social classification system . . . a system that organizes access to resources: age is connected to differences in power, prestige, and opportunities" (Unger & Crawford, 1992, p. 487). We turn now to the social context within which midlife women live out and attempt to make sense of their changing bodies. If we are to understand midlife women's feelings about, and attitudes toward their bodies, it is important to examine the messages promoted by the media, the beauty and fitness industries, and by significant others in a their lives.

FOREVER YOUNG: MEDIA MESSAGES

Research cited in the previous chapter suggests that older women also rely heavily on the written and visual media as sources of information against which they judge and make sense of their experiences (Mansfield et al., 1992). Women's magazines appear to be especially influential in shaping women's experiences and expectations "through providing mirror images for our judgement" (Ussher, 1989, p. 116). It is not just "traditional" magazines such as *Good Housekeeping* that reinforce an obsessive focus on size, shape, and appearance for women of all age groups. More "modern" women's magazines are also filled with advertisements and articles aimed at capitalizing on women's vulnerabilities about their aging bodies. For example, in recognition of the growing 40- and 50-something market, magazines such as *Cosmopolitan* are increasing their efforts to take advantage of the expendable income and insecurities of this segment of their readership (McMahon, 1996).

A quick review of this and other popular "women's" magazines suggests that many of the articles and the majority of advertisements are related to "products that enhance the physical attractiveness of women" (Rothblum, 1994, p. 84). And yet the reality is that images of older women are largely absent from these magazines. Rather, the attractive, blemish-free faces of *young* women stare out from the pages. They implicitly seduce the reader into thinking that if she purchases a particular product (e.g., facial cream, hair coloring, moisturizer), she, too, can look younger (like the model in the picture). Or the reader is presented with the image of an actress like Suzanne Summers. While clad in a little tank top and a pair of very short, shorts she extolls the virtues of the various machines aimed at shrinking the size of the thighs or tightening the muscles of the buttocks. The implicit message is that with the right equipment and enough self-discipline, even a middle-aged woman can look fabulous. As Leigh (1987) points out, "Wrinkles are not beautiful or sexy, Tina Turner is. Tina Turner is the living proof that in spite of our age we can (or rather should) be skinny, wrinkle free and have amazing legs especially if we 'look after ourselves,' and this is the catch, if we are not skinny and wrinkle free it's OUR fault" (p. 22). "On the few occasions when [older women] are not invisible by complete omission—they are exhorted to stay young and beautiful, to do things to their bodies to achieve this, and to wear make-up, hair products and clothes to conceal their real age" (Itzen, cited in Ussher, 1989, pp. 116–117).

The pervasive message promoted in virtually all forms of the media (*The Golden Girls* notwithstanding) is that a woman's most important asset is her appearance. Women are led to believe that without considerable energy being directed at preventing the march of time, aging will rob us of this. As a result,

> many middle-aged women have no clear idea of what it means to look one's age. Clothes, make-up, hair styles are all modelled for us on much younger women. By showing us that this is the way we are *supposed* to look, we are told, over and over, that age is an enemy to be conquered. This is to strengthen us for the battle but it also serves the purpose of

> emphasizing the horror of ageing—not only to women but to everyone else. It is implied that any middle-aged woman could look like this model, this actress, if only she *cared* enough. The truth is that the role models shown to us—ageing actresses or winners of cosmetic manufacturers' contests—are individuals who, by dint of exercise or cosmetic surgery or genetics (or all three), do not look their age. (Cobb, 1988, p. 157)

In their recent review of aging women in popular film, Bazzini, McIntosh, and Harris (1997) underscored how older women are largely "underrepresented" in this medium. Those that do appear are presented as "unattractive, unfriendly, and unintelligent" (p. 531). The only role models and images of "successful" aging that are presented in the media are the artificially/surgically constructed 50ish actresses like Jane Fonda, Cher, or Joan Collins. It should not be surprising, then, that middle-aged women might struggle to find a place of comfort and contentment with their aging bodies. It is understandable that women might labor to find a place between these extremes. The popular media sorely lack images that accurately reflect the diversity and range of shapes, sizes, colors, contours, and appearances that represent the physical realities of most middle-aged women. As such, it is difficult for women not to feel that they have somehow failed themselves, and others, when the images they see in the mirror do not resemble those celluloid images that they are bombarded with from television screens and newsstands on a daily basis.

HOURGLASS FIGURES, OR "TIME IS RUNNING OUT": MESSAGES OF THE BEAUTY INDUSTRY

The media reinforce feelings of insecurity and vulnerability in middle-aged women by misrepresenting or completely ignoring their reality. Similarly, the billion-dollar beauty industry—cosmetics, fitness, and diet—counts on women buying into the belief that they can, and should, make all efforts possible to retain a youthful figure and appearance. Rodeheaver and Stohs (1991) refer to this as a "culturally accredited set of rituals of rejuvenation." Women are seduced into believing that if we engage "in the appropriate symbolic behavior," we can gain "control over the phenomenon of aging." These include "wrinkle creams, calcium supplements, workouts, and implants" (p. 144). In an effort to maintain the appearance of youth, "women are exhorted to use magical creams to erase the lines of age, to wear restrictive corsets to hide the unattractive bulging flesh and, if all else fails, to submit to cosmetic surgery to rejuvenate [our] looks and return to a more youthful appearance" (Ussher, 1989, p. 118).

The beauty industry's continued success is contingent upon making their products palatable to the social consciousness of each new generation of women. It attempts to cater to the intelligence and maturity (and expendable income) of the current group of middle-aged women by presenting itself as being preoccupied not with "beauty" but with women's "health." Kilbourne (1994) notes how these products and services are not packaged as beauty "luxuries." Rather, they are promoted as "necessities" for every woman's health. For example, anti-aging creams are no longer endorsed primarily as a way to reduce wrinkles. They are now portrayed as necessary dermatological solutions to "repair" the damaging rays of the sun. Diet programs are no longer promoted for aesthetic reasons, but are currently being marketed as "nutritional education programs." These programs are aimed at reducing the amount of "bad" cholesterol and "fat" in our diets. Their purported goal is a reduction in the risk of heart disease. And exercise classes are no longer marketed as insurance against the effects of gravity. Instead, exercise regimes are promoted as essential for "cardiovascular fitness." These programs and preparations are frequently endorsed by megapersonalities such as Oprah Winfrey. After packing on all the weight she lost after a much publicized near-starvation diet, Oprah hired her own cook and full-time personal fitness consultant to help her lose weight more sensibly and really keep it off. "No more yo-yo dieting for her," she says, "only good nutrition and fitness." Paralleling the discourse of the 1990s, "deprivation" is clearly out and "wellness" (i.e., in the form of fiber and fitness) is in.

Certainly, attention to good health and nutrition are laudable pursuits at any stage of the life cycle, not just during midlife, when the effects of time and living become more overtly apparent. So, too, are efforts to protect the skin from the increasingly harmful effects of ultraviolet radiation. However, it has been convincingly argued by many writers and researchers (e.g., Fallon, 1990; Faludi, 1991; Kilbourne, 1994; Wolfe, 1991) that much of this marketing "hype" is motivated primarily by economics. Any improvements in the health and well-being of midlife women are only secondary gains. These and other writers argue that while the overt message may be one of good health, the "hidden agenda" is to capitalize on women's feelings of insecurity and shame about their aging bodies.

And yet women's insecurity can never truly be abrogated. However fervent midlife women may be in their efforts to ward off the signs of aging, they cannot possibly live up to the increasingly youthful standards of physical appearance.

> Women do not allow bristles to sprout freely or warts and wens to proliferate. Nevertheless the fifty-year-old woman knows that her body is not what it used to be. No matter how fit she is, or how flat her belly, her skin is thinner and less elastic, her muscle tone less firm. Estrogen replacement may slow down such changes, but it cannot stop them or undo them. (Greer, 1991, p. 302)

To the extent that women attempt to defy the laws of nature, they are destined to feel like beauty failures. In this way, any feelings of guilt and inadequacy they might have had are reinforced rather than being diminished. As Rodeheaver and Stohs (1991) point out, "The image of the older woman cannot be eliminated, because, try as we may, we cannot halt the aging process" (p. 144).

BETWEEN LOVERS: MESSAGES OF SIGNIFICANT OTHERS

Women are socialized in North America to fear the signs of aging and to interpret these as the passing of health and youth. Through a lifetime of training, most women, to a greater or lesser degree, learn to value physical attractiveness (Faludi, 1991; Ussher, 1989). Some argue that this is particularly true for heterosexual women, who must compete for the attention and affection of men. However, research suggests that lesbian women are also not immune to the effects of feminine socialization. Although they are generally not as preoccupied with their appearance as heterosexual women, lesbians report "greater concern with weight, more body dissatisfaction, and greater frequency of dieting than . . . gay or heterosexual men" (Brand, Rothblum, & Solomon, 1992, p. 253). Wooley (1994) questions "whether it is possible for women not to feel pathologically self-conscious" about their bodies and appearance, irrespective of their race, ethnicity, or sexual orientation. He questions whether it is possible for women to "ever feel comfortable with [their] bodies in a culture that is, on the one hand, flooded with idealized images of women's bodies; and, on the other hand, conditioned to see real (*really* real) women's bodies as being in need of change, repair, improvement, better 'health' " (p. 19).

Men, too, are influenced by the same cultural messages regarding the relationship between youth and attractiveness for women (Sontag, 1979). As mentioned earlier in this chapter, men are also subjected to discrimination based on ageism. However, the sexual "double standard" that Sontag refers to places the emphasis not on the middle-aged man's physical appearance, but on the appearance of his female partner. A man's ability to catch and hang on to an attractive woman is another testament to his success, irrespective of his own physical appearance. His status is socially enhanced by her beauty. As such, the antidote prescribed for a man's acknowledgment of his midlife reflection in the mirror is not necessarily diet, exercise, or plastic surgery. Rather, it is a youthful and attractive partner.

It is socially acceptable, and not uncommon, for a middle-aged man to enhance his own social status when he feels his current partner has not "aged well" by turning to a younger partner. The middle-aged woman, however, is not accorded this same privilege (Barbach, 1993; Kitzinger, 1985). It is not socially acceptable for an older woman to partner with a younger man. She does not gain in status or prestige. Nor does her younger partner. He, in fact, is seen to actually lose status by choosing to partner with an older woman (e.g., *Harold and Maud*). Her options are limited then. Kitzinger (1985) highlights this clear, sexual double-standard in her book *Woman's Experience of Sex*:

> A woman enters with a much younger attractive man. She is obviously in her fifties. . . . The man must be about 28. She is holding his hand across the table. Mother and son? The messages passing between their eyes are obviously erotic. This is an aging woman who has captured a much younger man. Disgusting! Or, perhaps, ridiculous. There is something almost obscene in thinking of that no longer young female body naked beside the young man's. (p. 238)

There is some evidence to indicate that midlife marks a point in our development where we are less influenced by the negative evaluations of others and more reliant on setting our own internal standards of acceptability (Apter, 1996; Baruch et al., 1983; Dowling, 1996; Greer, 1991; Kitzinger, 1985). However, the evaluations of intimate others still appear to be significant in shaping most women's self-perceptions. A woman may be in an intimate relationship with a partner who accepts and values her, irrespective of the extra few pounds she may be carrying around her stomach and hips, and in spite of the lines that are beginning to appear around her eyes and mouth. Her partner's acceptance will reinforce her own self-acceptance. Or she may currently be unpartnered and be content with seeing herself "through her own eyes" (Apter, 1996, p. 66). She may rely more on "her own judgments" (p. 72) of her middle-aged body and appearance.

However, if she is seeking a lover, or is in a relationship with someone who is subtly or overtly critical of her appearance, it will be more difficult for her to maintain a positive body image (Dowling, 1996; Tantleff-Dunn & Thompson, 1995). Research indicates that pressure from their intimate partners is instrumental in the motivations of many women who seek plastic surgery (Currie & Raoul, 1992). Women are led to believe that "a well-preserved older woman has a better chance of holding onto her husband than one who has 'let herself go' " (Bartky, 1990, p. 72). Some women may well feel that their efforts to preserve a youthful appearance are necessary prerequisites to ensuring the continuance of their intimate relationships.

BETWEEN WOMEN

A woman's reference group may also be very significant in the way she experiences and evaluates her appearance and her body during midlife.

Women friends, family members, and colleagues serve as role models for, and witnesses to, the way a woman adapts to, and makes sense of the bodily changes that accompany the aging process. These significant others also help women gather and organize information about how best to cope with these changes, whether to accept their inevitability and "age gracefully" (Rodeheaver & Stohs, 1991, p. 144), or whether to "fight aging every step of the way" (p. 143). "Other women are, after all, comrades in sharing the same potential for humiliation" (Sontag, 1979, p. 462). And, one might add, the same potential for enjoyment. As Choi (1995) notes, "Women learn about life experiences from watching other women. Those who are fortunate enough to be in the company of others who have a positive acceptance of aging are more likely to look forward to the experience" (p. 57).

The mother-daughter connection may be particularly significant in this regard. For example, men who are attempting to assess the long-term advisability of selecting a particular woman as a life partner are often jokingly advised to look at their wives' mother if they "want to know what she's going to look like when she gets older." Although there is a derogatory edge to this type of comment, it is common knowledge that genetics plays a role in how women (and men) weather the vicissitudes of time (Stevens-Long & Commons, 1992). From the age at which a woman's hair begins to grey, to the texture and tone of her skin, to the areas where she is more prone to put on weight, much is predetermined by her genetic endowment. When women perceive that their mothers have not fared well in response to the aging process, they may be less inclined to surrender to a similar fate. This point is brought home in the following words of a 46-year-old woman:

> "My mother looked haggard and worn out by the time she was 50. She really let herself go . . . She was overweight, tired, and wrinkled—to see her you would have thought that she was an old lady. And there is absolutely *no way* I'm going to let that happen to me. I don't care what it takes, diets, hair dyes, exercise—even if it means surgery. . . . I *refuse* to look old before my time!"

However, mothers may also serve as role models of successful aging, as in the case of the following 51-year-old woman:

> "My mother looked stunning well into her 70s. She was never a beautiful woman, and she certainly wasn't small or petite, by any means. In fact, by today's standards, you'd probably say she was overweight. But she was a strong and powerful figure. She always held herself upright and walked with dignity. She had her own style and took care of herself. She always looked and acted her age—and I always thought of her as beautiful. I always hoped I could pull it off

just like she did, that I could age as gracefully as my mother . . . and so far I think I'm doing OK, I feel good about how I look, and I don't feel like I have to live up to anyone else's standards, just my own."

The standards of acceptable appearance and behavior within a woman's reference group may also be influential in how she responds to, and copes with, the aging process. Each reference group has its own particular norms directing what is acceptable in terms of physical appearance for its membership. There are implicit and explicit norms about what measures are considered appropriate to meet these standards (Plummer, 1975, 1982; Weeks, 1985). For example, liposuction may be considered a very appropriate "solution" to the persistent problem of "saddle bags" for the socioeconomically advantaged, middle-aged, suburban homemaker. Friends and neighbors may be quick to recommend the "best" plastic surgeon or most effective weight-loss program. Cosmetic surgery would not likely be sanctioned, however, for members of a feminist, grassroots organization.

There are also norms among groups of women as to what constitutes "acceptable" reasons for pursuing particular solutions to women's dissatisfaction with their physical appearance. For example, certain types of plastic surgery may be considered more acceptable than other types, depending on the degree of disfigurement a woman is desiring to correct, and on whether "health" versus "vanity" appear to be motivating her decision. Plastic surgery to alter the effects of a mastectomy would likely be considered more acceptable among most groups of women than a "tummy tuck" or "face-lift." This point was brought home to me recently when a friend in her mid-50s told me that for Christmas she was "giving" herself the gift of a face-lift and tummy tuck. I found myself in a dilemma. I wanted to support her in a decision that she had not made lightly, and that I firmly believe is hers to make. Yet I also wanted to talk her out of the surgery based on my perception of her as already being a "beautiful" woman.

Rothblum (1994) talks about the norms for physical appearance in the lesbian community. These norms serve to help lesbian women identify each other within the dominant heterosexual culture and consolidate a separate and distinct identity among lesbian women. They may be very functional at one level, but like all rules of conduct, they may also be experienced as oppressive. In an article entitled "Growing Old Disgracefully," Sue Leigh (1987) laments the restrictiveness of the "hidden rules of acceptable behavior" she experiences as a middle-aged lesbian feminist. She comments on how these implicit and explicit codes of behavior limit individual choice. "It's OK to be a lesbian, more than OK to be a feminist, great to be anti-nuke, but in private life style, dress, behavior, musical/cultural tastes you should definitely have settled down by forty" (p. 21).

Wolf (1991) suggests that the reason the "beauty myth" is so successful in keeping women insecure is because of its divisiveness in pitting women against one another. She underscores the rivalry that is at the core of this myth—the "constant comparison, in which one woman's worth fluctuates through the presence of another." This forces "women to be acutely critical of the 'choices' other women make about how they look" (p. 284). It compels women "to be at once blindly hostile to and blindly envious of 'beauty' in other women" (p. 285). Rather than being allies, women's insecurities about their own bodies and their fears related to the aging process may make it more difficult for them to be accepting of each other's bodies, wrinkles, and choices. As one middle-aged woman pointed out,

> "When I make comments about another woman's size, or shape, or appearance, . . . whether she's 'too thin' or 'too fat,' . . . whether she wears high heels, or shaves her legs, wears makeup, or dyes her hair to hide the grey, I'm just prescribing another set of rules about how she *should* look and behave. Maybe the rules are different from the normal standards, but they're rules and expectations nonetheless . . . and when I do that to other women, what does that say about how I feel about *myself*? When I'm critical of other women, I'm really being critical of myself, and I'm turning away from the people whose approval I value and *trust* the most . . . other women!"

A woman's subculture necessarily shapes her perceptions and experience of her aging body. It influences the choices she makes in coping with, and responding to, the march of time. It can be liberating in honoring a woman's right to choose. Or it can be oppressive in limiting her choices. As Wolf (1991) points out,

> A woman wins by giving herself and other women permission—to eat; to be sexual; to age; to wear overalls, a paste tiara, a Balenciaga gown, a second-hand opera cloak, or combat boots; to cover up or to go practically naked; to do whatever we choose in following—or ignoring—our own aesthetic. A woman wins when she feels that what each woman does with her own body—unforced, uncoerced—is her own business. (p. 290)

Dowling (1996) concurs when she speaks of the "integrity, aggressiveness, and self-affirmation of women who are able, at midlife, to respect themselves." She talks about women who have the capacity "to be *among* women, to feel validated by them rather than competitive with them" (p. 14). The words of a 52-year-old woman in Apter's (1996) study underscore this perspective: "You just come to realize that all sorts of faces look good. It's a matter of seeing what's inside—all those little movements—surprise, amusement, doubt. I used to automatically erase those things, while I weighed up the shape of the nose and the mouth. Big deal! Even Madonna's face is going to fall to pieces that way" (p. 66).

SUMMARY: PROBLEMATIC MEANINGS

In 1979, Susan Sontag referred to aging not only as women's destiny, but also as their "vulnerability." It was her contention that "most men experience getting older with regret, apprehension. But most women experience it even more painfully: with shame" (p. 469). Paula Weideger, in 1978, similarly reflected on women's painful awareness of their changing bodies and appearance:

> Not long after her thirtieth birthday a woman begins searching the mirror for signs of age. . . . A few years pass and looking in the mirror becomes a game of darts. The eyes travel on beams of light directly to the signs of age, land for a split second, and flick away. . . . But however skilled a woman becomes at the game of mirror darts, a moment comes when she *knows* she has aged. (p. 206)

Almost 20 years later, feminine beauty continues to be identified with slenderness and youth (Seid, 1994). North American culture "still has not found an acceptable way to represent a whole woman . . . an intelligent, strong-willed, full-bodied woman" (Wooley, 1994, p. 46). However, over the past 20 years, women have more clearly defined themselves "by [their] actions and works" within and outside the domestic spheres. As such, many more midlife women are now able to "disavow and free [themselves] of male representations" and reclaim their "bodies and [themselves] as whole persons" (Wooley, p. 46).

Certainly, several writers (e.g., Apter, 1996; Greer, 1991) suggest that women of the current midlife cohort feel they look "far better—healthier, younger, more active and appealing—than did women of the same age in previous generations" (p. 74). In Apter's study, "most women at 40 and 50 and beyond" felt that they looked "far better than they had expected to look at this age" (p. 74). The hard lessons learned on the road to midlife appear to supply many women with the strength, clarity, and resources to live more comfortably in their bodies. Being socially released from the objectification of youth appears to provide women with a new freedom to set their own standards. "As a woman gains self-confidence, the disapproval of others loses the meaning it once had. This provides the freedom to get on with her life in ways younger women can, on the whole, only vaguely imagine" (Apter, p. 75).

Indeed, as the client quoted earlier in this chapter indicated, midlife women may eventually reach a point in their lives when they decide that they are "so far removed from the cultural ideal" that they can in fact say

"Well, to hell with it." However, it would appear that for many women, this resignation is preceded by a period of considerable struggle to reconcile themselves to their changing bodies. It is difficult, if not impossible, for any woman to reach middle-age without becoming increasingly self-conscious about the shape and appearance of her aging body (Wooley, 1994). As women's metabolisms change, it is not uncommon for women in their 40s and 50s to speak with frustration about their inability to control their weight or about the changing distribution of fat in their bodies. It is not uncommon to lament about the lines in their faces, the luggage under their eyes, or the loose skin around their necks. To a degree, women cannot help but perceive it to be a personal failure—a reflection of inadequate effort or willpower—when the normal bodily changes of midlife become apparent.

In a time of personal, social, and physical transitions, the bodily changes that women experience during their middle years leave many feeling that the homes they occupy have become a strange place (Leigh, 1987). Captured in the words of a midlife woman interviewed by Dowling (1996), "She was living in a kind of time warp. Something was out of kilter. When she looked in the mirror, she felt no congruence with the image she saw" (p. 69). And, indeed, as with any physical change, it takes time for a woman's internal perceptions—her body image—to catch up with her new external reality (Hutchinson, 1994). It takes time for her to become comfortable with this new reality and to incorporate this into her self-structure. Apter (1996) notes how "the steps a woman takes to repossess her own image are often slippery and uneven" (p. 67). It involves a process not just of "rejecting others' views; it also involves constructing one's own. . . . To emerge triumphant from this journey, a woman needs to lift the blind on her own new vision" (p. 68).

Many prominent women writers herald midlife as a time of growth and opportunity for women (e.g., Apter, 1996; Friedan, 1993; Greer, 1991; Steinem, 1992). No longer valued for sex appeal and freed from over 30 years of sexual objectification, midlife women are able to regain the boldness, honesty, and courage of their younger years. More sure now, of who they are, and who they are not, "if [they] can avoid the temptations of the eternal youth purveyors, the sellers of unnatural thinness and cosmetic surgery, [they] may be able to tap into the feisty girls [they] once were" (Heilburn, cited in Dowling, 1996, p. 35). As Friedan (1993) points out, "The attempt to hold on to, or judge oneself by, youthful parameters" can blind us to "the new strengths and possibilities emerging in ourselves" (p. 30). In the words of Woodman (cited in Dowling, 1996), "You know . . . you're going to go down that path whether you like it or not. You can go like a squealing pig towards the slaughter, or you can go consciously and with as much grace as you can muster. . . . The point is that the ego surrenders, opens the heart, and in that opening new energy comes in" (p. 67).

CHALLENGE AND CHANGE: CREATING NEW MEANINGS

If we are to assist midlife women with the process of integrating into their self-structures the physical changes brought about by the aging process, it is first necessary to confront our own fears about aging. We need to examine our own beliefs and values about women's use of beauty aids (hair dyes, skin peeling, cellulite stripping, collagen treatments, etc.) and services aimed at maintaining the appearance of youth (cosmetic surgery, weight-loss programs, fitness regimens, etc.). What makes it more acceptable to have a breast *reduction* than a breast *augmentation*? We need to ask why a face-lift or tummy tuck is less acceptable than surgery to remove a birthmark or to correct a harlip? To avoid passing judgment and imposing our own values about the choices women make regarding their bodies, we need to be cognizant of what these values are. "Among women, especially on the culturally loaded subject of our bodies, there is always a danger of diminishing each other's self-authority. Therefore, the point is not to give each other answers, but to share questions and experiences" (Steinem, 1992, pp. 240–241).

After years of seeing themselves through the eyes of others, it is not an easy task for women to reject "the limitations of an external vision" (Apter, 1996, p. 71) and to see themselves and their bodies through their own eyes. So where do women begin this process? In her book *Revolution from Within,* Gloria Steinem (1992) suggests that in working with midlife women on issues related to body image, it is necessary to work from "the inside out" (p. 232). We begin, then, by helping women to explore their thoughts and feelings about living in their changing midlife bodies. We help them to examine the personal and social meanings these changes hold for them in their lives. And we help them create their own visions.

There are a number of exercises and strategies that counselors might employ to facilitate this process. Several of the activities outlined in Chapter 9 to help women "in the prime of life" combat and overcome feelings of bodily inadequacy, can easily be adapted for work with midlife women. The mirror exercise and the use of metaphors, dance, and movement can assist in the assessment of women's perceptions of, and comfort with, their bodies. Early recollections, collages, family sculpting, and psychodrama can be used to help women identify and explore the sources of their bodily discontent and feelings of inadequacy. Body casting, positive affirmations, and inner-child work are only a few of the many other activities that counselors can use to assist women in rejecting the standards of others and in coming to a place of self-acceptance.

Other interventions aimed more specifically for work on body image issues with midlife women are presented here. Again, these are only examples of activities that may be of assistance in doing this type of work.

Readers are encouraged to refer to the books listed in Appendix B to expand their repertoires of clinical interventions. It is important that readers utilize their own therapeutic experience and creativity in developing other viable strategies for doing affirmative body work with midlife women.

The Reckoning

At some point, all midlife women come face-to-face with the reality that no amount of plastic surgery, exercise, hair dyes, or magical anti-aging creams will be sufficient to hide the signs of aging. At some point, women realize that try as they might, they cannot hang on to, or recapture, their fading youth. Every woman hits this "wall" at some point. For some, this reality happens later. For others, illness or disability may bring this reality into sharp focus. Eventually, all women must find a way to reconcile themselves to what can no longer be. Greer (cited in Cobb, 1988) notes how this

> isn't a gradual, imperceptible process, but happens in leaps and bounds. You can go on for years being the same age. Your face doesn't change much; your weight remains much the same. You never think of yourself as too old to learn the latest craze, can't wait to [get] off with the old and [get] on with the new. Then, crunch. You're polishing a mirror table and your realize your neck has gone. Just like that. (p. 16)

It is a point of reckoning. It is a point in time when a woman realizes that she has to let go. In a way, it can be very liberating. There is a definite freedom in not having to meet the unrealistic standards set by others. But there are also losses (the loss of attention, the loss of attractiveness, the loss of youth, the loss of control, the loss of power, etc.). Some women may acknowledge and appreciate these gains in setting their own internal standards of attractiveness and acceptability (Apter, 1996). For others, the losses associated with fading youth and waning physical attractiveness are difficult to overcome.

To help women identify these losses, it is important to explore what meanings youth and aging hold for them. In a simple exercise that can be undertaken individually or in a group, women can be asked to create two lists. One list should be entitled YOUTH and the other, AGING. Under each, women can be asked to list the *losses* and *gains* they perceive to be associated with youth and with aging for women. Most often, the lists are fairly skewed. Many women find it easy to identify a number of gains associated with youth (attractiveness, energy, vitality, power, fertility, sexual desirability, etc.). It is often more difficult, however, for midlife women to identify the benefits associated with aging. Correspondingly, women generally identify few losses associated with youth but many with aging (e.g., loss of energy, vitality, attractiveness, sexual desirability, fertility, health, etc.). It is important that counselors not deny or downplay the physical and social losses that some women experience with aging (e.g., loss of a youthful appearance, loss of attention, loss of fertility, less ability to control one's weight, etc.). Rather, women should be provided with the opportunity to acknowledge and work through these losses. For example, some women may find it difficult to become sexually invisible, and may struggle to give up their hair dyes and high heels. Others, who have battled for what seems like a lifetime with maintaining control over their weight, may find it particularly difficult to watch the scales slowly inch up with each successive year. It is also important to explore the meanings these experiences hold for women and without discounting clients' feelings, also validate the positive aspects of women's midlife experiences (e.g., greater freedom to set one's own standards, stronger sense of self, greater self-confidence, more self-knowledge).

Every Picture Tells a Story

Another way counselors can assist in this process of understanding the significance of body image at various stages throughout their lives is by asking women to engage in what might be referred to as a physical "life review." The review essentially involves guiding women through an exploration of their personal body image histories. Using a modified lifeline and family photo albums, women can be asked to create a pictorial of themselves beginning in childhood and progressing throughout the years to the present time. In undertaking this exercise, women are directed to select one picture that is most representative of how they looked, for each 5-year block of time (0–5, 6–10, 11–15, 16–20, etc.). A scrapbook or journal is usually best for this exercise. Once these pictures have been gathered, women are instructed to glue one picture to each page of their scrapbook. Next, they are asked to place a one-word description under each picture reflecting how they *perceived* their bodies and appearance. This should be followed by one word that describes how they *felt* about their appearance at each point in their lives. For example, under the 11- to 15-year-old picture, a woman might describe herself as looking "gawky" and feeling "self-conscious." Under the 16- to 20-year-old picture, she may describe her appearance as "sexy" and her attitude as "cocky." Once the pictorial is completed to the present, women can be asked to share their body image histories and to tell the story behind each picture (this is particularly powerful if undertaken in a group format). Women should be encouraged to take time to discuss the periods when they felt particularly "good" about their bodies. They should also share the times they were dissatisfied with their appearance. It is important to explore the reasons for, and context of, these positive and negative self-evaluations. Emphasis should be placed on identifying body image *themes* that seem to reoccur throughout their lives.

Women commonly identify early childhood as a time of positive body image. As well, they positively highlight times during their lives when they most closely approximated the cultural ideal. However, in looking back at the words they associated with each picture, they are often surprised at the incongruence between their external images at the various stages of their lives, and their internal feelings about their bodies and their own self-worth. For example, during periods when they "looked" attractive by cultural standards, women often indicate that they felt very inadequate and unsure of themselves and their looks. Many are surprised to realize that their times of inner contentment and satisfaction frequently did not coincide with the times in their lives when their bodies paralleled external cultural standards. For many women, pregnancy is remembered as just such a time, when they felt less self-conscious of their appearance and more appreciative of their physical capacity to nourish and birth a child. For example, for one woman who had suffered with profound feelings of physical inadequacy most of her life, the experience of pregnancy and childbirth was instrumental in changing her bodily self-perception and meanings.

In taking this "walk down memory lane," women should be encouraged to look for continuity in their images over time. They should be assisted in seeing the links between their younger selves, and their older selves and in identifying those enduring physical characteristics that they like and value in themselves (e.g., their smile, their distinctive facial features, the power of their back and shoulders, the shape of their legs, the strength of their hands).

Women who suffer from illness, injury, or disability during midlife often struggle with a sense of betrayal and alienation from their bodies. Unfortunately, adequately addressing the needs of these women is beyond the scope of this book. Readers are referred to Bullard and Knight (1981) for some excellent suggestions on ways to help women who experience illness and disability to reclaim the disowned parts of their bodies. The references in Appendix F may also be useful in helping restore a sense of bodily acceptance and integration.

Unchaining the Shackles: The Freedom of Age

For midlife women to be able to appreciate the benefits of their renewed "subjectivity," it is necessary to confront their fears related to aging. These fears often become apparent from generating the list of "losses" associated with the aging process in the activity discussed earlier. This list can, in fact, be a useful jumping-off point in terms of more in-depth exploration.

Barbach (1993) suggests that the greatest fear of midlife women may be their loss of sexual desire and *desirability* during and following menopause. Certainly, most women raised in our youth-oriented North American culture associate aging for women with a loss of attractiveness and desirability. Irrespective of their race, ethnicity, or sexual orientation, most women feel some remorse associated with these losses. However, depending on each woman's particular history, there may be other, more significant, losses associated with the aging process. These may leave women feeling fearful of what the future will hold. For example, one 42-year-old woman lost her mother to breast cancer in her mid-40s, and her grandmother to this disease at a similar time of life. She experienced tremendous fear of losing a breast and eventually dying. Another 46-year-old woman had been diagnosed in her late 20s as having multiple sclerosis. Since then, she had not experience any signs or symptoms of the disease. However, as she approached her 50s, her image of her future possibilities was clouded by her fears of progressive physical deterioration. A midlife woman whose mother was diagnosed with Alzheimer's in her early 50s reported always feeling the dark shadow of mental incapacitation hanging over her as she contemplated her own future.

For some women, the fear of lost youth and attractiveness may be their "worst fear." However, it is important that counselors not assume that the loss of physical desirability is the *primary* concern of women as they enter midlife. Rather, it is necessary to explore with each client her personal fears and to help her identify and face these fears. I find it useful to have women create a hierarchy of their fears associated with aging and the future. Once this task has been completed, counselors can assist women in addressing and working through their fears. It is generally best to begin addressing the *least* frightening item on the list, and to progressively work through to the *most* frightening. In some cases, this may involve challenging faulty assumptions. In other cases, it may be necessary to use progressive relaxation and systematic desensitization techniques to help reduce women's anxiety as they confront their fears. It can also be helpful to have women "play out" their worst fears in their minds. In this way, certain fears may lose some of their power. Alternately, this process can serve as a springboard to help women plan how they might cope should their worst fears eventually be realized.

Once they have identified and begun the process of confronting their fears, women will be more free to explore and expand upon the advantages and benefits of aging. It can be energizing and liberating for women to begin to open up their minds to the *possibilities* of this time of life. Again, the exercise discussed earlier can be used as a starting point in terms of identifying the benefits of aging. Alternately, women can be asked to brainstorm about the things that they are most looking forward to, or that they enjoy the most about being middle-aged. "Freedom" seems to be a central theme in women's reflections on the aging process [i.e., *freedom from* pregnancy, from the responsibilities of raising young children, from being treated like an object or being dismissed based on appearance, from the oppression of trying to live up to cultural images of beauty, from trying to fight gravity, from the baggage of other's expectation; *freedom to* be themselves, to chart their own course, to act in their own self-interest, to be "outrageous" (Sheehy, 1992)]. Women might also appreciate the benefits of having more choice and freedom in midlife to pursue the things that are important to them. Helping women explore their options and supporting them as they act on their decisions (even if these decisions are not consistent with our own values), is an important component in reinforcing the agency and entitlement of the midlife woman. What she chooses to do with her body, and with her life, must be based on her own considered decision and values.

Changing the Lenses

Cobb (1988) contends that part of the work of coming to terms with menopause and aging for women is learning to let go of the youthful image women carry with them into middle age and replacing this "with a more mature, capable image" (p. 15). In reference to women's sexuality, Vance (1984) notes how "it is not enough to move women away from danger and oppression; it is necessary to move toward something: toward pleasure, agency, self-definition" (p. 24). The same may be said for body image. In asking women to turn away from a youthful vision or image of attractiveness and beauty, it is necessary to move toward another desirable image.

However, herein lies a potential problem for many women. As Greer (1991) notes, "All our heroines are young" (p. 22). For most of their lives, "women are well trained . . . to shy away from identification with older women" (Wolf, 1991, p. 283). Role models of middle-aged and older women are relatively invisible in our youth-oriented culture. As such, it is often difficult for women to change the critical lenses they have worn in assessing their own physical worth and appearance, and that of other women. It can be a real challenge to replace these with a different, more broadly accepting set of lenses. It can be very difficult for women to envision images of older women that do not merely reflect the "remarkable" and "unique" ability of a select few women who manage or appear to maintain the appearance of youth (e.g., Tina Turner, Jane Fonda, Joan Collins, Candice Bergen, Jane Seymour).

Part of the process of helping midlife women to change these critical lenses involves helping them to identify older women whom they admire. Women whose faces "show the lives they have lived" (Sontag, 1978, p. 478) can serve as role models, reflecting as they do, a more mature beauty and depth of character. So few media images exist of vital and attractive older women who have "let themselves age naturally and without embarrassment" (Sontag, 1978, p. 478) (with the possible exception of screen stars such as Joanne Woodward and Colleen Dewhurst). It may be necessary and useful, then, for women to turn to the real world of their own lives and families to identify positive role models of successful aging.

Women might begin by reviewing their family albums and making a concerted effort to look at the faces and appearances of the older women in their families. Or they might consider other women with whom they work or are acquainted. The goal of the exercise is to identify at least *one* older women whose image they perceive would fit well under the heading "A Life Well Lived." If a woman is unable to identify a particular person in her life that fits her ideal, she might turn to the visual or printed media (art, magazines, etc.) and create a composite of the characteristics of such a person. Women should then be encouraged to discuss why they have selected the woman in question. They should be asked to identify the characteristics that they most admire about this older woman. (In a group, it is useful to have women share their role model's picture with the other group members. Group members can gain from identifying and discussing the ways in which the characteristics of these older women differ from the youthful standards of beauty that are promoted in our culture.) This exploration can help to expand women's notions of feminine beauty, and can validate the possibilities of age.

Revisioning the Future

Women's attitudes and expectations about aging are implicated in their feelings of self-worth and self-esteem, and in their perceptions about the possibilities that are available to them (e.g., to continue to be sexually active; to engage in satisfying intimate relationships). Sheehy (1992) contends that during midlife, women "must make an alliance with our changing bodies and negotiate with our vanity." Realizing that "we are never again going to be that girl of our idealized inner eye . . . the task now is to find a new future self in whom we can invest our trust and enthusiasm" (p. 136). She suggests that it is vital for the midlife woman to "develop a future self in the mind's eye."

> She is our better nature, with bits and pieces of the most vital mature women whom we have know or read about and wish to emulate. If we are going to go gray, or white, we can pick out the most elegant white-haired woman we know and incorporate that element into our own inner picture. The more clearly we visualize our ideal future self, admire her indomitable skeleton and the grooves of experience that make up the map of her face, the more comfortable we will be with moving into her container. (p. 149)

Having completed the above exercise of identifying their role model(s) of a life well lived, women can begin the task of envisioning their future selves, using a guided fantasy exercise. In this exercise, the client is guided to a meeting with herself as she thinks she will be when she is approximately 60 years old. Initially, in this exercise, the client takes the role of voyeur or observer, watching her older self from a distance. She should take note of her appearance and presence in great detail. She should be sure to be cognizant of her physical characteristics—hair style and color, skin tone and texture, size, shape, weight, stature—as well as the clothing she wears. She should note the way she carries herself in the world—her mannerisms, her mobility, her style of walking, the "look in her eye," how she presents herself—and the statement she makes to the world through her self-presentation. Parts of this image may be drawn from her own pictorial (discussed earlier) and from the enduring personal characteristics she identified during that exercise. Some of it may be drawn from the image of her ideal role model. Some of it may be based on the characteristics of the older women in her own family that she most resembles or most admires. This does not have to be, and ideally should not be, a Pollyannaish picture that has no basis in reality. Each woman should be encouraged to base her fantasy on a realistic assessment of her own characteristics. For example, if she has a spinal cord injury, her wheelchair will be a part of her vision of her future self. However, it may not be a predominant part. It may be foreshadowed by other aspects of her body and appearance. If she is a woman of size, her vision of herself may be expansive. Her physical presence may be a significant and positive component of her future image.

Once these images have been created in their mind's eye, women should be encouraged to make them more concrete by drawing or painting them (perhaps in the pages of their pictorial book). They do not have to be artistically talented or accurate in their portrayals. Rather, they need only attempt to capture on paper the colors, contours, and dimensions of the image of their future selves that is in their mind's eye. Following along this line, women can envision themselves in 10-year spans, creating a somewhat older image of their ideal selves for each successive decade. They should take into consideration the normal physical changes that occur as part of the aging process. In addition to envisioning these ideal images, it can be useful for women to create a metaphor for each life stage to accompany their pictures. These metaphors should capture the spirit behind each image.

Finally, it is important to go one step further by assisting women in envisioning how they might best realize their ideal future images. It is important to ask what it will be necessary for them to do in their lives in terms of attending to their physical, psychological, and spiritual health to eventually realize these images. For some, this may mean taking care of their bodies through good nutrition and exercise (e.g., swimming, yoga, walking). For others, it may require paying greater attention to nourishing their intellectual or spiritual selves. Some will need to find new ways to replenish more regularly their depleted personal resources. For others, achieving their older ideal will require leading a more balanced life. It is important for counselors to emphasize that finding some peace and contentment with their inner selves may be the most significant factor in women achieving the external appearance that they would ideally like to see reflected in the mirror.

14

INTIMATE CONNECTIONS

Sexual Expression and Relationships

We come together shy as virgins
with neither beauty nor innocence
to cover our nakedness, only
these bodies which have served us well
to offer each other
"We are real," you say, and so we are,
standing here in our simple flesh
whereon our complicated histories are written,
our bodies turning into gifts
at the touch of our hands.

—MARCIA WOODRUFF, "Love at Fifty"

The biological and psychological changes that occur during midlife may well present some challenges to the sexual expression and satisfaction of women. As discussed in Chapter 11, hormonal shifts that occur during menopause often precipitate changes in women's sexual comfort and responsiveness. Many of these are temporary, and most can be fairly easily managed with herbal remedies, estrogen creams, and in some cases, with a sensitive and creative partner (Boston Women's Health Book Collective, 1992; Cole, 1988; Leiblum, 1990; Morokoff, 1988). Any potentially negative physical changes are also counterbalanced by the greater self-assurance, self-knowledge, and accumulated sexual experience of most midlife women (Apter, 1996; Greer, 1991; Kitzinger, 1985; Sang et al., 1991). The research is fairly consistent in reporting women's continued physical and emotional capacity for sexual expression and enjoyment throughout the life span (e.g., Barbach, 1993; Cutler et al., 1987; Leiblum & Swartzman, 1986; Sheehy, 1992).

The impediments to the achievement or maintenance of a positive sexual self esteem and sense of sexual agency for women do not appear to be physical or developmental. Rather, they seem to have more to do with social expectations and perceptions of the midlife woman. The current cultural ethos supports the continued importance of sexual activity for the maintenance of health and well-being throughout life. We might then expect that midlife women can look forward to several decades of some of the "best sex of their lives" (Sheehy, 1992, p. 140). Unfortunately, however, the standards of sexual eligibility for women have not become more inclusive and relaxed. Sexual desirability for women in North American culture has always been equated with physical beauty. And, as noted in Chapter 13, images of physical beauty have become increasingly younger. Very discrepant standards of sexual desirability and attractiveness continue to be promoted for midlife women and their male counterparts. Midlife women who are still interested in heterosexual intimacies face early social disqualification. "Women . . . even good-looking women, become sexually ineligible much earlier than men do" (Sontag, 1978, p. 465). Women in midlife whose faces and bodies, like canvases, reflect the rich contours of their lives, may find themselves "out of the (hetero)sexual game" at precisely the time in their lives when they are coming into "full flower" (Banner, 1992).

Midlife women's experience of their sexuality, the sexual choices they feel entitled to make, and their perceptions of their sexual desirability are powerfully influenced by social and cultural expectations. The messages of menopausal disease promoted by medical professionals are especially powerful. So, too, is the sexual invisibility in the popular media of woman who reflect their physical and social realities, and the communications of others in their lives with whom they choose to express themselves sexually. Closer examination of the expectations communicated by medical practitioners, the media, and significant others reveals some of the more significant social impediments to midlife women's sense of sexual desirability and entitlement.

THE SERVICEABLE VAGINA: MEDICAL MESSAGES

Gannon (1994) suggests that medicine has replaced religion as the authority to which women turn to maintain sexual "health" and well-being during midlife. She notes how, when religion was "in charge," sexuality was clearly linked to reproduction. This meant that there was no reason for the menopausal woman to be sexual. The medical profession reflected these conservative beliefs in reinforcing procreation as the *raison d'être* of sexual activity for women (Ehrenreich & English, 1978; Hubbard, 1990; Martin, 1987). As such, sex and menopause were anathema.

Currently, however, the medical profession supports the perspective that it is healthy and normal for women to enjoy sex. Medicine has moved from the stereotype of "the placid, asexual postmenopausal woman" (p. 105) to "implying that not to be sexually active is 'sick' " (Gannon, 1994, p. 114). As discussed in Chapter 11, intercourse is now considered to be an important prerequisite for maintaining vaginal health. Similar to the popular belief that men "need" sex, "the received opinion now is that the older woman should be having sex" (Greer, 1991, p. 303). An active sexual life is promoted as a way for the estrogen-deprived menopausal woman to "plump up her cells, boost her confidence, tone her muscles and flood her with the hormones of everlasting youth" (Kitzinger, 1985, p. 241).

> In the nineteenth century, menopause was seen as a sign that sexuality was at an end; women who felt healthy, vigorous and sexy enough to marry were labelled "sick" and advised to see their physician. Today, menopausal women who prefer not to be sexual are advised to see their physician for help in restoring their lost sexuality. (Gannon, p. 119)

In a rather ironic twist of circumstance, menopause and midlife changes are no longer viewed as *barriers,* to the sexual expression of women. Rather, continued involvement in sexual activity, and in particular, intercourse, is now considered an important requirement for women's health. Ironically, masturbation and orgasm are not sufficient. Intercourse is still promoted as "the *sine qua non* of sex" (Kitzinger, 1985, p. 244). Whether we use a penis, a vibrator, or (heaven forbid), as Barbach (1993) suggests, a cucumber, women are encouraged to do whatever is necessary to ward off the "vaginal atrophy" that results from the "shutting off" of estrogen at menopause. While some may say the new medical ethos is liberating, it appears to be very much a double-edged sword. The new mandate of intercourse as a prescription for sexual and psychological health in midlife "is probably experienced by women as a series of rather mocking demands on them, namely, that there should be someone in their lives who wants to have sex with them, and they should also be wanting sex with that person" (Greer, 1991, p. 303). Neither of these assumptions is necessarily valid or realistic.

Porcino (1983) refers to "sexism and ageism" as the "twin prejudices of most health-care professionals" (p. 162). Ageism is apparent in the disqualification of the sexual and health concerns of older women. Sexism is apparent in the differential attention paid to the health care needs of midlife and older men and women. Based on their review of the medical and psychological literature between 1984 and 1994, Rostosky and Travis (1996) underscore the overwhelming emphasis in the medical community on pathologizing and labeling the climacteric changes of women, while ignoring and normalizing similar changes that occur for men.

As noted in Chapter 11, research indicates that, despite changes in estrogen levels, most women retain the capacity to be multiply orgasmic throughout their lives. For men, however, the refractory period between orgasm and subsequent erection increases with age (Masters & Johnson, 1966, 1970). Men experience natural declines in sexual interest and difficulties in achieving and maintaining an erection, as well as in reaching orgasm. Despite the prevalent stereotype of "continued virility and potency, . . . in fact, after age 50, a diminished sexual potency in men is common and is probably due, at least in part, to declining androgen levels" (Gannon, 1994, p. 104). And yet it is "strongly recommended that middle-aged and elderly women take estrogen supplements in order to remain sexual while it is not recommended that men of similar age take androgens" (p. 110).

The medical language associated with midlife women's bodies and genitals is also very problematic in reinforcing negative attitudes (Rostosky & Travis, 1996). Pejorative terms such as "vaginal atrophy," "ovarian senility," and "estrogen deprivation" are all too common in the medical literature in reference to the changes precipitated by decreased estrogen levels (Kitzinger, 1985). However, no comparable terms (e.g., penile incompetence, testicular failure) exist to refer to the common declines in sexual performance on the part of men as they age (Boston Women's Health Book Collective, 1992).

> We do not have "testicular insufficiency" to match "ovarian insufficiency" or "senile scrotum" to match "senile ovaries." In the *Merck Manual of Diagnosis and Therapy*, the common physicians' handbook, in describing premature menopause, specific medical directions are given for "preserving a serviceable vagina." Do you think there is equal discussion of a "serviceable penis"? . . . Of course there isn't. (Reitz, cited in Ussher, 1989, pp. 108–109)

Cole and Rothblum (1990) underscore how we need to "discover alternative descriptive terms that do not pathologize women's normative and natural experiences. . . . It is untrue that a woman's skin decays as she ages, or that her vagina wastes away. We must stop, immediately, equating age with 'rotting' " (p. 510).

Certainly, some women experience the physical changes associated with menopause as problematic in terms of their sexual desire, comfort, and satisfaction. The medical profession has an important role to play in responding to their concerns and easing their discomfort. For some women, estrogen creams can reduce vaginal dryness. Hormone replacement therapy may ease the menopausal symptoms that can affect a woman's sexual desire and responsiveness (e.g., sleep deprivation, hot flashes). However, as several feminist researchers and writers have noted (e.g., Boston Women's Health Collective, 1992; Carolan, 1994; Cole & Rothblum, 1990; Gannon, 1994; Greer, 1991; Kitzinger, 1985; Rostosky & Travis, 1996), medicine fails to attend to the complex interactions between biological, developmental, and sociocultural factors in women's experiences of sexuality during midlife. A more "developmentally, holistically, and contextually sensitive" (Rostosky & Travis, 1996, p. 302) approach on the part of the medical profession is critical to a better understanding and appreciation of women's sexual needs and desires during the middle years.

ON THE DOWNHILL SLIDE: MEDIA IMAGES

Medical professionals may now promote the importance of continued sexual activity for women throughout life. However, the powerful cultural connection between a woman's sexual desirability and a youthful appearance persists undaunted in the media. The popular media's resistance to challenging this link is apparent in the virtual absence of images of middle-aged women as sexually vital and vibrant human beings.

In viewing television shows, movies, or magazine ads, it would appear that there are only two types of women. There are those who are young, beautiful, and therefore sexually desirable. And there are those who are too old and unattractive by today's standards to be considered sexually appealing. Sandwiched between these extremes are the few middle-aged "celluloid" women who have managed to maintain the appearance of youth (e.g., Goldie Hawn, Jane Fonda). These are air-brushed images of women in their 40s and 50s who, through the beauty rituals and services available to economically advantaged women, continue to look remarkably "young." Therefore, they continue to be portrayed as sexually desirable. Juxtaposed to these are the middle-aged women who, in their attempts to hang on to their fading youth and sex appeal, are caricatured as sexual buffoons (e.g., Peg in *Married with Children*; Roseanne, who appeared on the cover of a national magazine in a teddy and garter belt).

It seems a rather huge leap between the sexual rompings of the nubile young women of *Melrose Place* or *Friends,* and the asexual friendships and companionship of the women in the cast of *The Golden Girls* (aside from Blanche, who is portrayed not as sexually enlightened but sexually desperate). The middle-aged woman appears to fall into a sexual abyss. Referring to the power of the media to shape and reflect social perceptions and expectations, Greer (1991) notes how "women over forty are still usually shown as pains in the neck, mothers-in-law in silly hats. The sexy middle-aged woman is not even a gleam in the ad man's eye, even though she may have significant buying power. The ad man knows that to sell to her he may as well use a younger woman with whom she too would rather identify" (p. 303). There are few, if any, realistic female role models presented in the popular media, reinforcing the fact that a woman can still be sexually "attractive after the 'first flush of youth' has passed. Those who do exist . . . are seen as exceptions, rather than as representative of their age group or as real women" (Ussher, 1989, p. 118). These media portrayals serve to remind midlife women "that youth and beauty are synonymous, and that the best thing the menopausal woman can do is disappear gracefully (as the menopausal 'media woman' does)" (p. 119).

In her book on women coming into their own at 50, Dowling (1996) refers to midlife as "a vivid age when we are freer and more individuated than we were when we were younger. At last we are confident in our strengths, accepting of our limitations, and wise in our ability to adapt, be flexible, dance to the rhythm of our own needs" (p. 2). Where then, is the midlife woman to turn, to find sexual validation and support for the gifts of creativity, maturity, and humor with which time and life have endowed her?

LOVERS AND OTHER STRANGERS: MESSAGES OF SIGNIFICANT OTHERS

The expectations, beliefs, and behaviors of those with whom the midlife woman shares the intimacies of her life are also important in shaping her sexual self-perceptions. Women who have been partnered for several years are likely to experience normal changes in their patterns of sexual activity and levels of sexual passion and erotic desire. Reduced desire and frequency are commonly reported in long-term relationships (Barbach, 1984, 1988). Couples also tend to experience considerable pragmatic and social pressures at this stage in their lives. Far from finding the midlife years a time of peace and respite, many couples have young children at home, or adult children who have returned to the "nest." These days, they may be beginning new careers, or may find themselves at the height of their occupational responsibilities. It is also not uncommon for couples at this stage in life to be dealing with their own health problems, as well as those of their aging parents (Cobb, 1988; Stevens-Long & Commons, 1992). Far from being free to enjoy "midday sex on the dining-room table" (Dowling, 1996, p. 38), many couples find they have even less time or energy to indulge in sexual pleasure, even if the mind is interested and the body is willing. Couples often find it difficult to sustain their sexual desire in the face of these competing demands, and many experience frustration that their levels of erotic desire and responsiveness are not what they use to be. Barbach (1993) also notes how couples in long-term relationships often neglect the romantic and sexual aspects of their relationships, and fail to realize that sustained passion requires sustained effort.

The physical and hormonal changes that occur for both members of the couple during the climacteric may also add to the problems heterosexual couples experience in sustaining a satisfying sexual relationship. The research regarding changes in sexuality during the middle years suggests that these are "remarkably similar for aging women and aging men" (Gannon, 1994, p. 107). Unfortunately, however, few men or women are aware that these changes are a normal part of the aging process. Changes in men's levels of sexual desire and performance are not acknowledged in the dominant sexual discourse or sexual script (discussed in Chapter 10). As such, it is not uncommon for middle-aged men to blame their diminishing sexual drive or problems in sexual functioning on their partners. Women may accept the blame, believing that their aging bodies are no longer sexually desirable.

> If a man experiences changes without realizing that they are normal, he may begin to question his love for his partner. He may blame his slower response on the fact the *she* is aging, that *she* has gained a few pounds, that *she* is going through menopause. And she may accept the blame, feeling that a change in the way she looks or feels, a change in her femininity, is somehow at the root of the problem. He may then look to a younger woman to rekindle the excitement and response he fears he is losing. (Barbach, 1993, p. 128)

This serves the dual purpose of helping him to "deny his aging and confirm his virility" (p. 95).

On the other hand, some of these changes in sexual functioning and responsiveness can enhance rather than detract from couples' erotic pleasures. Kitzinger (1985) notes, for example, how "as a man gets older he takes longer to climax and there are times when he is satisfied without ejaculation. This makes him a better lover" (p. 240). With increased maturity and self-knowledge about what gives them the most pleasure, women may well find their sexual relationships to be more enriched in the middle years. In the words of one midlife man as he reflected on the changes in his intimate relationship with his wife of several years,

> What's entered our contract is honesty. . . . I can talk about feelings of disappointment, of wanting it to be more passionate between us, and as I'm talking, suddenly I'm feeling more aroused, more excited. Even as I'm speaking about how disappointed I am about missing passion, suddenly passion reveals itself. . . . I had never imagined it could be like this at my age. I had never imagined being able to cry while "doing it." (cited in Dowling, 1996, p. 105)

Midlife may well hold the possibility for deeper intimacy and more satisfying sex. However, the reality is that many midlife women, by choice or circumstance, do not have intimate partners (Anderson & Stewart, 1994; Dowling, 1996; Greer, 1991). The number of never-married women now entering middle age has increased dramatically over the last 20 years. Divorce rates are also high among the middle aged. "Since 1978 divorce has increased 50 percent for midlifers between 40 and 65. . . . In 1970, there were almost 1.5 million divorced and still unmarried people between the ages of 40 and 54. By 1991, the number had risen to 6.1 million" (Dowling, 1996, p. 107).

Being unpartnered does not appear to be the fate worse than death that women have traditionally been lead to believe. Current research suggests that many divorced and single women are very satisfied with their lives. The stories of 90 never-married, divorced, and widowed midlife women between the ages of 40 and 55, interviewed by Anderson and Stewart (1994) "tell of freedom, adventure, self-satisfaction, ease, and an increased capacity to appreciate moments of joy and discovery . . . a feeling of spiritual regeneration or transformation" (p. 132). However, this does not negate the fact that women without partners, referred to by Anderson and Stewart as "solo women," may find it quite challenging to include safe and satisfying sexual activities into their lives. They note how some single women make alternate sexual arrangements (e.g., taking weekend lovers). Some have no real desire for sexual intimacy (Cline, 1993). Some find other outlets for their sexual and creative energy (e.g., masturbation and fantasy, dance, art, music).

The other pragmatic reality as women grow older is that there are more older women than men. With middle-aged men frequently turning to younger women, the midlife heterosexual woman may find that her options are limited to older or younger men. Both options may have their problems. As noted in Chapter 13, sexual relationships between older women and younger men may be very difficult to sustain in a culture where such relationships are not socially sanctioned. The following words of a 48-year-old woman capture the essence of these difficulties:

> For two years I tried to maintain a close and loving relationship with a professional colleague twenty years younger than myself. The strain was too great. Everywhere we went together, people asked me if he was my son (they would never dare do that to a male who came in with young women on his arms). The second major problem was children. I already have three, and that's enough—but he deeply wanted to have a child of his own. And so, despite a very compatible intellectual and sexual relationship, we decided to separate. (cited in Porcino, 1983, p. 191)

Another problem in finding a suitable sexual partner may be caused by the midlife woman's lack of tolerance of "playing the games" that are often a part of heterosexual interactions. She may be unwilling to make her needs secondary to those of her partner (Dowling, 1996). Greer (1991) captures this change in attitude on the part of some midlife women: "Middle-aged women, having perforce cast off the narcissism of younger women, are quite likely to be more direct in their sexual advances and to make quite clear what it is they are after, especially if, for the first time in their lives, what they are seeking is not love but a fuck" (p. 283). No longer content always to follow the lead or desires of their male partners, midlife women may pose a considerable threat to men who find it difficult to accept an equal sexual partnership.

For women who manage successfully to negotiate a new sexual relationship, whatever the age of their male partners, the prognosis for sexual enjoyment is very good. The research suggests that "women involved in *new* relationships report very few sexual problems during menopause; in fact, they often find it is better than ever" (Cobb, p. 63; Dowling, 1996; Gannon, 1994). However, both men and women in our culture have been "nourished on a diet of inauthentic imagery of womanhood" (Greer, 1991, p. 302). As such, the insecurities many women feel about their aging bodies may result in women shying away from or avoiding physical intimacy, especially in new relationships:

> It becomes more and more difficult for a middle-aged woman to undress before a stranger, especially if he does not know her age and she does not know what he expects. She may resort to subterfuge, to soft lighting and luxurious underwear, or drugs or alcohol, to blur the first impressions that she feels are so crucial. (Greer, 1991, p. 302).

The dilemma of the midlife woman entering a new heterosexual relationship is that while she has gained in sexual maturity and knowledge, she is often painfully uncertain about the sexual desirability of her aging body (Dowling, 1996).

For lesbians, midlife changes do not appear to diminish the quality of women's sexual relationships. As noted in Chapter 11, many lesbians report sex at midlife to be "as good as or better than ever" (Cole & Rothblum, 1991, p. 193). One reason for this may be that, with lesbian women, sex is not as "intercourse or penetration focused as heterosexual women and therefore the physiological changes of menopause might not be so disruptive" (p. 192). Sexual desirability is also not as closely tied to a youthful appearance for most lesbians. There appears to be greater tolerance, understanding, and acceptance of the physical changes that are a normal part of their own development and that of their partner at this life stage (Sang et al., 1991).

Referring to the experiences of lesbians at midlife, Nestle (1991) discusses how time and the wisdom of accumulated years can be an "erotic ally." The following quotation captures the depth, richness, and honesty that may be the rewards of sharing lives that have been well lived and bodies that are well loved:

> As I have come to enjoy my own middle-aged sexual wisdom, I have also come to recognize it in the other older women I see around me. Gray hair and textured hand are now erotic emblems I seek out. . . . I still want strong lovemaking, I still want to play and pretend and seduce. But a moment comes when all of me is stark naked in body and imagination and then I know all of who I am and who I am no longer and I rise to offer this honest older self to my lover. As if to return the gift of acceptance, my body has rewarded me with new sexual responses. (p. 182)

Finally, some midlife women choose a celibate lifestyle for significant periods of their lives (Cline, 1993). For these women, the issue of sexual expression is often related to self-expression (e.g., masturbation), self-care, and self-nurturing. Their needs for relational intimacy are met in their nonsexual relationships. Often, these relationships are with other women. In the words of one midlife woman, "I am blessed with a few special women friendships. They are nonsexual, greatly sharing, mutually supportive conversational love affairs" (cited in Porcino, 1983, p. 195).

SUMMARY: PROBLEMATIC MEANINGS

The available literature supports the fact that menopausal changes may well influence midlife women's desires for sexual interaction, the ease with which they become sexually stimulated, their comfort with intercourse, and the frequency and intensity of their orgasmic responses. However, the majority of women, appear to be able to adapt to, and accommodate, the hormonal changes that occur in their sex lives during midlife (e.g., using vaginal lubricant, taking more time to explore and play prior to intercourse, discovering new erogenous zones). Midlife sex may not be what it use to be. But what we know from the available literature, and from the stories of women themselves, is that "different than" does not necessarily mean "worse than." Quite the contrary, "midlife sex can actually be freer, more tender, more inventive, and more emotionally satisfying than sex was when [women] were younger" (Dowling, 1996, p. 18). It can also be a lot of fun! Maturity, self-assurance, and an "accumulated wealth of sexual self-knowledge" (Loulan, 1991, p. 182) comes with age. Accordingly, midlife women may find themselves enjoying sex on their own terms, and on equal terms, for the first time in their lives. As 48-year-old Judith Rodin (cited in Dowling, 1996) remarks, "One of the things I like about [this age] is that I'm no longer trying to be what the man wants me to be, the way we did when we were kids. Now I'm implicitly saying, 'This is who I am—and it would be great if we liked each other' " (p. 33).

For women involved in new relationships (Gannon, 1994; Golub, 1992) and lesbian women (Rothblum & Cole, 1991; Sang, 1991), find that midlife sex is often actually more enjoyable and satisfying than they had ever anticipated.

If midlife sexuality has such potential and offers such possibility, what goes wrong? Why are women in long-term relationship ready to accept responsibility for the declines in their partners' sexual desires or performances? Why do some women feel sexually disqualified at a time of enhanced personal and sexual self-knowledge? Why do women feel sexually "inactive" or "abnormal" when they are unpartnered, when they are partnered with a woman, or when they are uninterested in intercourse?

It would appear that the contradictory messages communicated to midlife women about their sexuality are highly problematic. The implicit message is that to be menopausal is to be asexual. Women are encouraged to believe that continuing to have an "active sex life"—meaning intercourse and orgasm—is a necessary prerequisite to maintaining a healthy vagina.

Women are continually bombarded with images and messages that underscore the importance of continued heterosexual activity. At the same time, their sexual desirability and entitlement are disqualified. Sexual disqualification and the sexual imperative coexist (Gannon, 1994; Kitzinger, 1985; Ussher, 1989, 1992a).

Is it any wonder, then, that many women approach this time of life with some fear, apprehension, and confusion about what awaits them when youth has faded, estrogen has been "shut off," and they have been rendered sexually invisible? "What many women fear most when they think of menopause is an end to their sexual desirability and their sexual pleasure" (Barbach, 1993, p. 108). In a society that ties women's "sense of sexual vitality to youth and vigor," as their youth and fertility begin to wane and their bodies start to show the inevitable signs of aging, many women fear the loss of their "sexual selves" (p. 95).

In arguing for the eroticization of our whole lives beyond puberty, Grant (1994) observes how

> we live in a society in which single, divorced, and separated women over the age of forty are doomed to sexlessness because our phallic culture has turned the young girl into *the* cult object of desire. So many people are sexually off-limits— the old, the disabled, the ugly. For Madonna, the one perversion she draws the line at is sex with a fat person. When a man looks at an older woman, he sees how time ravages youth. When a woman looks at an older man, she sees maturity and, in it, his history. We need to defeat the male gaze. Time can be an erotic dimension. (pp. 255–256)

CHALLENGE AND CHANGE: CREATING NEW MEANINGS

How can we help women deal with the developmental challenges of the middle years while continuing to affirm their sexual agency and vitality? How can we assist women in responding to the confusing and often contradictory messages that are communicated regarding their sexual desirability and invisibility? We need to begin by examining and challenging our own expectations and attitudes about what constitutes sexual desirability and healthy sexual expression throughout the life span. We need to help the women we work with to do the same. As Cole and Rothblum (1991) note,

> It is possible that if all women, lesbian and straight, could be free of heterosexist hangups about sexual functioning and the aging process, if all women were not handicapped by fears of aging, partner expectation and the extolling of youth, there would be many more reports of unchanged or better, more rewarding sex and deeper relationships, in our fifties, sixties and beyond. (p. 193)

Breaking the cultural link between sexual desirability and a youthful appearance is a critical step in affirming the sexual vitality and eroticism of midlife women. If women are to be freer to express their sexuality fully and spontaneously, on their own terms, it is necessary for them to feel comfortable in their midlife bodies.

It is also important to help midlife women "expand their vision of sexuality and sensuality beyond demanding and goal-oriented notions of sex." It is important to help them create alternate visions "that might include new kinds of touch, fantasy, play, and discovery." Counselors need to convey the message that there is no right way to be sexual. It is important to give women permission to have "a different, more mature kind of sex life than they had at an earlier age, a sex life that is neither better or worse, but simply different" (Cole, 1988, p. 166). As Gannon (1994) points out, "In the absence of any reason to the contrary, I suggest that the proper, correct, psychologically and medically healthy manner for menopausal and postmenopausal women to express their sexuality is exactly as they please" (p. 115).

To be of assistance in dealing with the concerns of women during this life stage, counselors need to be aware of the ways in which menopause may affect the sexual responsiveness and desires of women. It is our responsibility as mental health practitioners to know the common sexual complaints of midlife and menopausal women, and to normalize these concerns (Cole, 1988). It is important to exercise caution in the language we use in addressing the sexual concerns of women. We must be careful not to reinforce notions of sexual disease, decay, and deterioration (Cole & Rothblum, 1990).

For women who are sexually active but are not in a long-term relationship, it is important for us to help them incorporate safe sex techniques into their love making, without increasing their fears or creating a sense of sexual disentitlement (Barbach, 1993; Loulan, 1987). We also need to help women who are unpartnered, or who do not desire phallocentric sex, to find satisfying alternatives to intercourse. "Massage, sensual baths, backrubs with creams and lotions" are examples of alternatives that "can provide physical intimacy without failure" (Leiblum, 1990, p. 506). Similarly, Tiefer (1996) reinforces the importance of masturbation education as a "centerpiece of women's sex therapy. As a metaphor for empowerment, as a technique for teaching about orgasm, as a reframing of the purposes of sexuality, as an opportunity to learn about oneself from fantasy, and as a site of emotional sexual experience, masturbation remains the premiere *in vivo* therapeutic opportunity for both bodywork and mind work" (p. 59).

She also promotes the value of solitary pleasures such as mental masturbation. This erotic and sexual experience is "closely connected to sexual fantasy," and may afford able-bodied and disabled women alike "a rich and rewarding form of sexual experience" (pp. 60–61).

Cole and Rothblum (1990) also underscore the importance of removing the word "foreplay" from our sexual vocabulary. This word assumes that other pleasurable sexual activities are precursors to the main event of intercourse. It implicitly reinforces the centrality of coitus in our notions of sexuality. It is particularly important that women who are not having intercourse are not allowed to "be convinced that without the psychic release of sex [they] will become a 'frustrated,' bitter, cruel, dried-up, envious old stick. The symptoms of the climacteric should not be misinterpreted as signs of mental imbalance or emotional disturbance caused by sexual deprivation" (Greer, 1991, p. 304).

In their book *Flying Solo: Single Women in Midlife,* Anderson and Stewart (1994) also emphasize the importance of counselors helping single women at midlife to reject the idea that they are temporarily between men. Women who are not partnered, whether by choice or chance, may need assistance to mourn the losses associated with the "happily-ever-after" coupled vision of the future. They may need help to create new, more realistic and positive visions of personal fulfillment and sexual satisfaction outside of a long-term committed relationship. Unpartnered women may need assistance in exploring and discovering other creative and satisfying avenues for the expression of their sexual vitality and energy.

We need to help women nurture their sexuality as a central and vital part of their personhood. Wolf (1991) emphasizes

> the importance of cherishing, nurturing, and attending to our sexuality as to an animal or child. Sexuality is not inert or given, but like a living being, changes with what it feeds upon. . . . We can seek out those dreams and visions that include a sexuality free of exploitation or violence, and try to stay conscious of what we take into our imaginations as we now are of what enters our bodies. (p. 279)

Midlife can be a time of personal and sexual renewal for women. It can be a time of "great potential, a time of coming into their own, . . . an era dominated by the delicious task of figuring out what they have always wanted and going after it with a vigor and a certainty of purpose they did not have when they were younger" (Anderson & Stewart, 1994, p. 131).

Counselors have the opportunity to assist women in their journey of personal and sexual discovery. The activities described here may be useful examples of ways to facilitate this adventure. Some of the activities discussed in Chapter 10 may also be adapted for work with midlife women. In particular, the "Sexual Self Box" and the "Animal Metaphor" activities, as well as the "Inner-Child Guided Fantasy" by Walker (1992) may help women in redefining and reconnecting with their mature sexual selves.

Lifting the Cloak of Invisibility

An important first step in working with midlife women on issues related to their sexuality and sexual expression involves helping women to examine popular attitudes about what constitutes sexual attractiveness in general for women. It is also important to help them explore and challenge the myths and assumptions they personally hold regarding the sexual desirability and "normal" sexual expression of older women. This type of exploration can be undertaken in individual counseling. However, as I have reiterated throughout this book, it can be very empowering for women to talk about their sexual fears and expectations in groups with other women. Group work helps to diminish women's sense of isolation and normalize their feelings and behaviors, and it provides a forum for the sharing of information. The authors of the book *The New Our Bodies, Ourselves* (Boston Women's Health Book Collective, 1992) note how "in a group, we can discuss factual information; explore our feelings; talk out problems; practice communicating (verbally and nonverbally); get help deciding how, when and with whom to share sexual feelings; and learn alternative ways to get what we want sexually" (p. 59).

Individually, or within a midlife sexuality group, participants can turn first to the media to examine the attitudes and messages that are typically conveyed in North American culture about the sexuality and sexual expression of women. In a simple homework assignment, women can be asked to bring to the next session magazine advertisements, film clippings, videos, pictures, stories, and so on, that most powerfully portray popular images and messages about the sexuality of women. These images are abundant, and women generally have little difficulty in finding a plethora of material in response to this request. In reviewing this material, women should be encouraged to consider the following questions: "*What do these images tell us about women's sexuality and sexual expression, in general?*" and "*What do these images tell us about the sexuality and sexual expression of midlife women, in particular?*" In response to the first question, this exercise underscores the strong cultural link between a woman's appearance and her sexual desirability. Only those women who meet the cultural standards of physical beauty—young, slim, physically "unflawed" women—are considered sexually attractive. It becomes readily apparent in this review that *young* women's bodies and body parts are presented as the symbols of women's sexuality.

As for the sexuality of the midlife woman, women quickly come to realize that it is notable in terms of its virtual absence in most media portrayals. Women often find it difficult, if not impossible, to find any popular images of a healthy and vital midlife sexuality for women. When represented at all, it becomes apparent how the midlife woman's sexuality is usually presented as an aberration or anomaly (e.g., the "black widow spider" version of the temptress who embodies grave danger for the unsuspecting male that gets caught in her web—Mrs. Robinson in *The Graduate*, Glen Close's character in *Fatal Attraction*).

This exercise can serve as a springboard for women to engage in an exploration of their own fears and expectations about the potential sexual losses associated with aging and with the menopause (e.g., loss of sexual desirability, loss of sexual desire, loss of the ability to enjoy sex, loss of a suitable partner). Women need to confront their fears and expectations regarding the potential sexual wasteland that awaits them in mid- and later life. Counselors can serve an important role in providing accurate information about the sexual changes that are most frequently reported by women during the menopause. They can discuss the physical changes that typically occur in women's reproductive and genital areas as a result changing levels of estrogen. They can also differentiate these from societal expectations and myths regarding the absence of midlife women's sexual desires and responsiveness. Counselors can provide information and simple suggestions for addressing some of the more common sexual concerns reported by midlife women. They can also gently challenge those assumptions and expectations held by women that are erroneous or self-defeating.

In beginning to break the link between sexual desirability and youth, it is helpful to assist women in creating their own, more empowering and vital images of the sexuality and sexual expression of older women. They may turn away from the celluloid and airbrushed images of younger women. However, it is important that women have images to turn toward—images that validate, rather than deny, the sexual maturity and eroticism of midlife women. In this regard, the relative absence of images in popular culture may actually make it easier for women to construct their own images of midlife sexuality and eroticism. Counselors can ask women to look within their own families and lives for images of older women whom they perceive to represent an image of midlife sexual vitality. When they have identified a woman or women who seem to radiate sensuality and eroticism, they should be encouraged to explore and to describe what it is about these women (e.g., their features, their attitude, their manner) that strikes them as embodying these characteristics. For example, one client brought in a picture of her grandmother, taken when she was in her mid-50s. She commented on the combination of self-assurance and playfulness that was apparent in her grandmother's eyes and facial features. She was not a thin or particularly beautiful woman, but she radiated a kind of mature sensuality and eroticism that was quite captivating. This woman was widowed at an early age. She never married again. To the best of the family's knowledge, she never took a lover. However, she had a way about her that exuded a raw sensuality and sexual confidence. Another woman brought in a picture of an aunt whose sexuality was expressed in her artwork, and, in particular, in her images of the powerful bodies of older women.

In Search of the Healthy Vagina

Counselors need to help women confront the assumption that vaginal health is contingent upon the continued experiencing of orgasms and intercourse. It is important to counter the message that underscores the importance of women having "regular" orgasms to maintain the flow of blood to the genital tract. It is also essential for women to be liberated from the belief that intercourse is "the *sine qua non*" (Kitzinger, 1985, p. 244) of sexual expression, and that a woman cannot be sexually healthy or fulfilled without the presence of something in her vagina. Thoroughly debunking the "phallus = vaginal health" equation is important if women are to be free to explore the wide range of sensory and sensual experiences and possibilities that are available to them, whether or not they are partnered. This may be particularly important for women who have physical disabilities that preclude the possibility of enjoying or engaging in intercourse. As Romano (cited in Thornton, 1981) notes,

> We must remember that the disabled woman is first a woman and second disabled; she has desires, needs and feelings just like any other person and has the right to express them in ways that are acceptable to her. Sexuality is composed of may things, has many ways of expression, and requires the possibility of compromise just as other facets of life do; it offers satisfaction in giving, as well as getting. (p. 157)

This does not discount the fact that many women enjoy intercourse. These women may require information on ways they can ensure their sexual comfort and pleasure during coitus (Barbach, 1993; Cobb, 1988; Cole, 1988; Leiblum, 1990). Counselors need to be aware of medical specialists in their communities who can deal sensitively and affirmingly with menopausal women's physical discomforts. It is important to be aware of local therapists who are skilled in working with the sexual concerns of heterosexual, lesbian, and bisexual women, whether or not they are partnered (Barbach, 1993). Counselors may also need to assist women with disabilities in finding effective ways of dealing with such problems as catheters and urinary leakage during intercourse (for information on counseling women with spinal cord injuries and disabilities, see Bullard & Knight, 1981; Kitzinger, 1985; Sandelowski, 1989; Thornton, 1981).

If women are to begin to challenge the centrality of intercourse in defining sexual contact and pleasure, they may need assistance in exploring the meaning and experience of orgasm and intercourse in their lives. There are several ways that this may be accomplished. One approach involves a simple word association. In this activity, women are asked to spontaneously respond to the cue words "penis," "intercourse," and "orgasm." The word "intercourse" often generates mixed reactions. This word sometimes elicits feelings of being overpowered and subsumed. Sometimes it is associated with feelings of mutuality, connection, warmth, and intimacy. Responses to the word "orgasm" are also usually somewhat mixed, although generally more positive overall. Orgasm can be associated with feelings of surrender. It can engender feelings of being temporarily out of control or exposed. Or it may be associated with feelings of guilt and shame. Many of the associations related to orgasm, however, tend to be quite affirmative. These include reactions indicating feeling ecstasy, bliss, delight, a high, a rush, and fantastic.

In completing this exercise and debriefing their responses, women often indicate that it is not the act of intercourse per se that they perceive to be the most positive or significant part of their sexual lives. Rather, the experience of connection and intimacy that is "sometimes" but not always a part of their experience of intercourse is often most meaningful and memorable. Women frequently indicate that the experience of orgasm is highly pleasurable and relatively uncomplicated. It is also one significant aspect of their sexual pleasure that does not require the assistance of a partner. Women often appreciate that experiencing orgasm is within their own control, although sharing this with a significant other can add another dimension of pleasure to this experience. Similarly, many women suggest that intercourse is less about the satisfaction of sexual needs and desires, and more about the satisfaction of needs for intimacy and affection. With an increased awareness of the meanings of intercourse in their lives, women can begin to explore other ways these needs might be met in other forms of self- and intimate expression.

Another exercise that is useful in helping women to expand their notions of sexual pleasure and enjoyment involves a guided fantasy. In this exercise, women are asked to picture a movie screen on which the images of their most intense and satisfying sexual encounters throughout their lives flash before their eyes. The movie begins with their first experience that involved intense sexual pleasure and moves forward through their various sexual relationships and encounters. For women who have been committed to one sexual relationship, it progresses through the various periods and circumstances of their relationship that they would classify as highly stimulating and erotically intense. Women should be asked to pause the movie in their heads briefly at each encounter to ask themselves what made this particular situation or encounter so electrifying. What was it about this particular context, this relationship, this activity, or this person that ignited their sexual senses and passions? In debriefing this exercise, women are often struck by the importance of state of mind, contextual factors, and relationship dynamics in creating the experience of sexual heat. For those who find it difficult to envision their lives in this type of fantasy, counselors might use a guided autobiography technique instead to identify salient sexual and erotic themes and experiences.

Nongenital, sensate focus exercises are also quite effective in removing intercourse as the goal of sexual contact. These can help women to expand the boundaries of their sexual and sensual pleasure in connecting with the sensuality of the other parts of their bodies (see Kaplan, 1981, and Kitzinger, 1985, for detailed explanations of sensate focus exercises). In her section on revitalizing women's sex lives, Kitzinger notes how nonintercourse-focused massage and sensate focus serves as a "kind of psychophysical relaxation . . . to unbuckle the muscle armor in which we try to shut ourselves off from sensation and to hide and guard ourselves." She underscores the importance of daring to let the "mental and physical barriers down and . . . discover that inside, though soft, vulnerable and exposed, we are filled with sexual vitality and the richness and color of sexual experience" (p. 151). In completing sensory exploration and nongenital touching exercises, women are often surprised at the level of sexual excitement and pleasure that they are able to experience without intercourse. In fact, Hyde (1990) notes how some disabled and spinal-cord-injured women "develop a capacity for orgasm from stimulation of the breasts or lips." Many are "able to cultivate a kind of 'psychological orgasm' that is as satisfying as the physical one" (p. 263).

Owning Our Bodies, Owning Our Sexuality

In completing the aforementioned exercises, women may begin to realize that sexuality is not a gift that is bestowed upon them by men or by their relationship status. Rather, it is an integral part of each woman's personhood. With this realization, women can begin to explore the various aspects of their sexual selves and the many ways that their sexuality takes form and expression in their lives.

To begin to explore their sexual selves women can be asked, while in a relaxed state, to engage in a guided fantasy exercise. During this exercise, women should consider the times in their lives and the circumstances in which they recall feeling particularly sensual—when their erotic energy was at its peak and they felt they exuded sexual vitality. Once they are able to capture this image of themselves, they should be asked to stay with the image and to "get inside" and connect with this aspect of themselves and their sexuality. They should try to feel the sexual energy and vitality within their bodies and to attend to every sensory detail of the experience. Some questions that are helpful in guiding this exploration include the following: "What does this energy feel like as it flows through your body?" "What parts of your body are most affected by this energy? What color is this energy?" "From where in your body does this energy emanate?" "Where/what is its source?" "How does it make you feel?" "What do you want to do with this energy?" After staying connected to this feeling for a time, women can be asked to step outside of their sensual images and becomes observers of their own sexuality. As they watch themselves emanating sexual energy and confidence, they should be asked to consider how their sexual energy is embodied and communicated in these moments. They should consider the contexts within which they feel safe and comfortable in allowing this part of themselves to be shared with others.

When the fantasy is completed, the next step involves having women engage in a visceral activity that allows them to transfer the sexual energy from their fantasy to the present. This may take the form of dance and movement, or perhaps artwork. Finger painting is a wonderful sensory medium for this type of communication. Remembering their answers to the above questions, women find it quite pleasurable and usually quite easy to paint their sexual energy—with its colors and contours. For some, the painting is a mass of vibrant colors, whereas for others, a particular pattern of colors emanates from, and is sometimes restricted to, a particular part of their bodies. As women participate in this part of the exercise, it is important that they have an opportunity to share their painting and debrief their experience. If the activity is undertaken in a women's sexuality group, then it is recommended that group members share their work and discuss their experience first with one other group member prior to sharing their work with the entire group. An exciting extension of this exercise involves having women use clay to sculpt their sexuality.

In further exploring their own eroticism, women can be asked to consider how they nurture and communicate this. How do they dress when they want to feel sexual? What things enhance their sense of sexual vitality? For example, some women find that wearing attractive lingerie or a particular fragrance makes them feel very sensual. Others find that they are most in touch with their sexual energy when working up a sweat through dancing, running, or working out. In owning their own sexuality, it is useful to help women identify those things, people, or experiences that reinforce their sensual selves. It is important to validate their entitlement to nurture and delight in the enjoyment of their own sexuality in their everyday lives—purely for their *own* pleasure. For writer Joan Nestle (1991), a black slip and hose became the emblem of her midlife sexuality:

> When I was 47, fighting the depression of illness, I found the ground I could stand on. Gay Women's Alternative of New York asked me to read some of my erotic stories. I realized that I did not want to read about sexual desire in everyday clothes, that I wanted some way to mark the specialness of the language, so I decided to wear a black slip and black stockings for the reading. I wanted the audience to see a large older woman's body as I said the words of sex. This wearing of the black slip became my signature. I had found a way to transform perceived losses into newly acquired erotic territory. (p. 181)

Most midlife women are not as comfortable as Joan in making such a bold statement about their sexuality. However, with a bit of exploration, most can nonetheless identify a symbol of their own eroticism. Most can identify something that they do or wear when they want to nurture and celebrate this aspect of themselves. One midlife client finds toes "exquisitely sensual." When she wants to nurture her sexuality, she gives herself a pedicure and paints her toenails bright red. When she wants to communicate her sexuality safely, and on her own terms, she wears a particular pair of sandals that show off her painted toes. Another client buys silk or satin lingerie when she wants to nurture her sexuality. She delights in the private knowledge that she wearing something very sensual.

Another important part of the midlife woman's ownership of her sexuality involves accepting her midlife body. Without an acceptance and appreciation of her body, it is difficult for any woman to feel "at home" with her sexuality or to feel comfortable in expressing and sharing this part of her with another. For example, in Dowling's (1996) book on midlife women, she talks about one single friend who tries "to leave on as many clothes as possible for as long as possible" when she is becoming intimate with a new partner. She fears that he will be disgusted or turned off by her "stomach hanging over him" (pp. 168–169). Part of the work of counseling necessarily involves facilitating bodily acceptance. Several of the exercises discussed in Chapter 13 help achieve this goal. Also, counselors may want to encourage women to become actively involved in caretaking and appreciating their bodies. In Chapter 6 of her book, *Body Love,* Rita Freedman (1988) provides several suggestions for sensory and self-touch exercises that can help women become more tuned in to their sensory and sexual hungers, and become more intimate with their own bodies. Robyn Posin (1991) also talks about her struggles to accept the dimples on her thighs rather than perceiving them as symbols of her own personal failure to adequately care for her body.

> As I sat there, my eyes and heart softened. I continued with my morning ritual of massaging lotion into my body, being especially loving as I lotioned my thighs. I forgave them for showing the inevitable signs of being part of my temporarily able, almost 50-year-old body. I thanked them for their strength and dependability, for serving my mobility so long and without complaint. I thanked them for enabling me still to delight in my yoga, tai chi and daily wanderings in the canyons. Rather than launching into some program to change them, I lovingly included by thighs, dimples and all, in my life as I continued putting my time and energy where it feels the most appropriate and rewarding at this stage of my unfolding. (p. 144)

It is also important to help women work through any discomfort they feel about sharing their bodies with another. Women are socialized to be critical of their own bodies and the bodies of other women (Wolf, 1991). As such, it can be useful to "turn the tables," so to speak. Men's bodies also show the signs of aging. Yet they appear to escape the harsh criticism to which women subject themselves. It can be very liberating for women to recognize how they frequently overlook and accept the sagging pecs, "love handles," and disappearing buttocks of their aging male partners, or the "sagging tummies" and "layered chins" of their female partners. In this recognition, they may become more accepting of their own aging bodies.

The Best Years: Sexual Reawakening and Pleasure

As in other aspects of their personal lives, it is important for women to realize that midlife can be a time of sexual reawakening. The literature suggests that for midlife women, sex can be richer and more honest, that in taking on less urgency, there is opportunity for greater depth and intensity. Steinem (1992) suggests that older women "are more free to explore sensuality and sexuality as part of the pleasurable language of love." Citing Marilyn French, she goes on to say that "pleasure—which includes erotic joy but is not limited to it, is the opposite of power, because it is the one quality that cannot be coerced. . . . Pleasure is an expression of the true self" (p. 283).

Rather than focusing exclusively on the sexual losses associated with moving into the next stage in life, counselors need to help women explore and assess the gains of their midlife sexuality. Instead of emphasizing what women are leaving behind as they move from young adulthood into middle age, it is important to help them attend to what they are bringing with them into this life stage. In an exercise called "Sexual Treasures," women can be asked to go on a mental treasure hunt. They should mentally review their sexual lives and fill their treasure chests with all the sexual knowledge, wisdom, passion, experience, pleasure, self-assurance, and erotic joy that they have accumulated over their lifetimes. Nestle (1991) poignantly refers to the "accumulated wealth of sexual self-knowledge" that midlife women bring to their sexual relationships:

> The desire I experience as a 50-year-old lesbian woman is not the same as the passion I pursued in earlier years; my desire has deepened and I experience it as a gift I bring to my lover. Stretched out on the bed, waiting for her, I sometimes feel as if I am bursting with sexual knowledge that, carried in the fullness of my breasts and hips, is all the wisdom I have gleaned from pursuing the touch of women for half a century. I do not feel arrogant or invulnerable to rejection, but I do know the ground I am lying on. (p. 182)

In rummaging through their sexual treasure chests, and taking a mental inventory of their sexual strengths and gains, women can feel more empowered by the gifts they bring with them into this life stage. They need not be unnecessarily burdened by what they have left behind. In fact, it can be liberating for women to realize that as they enter their middle years, they are leaving behind a sexual self that was less aware, less knowledgeable, and less certain.

Been There, Done That: Writing New Sexual Scripts

It is important to help women become the authors of new sexual/erotic scripts that are more reflective of the realities of their lives. These need to be based on their own visions of sexual pleasure and fulfillment. For women who are partnered in more long-term relationships, this may mean putting energy into regenerating the sexual passion that time, familiarity, and the stresses of everyday living have caused to wane (see Schnarch's 1997 book, *Passionate Marriage: Sex, Love and Intimacy in Emotionally Committed Relationships*; also see Barbach's books, *For Each Other: Sharing Sexual Intimacy,* 1984, and *Erotic Interludes,* 1988; couples can also be encouraged to incorporate fantasy and erotica into their sexual lives as a way to rekindle passion). For women who have experienced health problems, disabling injuries, or disfiguring surgery such as a mastectomy or colostomy, this may mean exploring ways to increase their sexual comfort, spontaneity, and pleasure. Women who are unpartnered may require assistance in writing sexual scripts that incorporate safe-sex techniques. They may need permission to explore the depths of their erotic desires and how these can be realized in their relationships with their own bodies. And women who are celibate may need to write sexual scripts that emphasize the diverse ways in which their sexual energy and creativity might be expressed in their lives.

Whatever their unique situation, it is useful to ask all women to construct and write about their "ideal sexual experience or encounter." Counselors can encourage women, within the context of their present life circumstances, to imagine in explicit detail what this ideal sexual experience would be like. Women should attend to the place it would occur, the individual or individuals involved, the sounds, the smells, the tastes, the activities, and so on. They should be encouraged to be as creative as possible. They should allow their imaginations to "take flight," without limiting their imaginings based on social or moral conventions. This might include participating in, or observing, erotica. It may involve bisexuality or group sex. Or it may involve venturing into the realm of unconventional sexual practices (e.g., S&M, fetishism, voyeurism, exhibitionism). When women have completed their scenarios, it is important that they consider whether they would actually like to realize their desires or if maintaining the fantasy is sufficient. In the former case, it is important to explore what steps they would need to take to realize their erotic desires and ensure that this would be a satisfying experience. For example, for one woman in a long-term relationship, it was necessary for her to "take charge" of the sexual encounter rather than letting her partner initiate their interaction (including the setting, the time, the activities, etc.). For a celibate woman, acting on her ideal sexual experience involved assuming responsibility for her own pleasuring, and giving herself permission to incorporate erotica (pictures and literature) into her sexual fantasizing. Realizing her ideal sexual script for another woman involved exploring her sexuality with a woman. For another, it involved orchestrating and participating in a *ménage à trois*. Whatever women's preferences, it is important for counselors to underscore that "all is normal within a loving relationship so long as one's actions are informed by kindness" (Nickerson, 1992, p. 213), safety, and mutual respect. Those whose life circumstances preclude the realization of their ideal experience, or those who have no desire to fulfill their fantasy, can be encouraged to keep it in their minds as a part of their personal erotic repertoire—to be turned to as they desire for their own erotic pleasure and satisfaction.

Fantasies: "The Poetry of Sex"

There are many erogenous zones in a woman's body, not the least of which includes the mind. Certainly, an entire oasis of potential sexual and erotic stimulation in the form of images exists within the confines of women's minds. These are limited only by women's imaginations, and by their comfort in, and willingness to, indulge themselves in the world of fantasy (Tiefer, 1996). Referred to by Kitzinger (1985, p. 90) as "the poetry of sex," sexual and erotic fantasies are an important and "legitimate form of sexual expression." Virtually all women have these available to them, irrespective of their relationship status or their state of physical health and well-being.

> Fantasies are part of this life of the imagination. . . . Fantasies may never have actually happened and probably never will, but have the same power to stir emotion. Sensual images can be conjured in a profusion of shapes, colors, cadences, tastes, which can in a second flood us with erotic arousal. . . . They provide the imagery which gives [sex] different flavors. Sometimes this poetry is lyrical, sometimes it has the beat of jazz or blues, sometimes it has a heavy rock rhythm. (p. 90)

Women can be encouraged to nourish this powerful and safe avenue of sexual pleasure in their minds, or through reading or writing erotic stories. Counselors can help women to broaden their understanding of sexual fantasy beyond the male fantasies of female sexual submission by exposing them to other forms of erotica (e.g., stores that specialize in erotica can provide a veritable cornucopia of erotic films, literature, and products). Some women are aroused by fantasies that are explicitly sexual. For others, the content of their fantasies are more sensual and erotic. In either case, sexual fantasies can be a "rich and rewarding form of sexual experience" (Tiefer, 1996, p. 60).

CONCLUSION

In discussing the benefits of middle age for women of the current generation Fleming (1994) comments on how "getting older for most of us was a blessing, because we were able to let go of a lot of things, to live with men on our terms or without them if need be, to be accomplished without apology and raucous without restraint in a country deeply ambivalent about women" (p. 253). Reclaiming sexuality and sexual entitlement during midlife is not an easy task for women in a culture that disqualifies our sexual desirability. However, midlife women have both the space and the unique opportunity to turn their creative energies and sexual wisdom toward the task of envisioning and living more sexually self-affirming and satisfying lives. As counselors, we can help women write "the poetry of [their] own eroticism" (Fleming, 1994, p. 247) during midlife and beyond.

15

COMING FULL CIRCLE

I am open
To you, Primal Spirit, one with rock and wave,
One with the survivors of flood and fire,
Who have rebuilt their homes a million times,
Who have lost their children and borne them
  again.
The words I hear are *strength, laughter, endurance.*
Old Woman I meet you deep inside myself.
There in the rootbed of fertility,
World without end, as the legend tells it.
Under the words you are my silence.
—MAY SARTON, "When a Woman Feels Alone"

Later life is clearly a time of many changes and transitions; of losses and gains. These changes inevitably affect a woman's sexual self-perceptions and the ways in which she expresses her sexuality. Rotberg (1987) contends that in the final analysis, however, the most important determining factor regarding the sexual expression of older women, other than physical health and fitness, may well be "the attitudes that women hold" (p. 8). To a degree, these attitudes are a product of our culture.

> The feelings a woman has about her body and about herself as a sexual being derive from the way in which she sees herself reflected in the eyes of others. Her self-image is bound to this reflection. Throughout her life she has been trained, as a woman, to study that reflection and to value herself in terms of it. When it tells her she is old and unwanted she feels completely discarded and drained of vitality. (Kitzinger, 1985, p. 242)

According to Rodeheaver and Stohs (1991), "double jeopardy and the double standard . . . are conceptually important in describing the context in which women grow old" (p. 146). It is to this context that we must turn to understand the formidable obstacles women face in attempting to maintain a sense of sexual entitlement and agency in their later years.

OVER THE HILL: MEDICAL MESSAGES

Sexist and ageist assumptions held by members of the medical profession have resulted in the sexual health needs of older women being poorly understood. Citing the 1985 United States Public Health Service Task Force on Women's Health Issues, Nickerson (1992) reports that

> women are treated with less respect within the health care system, and receive poorer medical care than men. . . . The illnesses of women, especially "old" women, are seen to be of less importance, and prevention is often not deemed worth the time it takes the doctor to explain. Men are deemed to have "real" illness; women are regarded as neurotic and troublesome, and old women hardly worth treating. (pp. 137–138)

This double-standard appears to be especially prevalent where issues of sexual functioning and satisfaction are concerned. What little information we do have regarding "the attitudes and preferences of the sexually active post-menopausal woman . . . come from a medical profession which sees mainly sick or impaired women, assumes they are asexual, and generally approaches ageful women as ailing women" (p. 207).

Most older women have been socialized to unquestioningly bow to the "wisdom" of their doctors. Dismissing and sexist attitudes on the part of medical professionals make it difficult for older women to feel that sexual needs and erotic desires are *normal* at this stage in their lives. Although the proportion of women physicians is increasing, the majority of medical practitioners, particularly older physicians, are men. Discussing sexual concerns with a male doctor may be difficult for women at the best of times (Kitzinger, 1985; Porcino, 1983). For women who grew up during a time of severe sexual repression, however, raising concerns about "vaginal dryness" or "orgasm," much less "condoms" and "safe sex" may be especially problematic. This difficulty can be compounded by members of the medical profession when they do not extend invitations to broach the subject of sexuality with their older women patients. Whether male or female, younger physicians may be very uncomfortable in discussing sexual issues with their patients. An older woman relayed the following experience in reference to her queries regarding alternate forms of sexual expression: "I asked a woman gynecologist with an excellent reputation, 'Does it have to be intercourse? What about widows, or divorced women, or lesbians, or women whose husbands aren't too interested in sex or are ill?' I couldn't get a straight answer from her" (cited in Boston Women's Health Book Collective, 1992, p. 534).

A lack of attention to the sexual needs of older women can also be seen on the part of the pharmaceutical industry (Boston Woman's Health Book Collective, 1992; Kitzinger, 1985). For example, Jean Nickerson (1992), author of the book *Old and Smart,* was dissatisfied with the lack of a safe and effective vaginal lubricant to help deal with the vaginal dryness commonly experienced by older women. She took it upon herself to contact three large pharmaceutical companies and a major cosmetics chain to "draw their attention to the older woman's need for a suitable, easily applied, non-irritating vaginal lubricant" (p. 225). She reports that none of these companies demonstrated any interest whatsoever in helping older women achieve more satisfying and comfortable sex lives.

> One company said it was not necessary to develop such a product, another said they are doing "all kinds of things to improve the lives of women, but this was not deemed in the best interest of the company," and the third said K-Y Jelly was adequate. . . . Even a self-proclaimed sensitive and progressive cosmetics chain said they didn't see a need for such a product at this time. (p. 225)

"To the extent that our society defines the sexual interest and activity in older persons as deviant behaviors, persons in whom sexual interests and activities continue will suffer" (Koadlow, cited in Kitzinger, 1985, p. 245). By denying, ignoring, or dismissing the sexual needs and desires of older women, medical professionals do a tremendous disservice to those women who have the courage to seek their assistance and advice.

ROCKING CHAIRS AND APPLE PIES: MEDIA MESSAGES

The older woman who is seeking some validation for the normality of her erotic desires and feelings will find no solace in the popular media. Acknowledgment of the sexuality of postmenopausal women is virtually absent in books and magazines, on television, and in the movies (Bazzini et al., 1997). In a culture that worships youth, when older women are portrayed at all, they are portrayed as nurturing, loving, and sometimes wise caretakers. Or they are depicted as harsh and vindictive matriarchs who obsessively control the lives of those around them. They are good or they are evil. They are rarely sexual.

In the few instances where the sexuality of the older woman is acknowledged in the visual media, these women are portrayed as eccentric or comical creatures (e.g., Maude from *Harold and Maude*), or as being from another planet (e.g., Roxanna Troy from *Star Trek: The Next Generation*). Other than a few novels (e.g., Dorris Lessing's 1995 book, *Love, Again*), there is a dearth of positive and accepting media portrayals of older women engaged in sexually vital and passionate relationships. It is interesting to note that the older characters in the popular movie *Cocoon* recaptured their sexual passions only after they recaptured their youth. The absence of examples of the possibility of sexual passion and fulfillment in the lives and relationships of older women makes it more difficult for women to envision these possibilities in their own lives.

Messages of the advertising industry further compound the sexual invisibility and insecurity of older women. They continue to reinforce the link between physical attractiveness and sexual desirability for women but not for men. In an stark example of this sexual double standard, Sean Connery, a man in his mid-60s, was recently voted the "Sexiest Man Alive" by the readers of *People* magazine. Certainly, women such as Sophia Loren and Elizabeth Taylor continue to be presented in the media as images of aging beauty. However, it is difficult to imagine either of these women, or others of their cohort, receiving a similar designation (i.e., "The Sexiest Woman Alive") in the popular press. Aldrich (cited in Page, 1993, p. 20) refers to the "rule of youth" in North American culture, as "the single most soul-destroying, pleasure-denying, love-shrivelling consequence of living under the domination of American beauty." He laments on how this:

> blinds us to the loveliness, the libidinous loveliness, of the fully lived life. A people who do not see the sexual allure of Jeanne Moreau's love-spent face, who do not respond to the magnificent ripeness of Sophia Loren, who cannot hear the erotic agony in the voice of Maria Callas—such a people deserve their subservience to the image of Christie Brinkley. (p. 201)

Body image concerns haunt women most of their lives. Unfortunately, "the standards for the appearance and performance of the body seem to be increasing with each subsequent generation." These standards may well "extend beyond the reach of older women in the future" (Rodeheaver & Stohs, 1991, p. 146). As Nickerson (1992) notes,

> It isn't an accident that the bleachers are full of opportunists ready to create and profit from our discontent. They come offering new potions, magic elixirs and exotic concoctions which, if we pay the price, will miraculously stop time, turn us back into Marilyn Monroe with liver spots. Our common sense tells us these expectations border on foolishness; our yearning makes us vulnerable. (p. 74)

INTIMATE RELATIONSHIPS: MESSAGES OF SIGNIFICANT OTHERS

Changes in interpersonal relationships can also significantly affect the sexual behavior and satisfaction of women in later life. For women in long-term relationships, the nature and character of their sexual interactions with their partners often change over time. Some older couples are quite glad to abandon intercourse altogether, and draw comfort from other forms of intimacy and companionship within their relationships (Kitzinger, 1985). Others find that "sexuality doesn't die" but "is transformed from the frightening urgency of youth into a warm and mellow exchange of intimacy between loving partners who know and understand each other" (Nickerson, 1992, p. 213). Certainly, for many couples who have been together a long time, sexual intimacy often takes on a different meaning in their relationships. "Sensuous, loving touch, tenderness for the other person, the joy of shared memories, the same sense of fun—all these play a dominant part in sex when a couple have been together a long time, and the relationship is a good one" (Kitzinger, 1995, p. 243). The following quotation captures the richness and depth of one couple's lifetime love affair:

> I am seventy-four years old and have been married for fifty-two years. We are fortunate to have good mental as well as physical health. This is not entirely a matter of luck. We have worked at it. Our good times have been more numerous than our bad times. The medical profession has only recently discovered the healing power of laughter. In our fifty-two years together we have had a lot of laughs. A sense of humor is as important as food, especially within the confines of marriage. For us the sharing that comes with having a warm and loving sex life over so many years deepens our joy in one another. (Boston Women's Health Book Collective, 1992, p. 535)

However, not all couples are fortunate enough to be in good health, and some are not able to sustain satisfying sexual relationships. Some women may be in relatively good health themselves and still be very interested in maintaining active sexual lives. Their partners, however, may have lost interest in sex or may be experiencing poor health or physical decline (Sheehy, 1992; Unger & Crawford, 1992). Differences in levels of sexual desire, side effects caused by such common drugs as high blood pressure medication, or long periods of ill-health, make it difficult for couples to maintain a level of sexual intimacy and activity that is mutually satisfactory.

The other pragmatic reality for older women is that many who do have sexual needs do not have partners. "Women are four times more likely than men to be widowed, are more likely to be widowed at an earlier age, and are more likely to remain widows with many years of life ahead of them. Nearly two-thirds of women over the age of 65 are widows" (Dowling, 1996, p. 119). Citing Walsh and McGoldrick, Dowling notes that over 75% of men older than 65 are married, whereas only 33% of women over 65 are. "In the United States, by the year 2000, there'll be two unmarried women for every unmarried man over age 65" (p. 119). With their longer life expectancy, married women can expect to face almost two decades of late-life widowhood. On the basis of these statistics, Walsh and McGoldrick refer to the later part of women's lives as the "for women only" phase.

Many older women miss the physical aspects of sex and orgasm. They miss the physical and emotional closeness, the pleasure of touching, holding hands, and gently caressing another. They miss the excitement and romance that is a part of many sexual relationships. They miss the intimacy (Troll, 1994). These sentiments are captured in the following words of a woman in her 70s: "It's the intimacy that I miss more than the actual sex act. Shared jokes—you know. I'm finding this with a number of women as well as with men, but the whole romantic aspect of my life seems to have gone by. I miss that" (Boston Women's Health Book Collective, 1992, p. 534).

Many older women have rich social support networks. Their continued contact with friends, neighbors, and family members can help to meet some of their needs for intimacy, closeness, and connection (Dowling, 1995; Roberto, 1996; Rotberg, 1987; Unger & Crawford, 1992). Some find contentment in a celibate life, like one of the older women in my research group (Daniluk, 1993):

> "I've come to the stage in my life when I don't need relationships with men. I've been celibate for a long time. I'm finding it incredibly comfortable. I actually worry about the fact that I find it so comfortable. The only men that I want relationships with are my son and brother and brother-in-law, and the people that are already close to me. . . . My relationships with them are so rich. As for sexuality, I guess I still think that I have sexual energy but I don't seem to need to act on it anymore. There were very intensely involved sexual years and now . . . I'm very comfortable letting that part of my life go. . . . It was wonderful, but it's part of my past."

Women may also turn to one another for comfort and companionship. Those who are not content with a celibate life may seek sexual intimacy and fulfillment in the arms of another woman (Starr & Weiner, 1981). Or they may find their needs for sexual expression satisfied in a new relationship with a male partner.

New sexual relationships can be exciting and rewarding at any time in life. For example, Nickerson (1992) quotes one 62-year-old woman who thought she had "dried up years ago." When she met an "interesting widower," she was delighted to find that this was not the case: "I was surprised when I found a pleasant, rosy feeling building up in my loins, and my female juices flowing like a teenager. This is the best time of all. I'm finding out what sex is all about, and I don't have to worry about getting pregnant" (p. 223). However, women in new sexual relationships may find it especially difficult to overcome their insecurities about their aging bodies and appearance (Kitzinger, 1985).

Women who are fortunate enough to meet new and interesting partners may also find themselves faced with considerable resistance to these new relationships. Adult children, in particular, are often resistant to their parent becoming involved with a new partner. Rotberg (1987) notes that when one parent dies and the surviving parent becomes interested in someone else,

> the sons and daughters often become uncomfortable with their parents sexuality and see this need for romance and intimacy as a threat to their inheritance and to their ability to manage their parent. There seems to be little social tolerance, especially among family members, for sexual and social liaisons between widowed and/or older persons. (p. 8)

Adult children's denial that their parents have sexual needs can make it extremely difficult for some older women to sustain their new relationships.

Women in care facilities may also find pragmatic problems in having their needs for sexual intimacy met. More nursing homes and intermediate care facilities are beginning to acknowledge the needs of older women and men for physical contact (Kitzinger, 1985; Nickerson, 1992; Stevens-Long & Commons, 1992). However, many still have policies that reflect institutionalized ageism and sexism. Few respect or support the needs or rights of the elderly to be sexually active by ensuring that their tenants are provided with adequate opportunities and the privacy that is conducive to sexual intimacy.

> Some nursing homes discourage any sexual contact, even to the extent of separating husbands from wives. They seem unable or unwilling to recognize elders' need for closeness, companionship and mature love. Through the ignorance of society, this lovely, natural expression of human compassion between older people is turned into something disgusting and unclean. (Nickerson, 1992, p. 222)

SUMMARY: PROBLEMATIC MEANINGS

Women in later life face some very real impediments to sexual pleasure and enjoyment, including poor health, poverty, and lack of a desirable or willing and able partner. Demographic realities and the natural aging process "put the brakes on some activities" although it may also "open up the possibility of others for those who are prepared to look for them" (Kitzinger, 1985, p. 242). While these realities need to be accommodated, they are not insurmountable. As Tiefer (1996) notes, women can experience sexual and erotic pleasures irrespective of whether they have a partner or have the full use of their bodies. Although changes in health and circumstances may challenge traditional notions of sexuality and sexual pleasure, they do not preclude other, rich and satisfying avenues to the expression and experiencing of women's sexual desires and energy. That part of the self that is women's "erotic lifeforce" (Lorde, 1984, p. 55) can still be a powerful source of pleasure and enjoyment.

The ageist and sexist attitudes in our culture that deny and invalidate the sexual needs, desires, and expression of older women appear to be a more significant impediment to the sexual self-esteem and sexual expression of women in later life. Societal expectations are critical in understanding the sexual self-perceptions and experiences of older women (Rotberg, 1987). In North American culture, "geriatric sex is considered peculiar, laughable, often disgusting and obscene" (Kitzinger, 1985, pp. 243–244). The elderly are suppose to be "past all that." Their minds and bodies are suppose to have turned to other things such as volunteer work, tending to grandchildren, hobbies, or their ailing health.

When it becomes apparent that some elders still have an interest in sex, society's willingness to accept this reality differs greatly for men and women. The "silver-haired" older man is often secretly "admired for his voracious sexual appetite in old age" (Kitzinger, 1985, p. 245). Nudge, nudge, wink, wink—"the old devil" can still get it up. Similar tolerance and admiration are not extended to a woman of the same age who seeks sexual gratification. Overt, or even subtle, expressions of sexual interest or activity on the part of older women are considered "indecent, and somehow very threatening to the young" (p. 245).

> The image of the postmenopausal woman common in Western cultures has taken two forms. The first is the grandmotherly matron, somewhat overweight, who occupies her time knitting and cooking; and the second is the irritable, depressed crone who occupies her time meddling in others' lives and gossiping. For both stereotypes, sexuality is conspicuously absent—the grandmother has fulfilled her sexual role in the form of maternity and no longer desires sex, nor do others find her sexually appealing; the crone has always been and continues to be sexually dissatisfied and unfulfilled. (Gannon, 1994, p. 116)

After years of being defined by their sexuality, for women in later life, the chorus of voices stops. Older women are faced with a deafening silence. They are no longer defined by their sexuality. Instead, they are defined by its absence. In her article entitled "No Country for Older Women," British journalist Katherine Whitehorn (cited in Kitzinger, 1985) talks about how the crone is the only alternative for being a sexy and young woman in our society. "There are other words for women of this age, but all of them are equally unattractive: matriarch, harridan, hag, battle-axe and old bag" (Kitzinger, 1985, p. 241). As Koadlow (cited in Kitzinger, 1985) notes, the "denial of late-life sexuality has a destructive effect that goes far beyond its negative impact upon the aging person's sex life and self-image. It complicates and distorts interpersonal relations" (p. 245).

CHALLENGE AND CHANGE: CREATING NEW MEANINGS

Beyond the social invisibility of the sexual older woman, there may indeed be opportunities for continued sexual pleasure and adventure. With the knowledge and confidence she gains over a lifetime, new space may open up for the older woman to explore creatively and experiment with aspects of her sexuality that have long been denied or suppressed (Sheinkin & Golden, 1995). To assist women in embracing the possibilities of sexual adventure and pleasure well into their later years, mental health practitioners first need to confront our own ageist assumptions regarding the sexuality and sexual expression of older women. "As therapists, we owe our clients a sensitivity to their sexual needs and desires. We [also] owe ourselves an honest approach to our personal feelings about growing old" (Rotberg, 1987, p. 3). This includes facing our own concerns about physical deterioration and mental decline, and our fears of ending up alone and discarded. We cannot expect to divest ourselves of all of our ageist attitudes and beliefs overnight, any more than it is realistic to expect that older women will themselves be free of these attitudes. However, it is important for us to recognize and confront our own ageist attitudes and beliefs about elder sex and passion in all its varied forms of expression.

It is also important that we become comfortable addressing issues of sexuality directly with older women. We need to invite them to talk openly about their sexual needs and concerns. We should not wait for them to initiate this type of exploration. Rather, we need to provide opportunities for them to share their fears and feelings about the changes that are occurring in their sexual lives and in their sexual self-perceptions as they age. In working with older clients, we should also remember the therapeutic and healing value of human touch. Many older women live alone and have limited physical contact with others. In becoming comfortable with touching our elders in gentle and unobtrusive ways, we can communicate validation, reassurance, and support.

In our selection of interventions, we need to be sensitive to the fact that the present cohort of older women was raised during a time of tremendous sexual repression. We cannot expect elder women to feel comfortable examining their bodies. We cannot expect that they will begin masturbating if they have never done so before. As Nickerson (1992) notes, "The pleasures of masturbation were denied us, and for many of us the shame persists" (p. 211). Because of poor sex education and the taboos of their early years, many older women may know little about the functioning of their own bodies (Kellett, 1991). Launching into an exploration of the sexual intimacies of women's past or current lives, suggesting body exploration exercises, or assigning homework aimed at increasing their sexual awareness or comfort may not be appropriate with some older clients.

If women are to develop and maintain a sense of sexual entitlement and esteem throughout their later years, it is important that we validate their sexuality. We need to help them become comfortable with their changing bodies and appearance as they age. Many older women are faced with physical disabilities and health problems that impair their sexual expression and enjoyment. It is important to normalize the physical changes in sexual responsiveness that occur over time and to help women expand their definitions and notions of sexual expression and intimacy. "Women now in their older years must shed years of training to act on the knowledge that there are alternatives to intercourse and that they can initiate sex . . . to break through old patterns, assumptions, misunderstandings and miscommunications" (Boston Women's Health Book Collective, 1992, p. 535).

Using the exercises presented here (as well as those discussed throughout the book and in particular in Chapters 13 and 14), counselors can assist women in exploring and discovering new avenues for sexual expression, intimacy, and love (Rotberg, 1987). In the words of Nickerson (1992) "Sex after sixty is much like any other activity—you get back what you put into it" (p. 207). Perhaps Kellett (1991) states it best when she says that the goal in working with older women is to help them to "feel free to alter their sexual practice to suit themselves" (p. 147).

> Human beings have the choice of continuing intimate sexual contact through ageing until death, though many will respond to declining libido or loss of a partner by giving up this aspect of their lives. Our role as therapists, however, must be to avoid putting pressure on patients to conform to our ideals. Equally, we should prevent others from destroying this intimacy by interventions which ignore the sexuality of the patient. The elderly have earned the right to decide for themselves. (p. 154)

Together, counselors and the older women with whom they work can embark on a journey of discovery that may well enrich both of their lives.

A Walk Down Memory Lane

An important first step in understanding a woman's current sexual self-perceptions involves exploring her sexual history. This usually involves detailed questions and answers. However, some older women may find this type of inquisition format too invasive. The questions may be too uncomfortable. Alternately, counselors can ask women to "take a walk down memory lane." Women can review their sexual histories from childhood to the present, through the use of questions such as the following:

What is your earliest memory of being conscious of yourself as a sexual person?

How old were you when you started to menstruate, and what do you remember about that experience? How did you feel? How did others react?

How did you learn about sex, menstruation, making babies, and so on?

How did you feel about your body when you were a child, a teenager, a young woman, middle-aged? How do you feel now?

How comfortable were you with touching and exploring your own body? How comfortable are you now?

What was your first sexual experience with another person like? Overall, what has sex been like for you over the years? When it was good, what made it good? When it was bad, what made it bad? How do you feel about sex now?

Did you have, or want to have children? What was that part of your life like for you? What were the losses? What were the gains?

What was menopause like for you?

When you look back over your reproductive and sexual life, what has been the best part of being a woman for you? What has been the most challenging part?

If you had your life to live over again, what would you do differently in terms of your reproductive choices, your intimate relationships, and the ways you have chosen to express yourself sexually?

If you were to take this life journey again, what would you hope to take with you that you did not have the first time around (e.g., information, confidence, self-assurance, etc.)

If you were talking to a young woman who had her whole life ahead of her, what advice would you give her about her sexual relationship(s), her relationship with her body, and her reproductive choices?

Other questions can be added as relevant. The intent is to guide women in their explorations and reviews of their sexual lives. This activity can be undertaken in a guided fantasy, in which case, it should be followed by the completion of something more concrete. A lifeline might be used upon which women mark and discuss significant events in their sexual and reproductive lives. Or they may wish to engage in this exploration in a narrative form. Some women find journaling to be an effective medium for this exploration. For others, the manual dexterity they require to write is compromised by chronic illnesses such as arthritis. They might review photo albums and share pictures of themselves, their partners, their children, their grandchildren, and so on at various stages in their lives.

As they review and discuss their personal histories, women can be ask questions that deepen their exploration of issues that seem particularly significant to their sexual self-constructions and expectations. In the process, they may learn a great deal about their values and unique life circumstances, and about their sexual needs, experiences, and comfort. This information can be especially helpful in guiding the timing and selection of appropriate interventions. It is unlikely that most older women have had an opportunity to discuss these issues in detail with another woman before. Most have not had the opportunity to undertake this type of review of their reproductive and sexual lives in terms of significant moments, events, and circumstances. As such, this activity can prove to be quite significant in helping women to identify the patterns of their lives and to see the continuity and disjunctures of their journeys from a more objective perspective.

Never Too Old to Feel

As indicated earlier in this chapter, the ageist and sexist attitudes that are so pervasive in North American society are not limited to the young. Older women have also been socialized to believe that their sexual needs and desires are somehow perverse. In the absence of viable images of healthy later-life sexuality, and given the sexually repressive period that the current cohort of older women grew up in, it is likely that, to varying degrees, they will have incorporated these ageist assumptions. These can be as debilitating in preventing women from knowing and acting upon their own sexual needs and desires as any externally imposed constraints. It is important, therefore, for counselors to help women explore their attitudes about the physical and sexual realities of aging. It is necessary to provide accurate information, and to gently challenge sexist or ageist assumptions that appear to be preventing women from knowing and acting on their sexual desires. It is especially important that counselors help older women to reject the myths of diminished capacity, decrepitude, and uselessness that are so prevalent in our society. As Nickerson (1992) notes, "Women who believe in themselves are enhanced by the sum of their years" (p. 22).

Exercises have been presented throughout this book that are aimed at assessing and challenging popular myths and assumptions about women's bodies and sexual functioning (word associations, true–false statements). Any of these could be easily adapted for working with older women. Another example of this type of activity involves having women read brief vignettes about older women in a variety of situations. These vignettes should include women who are partnered and women who are unpartnered. They should include women who have elected to abstain from sexual activity, women who have taken a lover later in their lives (male or female), women who have active sexual fantasy lives, women who masturbate regularly, women who are having unprotected sex with a new partner, and so on. The purpose of the vignettes is to allow women to examine their beliefs and attitudes from a safe emotional distance.

Counselors should normalize and validate the rights of older women to engage in whatever form of sexual expression they desire and feel is comfortable for them. This opportunity can also be used to help women explore their sexual interests and desires, and how these might be met (e.g., masturbation, taking a lover, sexual fantasy, erotica). What do they find stimulating and erotic? What, for them, constitutes a satisfying sexual encounter? It is also useful to explore the possible barriers to having these desires fulfilled (e.g., What keeps women from acting on their desires?).

This exploration can provide a springboard for women to discuss issues such as safe sex, lack of a suitable partner, etc..

Role plays can also be useful. They can help women become more comfortable in asking their physicians for information or assistance with remedies to increase their sexual comfort. They can help women to communicate more easily their sexual needs and desires to their partners, or to initiate a sexual encounter with someone they are interested in pursuing in a sexual relationship. And they can assist women in responding to the queries, concerns, and the potential discomfort of their adult children regarding their intimate lives and choices.

I Am Woman, I Am Invincible, I Am Tired: Necessary Losses

As discussed in Chapter 11, loss is a significant theme in the lives of the elderly. Many older women experiences a host of losses that inevitably have a short- or long-term impact on their sexual self-esteem, self-perceptions, and relational possibilities. It is important for counselors to help women identify and acknowledge these losses. Information and suggestions should also be provided on how women might cope with these changes in their lives.

Counselors can begin by asking women to examine and consider the significant losses that they have experienced in their lives, especially recent losses. Specifically, women should focus on the losses they feel have affected their sexual self-esteem and the way they express themselves sexually. These may include the loss of health, vitality, or mobility through illness or injury; the loss of energy through the aging process; the loss of a life partner through divorce or death; the loss of friends and family members who have moved or passed away; the loss of economic resources and security; or the loss of familiar surroundings due to desired or forced relocation. It is important to validate the significance of any and all of these losses in terms of their impact on the sexual self-esteem and expression of older women. It is also important to help women appreciate the connection between their sexual feelings and desires, and the changing circumstances of their lives. Certainly, it may be difficult for a woman who has gone to the beauty salon every Saturday for the past 40 years to continue to feel attractive and sexually desirable when she can no longer afford this luxury due to a change in her economic circumstances. Also, a woman who is grieving over the loss of her life partner may feel emotionally and sexually dead, or she may find that her sexual and erotic appetite is heightened during her grief. As Kitzinger (1985) points out, there is no one "typical" response to grief in terms of women's sexual feelings and desires. Women may well need validation for the normalcy of their sexual urges, or for their absence, during times of grief and loss. Suggestions on how women can continue to satisfy their erotic appetites in ways that are acceptable to them (fantasy, self-stimulation, etc.), can be very helpful.

It is also important to validate women's continued needs for intimacy and nonsexual contact. As Rotberg (1987) notes, "The need for a loving relationship is vital and necessary for life at every age. This loving relationship can satisfy the need for friendship, acceptance, and intimate exchange with another person, without necessarily being sexual" (p. 10). Counselors can assist older women in finding ways to have their needs for intimate connection met (e.g., nurturing a platonic relationship with another woman or with a man; spending time with children or grandchildren). "Female friendships along with strong family networks and neighborhood support systems" often are instrumental in satisfying some of "the older woman's love and belonging needs" (p. 9).

For women who are experiencing deteriorating health, or who are disabled, counselors can provide information and assistance on how they can continue to enjoy their sexuality in spite of their physical limitations (see Bullard & Knight, 1981; Kitzinger, 1985; Sandelowski, 1989; Thornton, 1981). Exercises such as those discussed in Chapter 14 (e.g., Fantasies: "The Poetry of Sex"; Writing New Sexual Scripts; Owning Our Bodies, Owning Our Sexuality) can be especially useful in this regard. Also, information on nutrition and physical exercise can be important for women whose life circumstances or grief have resulted in their not attending to their own health (Boston Women's Health Collective, 1992). Nickerson (1992) underscores the immeasurable value of regular exercise and movement to maintain the physical and psychological health of older women. "With exercise we flower and become. Without it we wither and die. Exercise may be our *best* medicine. The human body was created to move, to do, to act, and when we stop doing, the bones, joints, and circulation more or less seize up. It may even be that women live longer than men because of our ongoing activity" (p. 178).

It is also comforting for women who are grieving to know that these feelings will pass in time. This may be an age-old adage, but it is one that bears repeating and reinforcing when a woman is in the throes of depression or despair at the loss of a significant person in her life. The goal is to help women "create the best old age" they can, whatever their life circumstances.

Badges of Honor

Body image problems are not uncommon for women in later life. This is particularly the case when women have experienced disabling or disfiguring health problems, or when they are considering entering a new sexual relationship. Women in long-term relationships who recently have had a mastectomy may find it difficult to accept their own bodies or to allow their partners to see or touch the bodies they perceived to be "disfigured" (Dackman, 1990; Kitzinger, 1985). It is also not an easy task for older women, particularly the present cohort of older women, to feel comfortable in their aging bodies and in their nakedness when they are with other women in nonsexual situations (e.g., in a swimming pool changing room), much less when they are with a new lover. This is similar to the midlife woman, discussed in the previous chapter, who wore clothes to bed when with her new lover for fear that he would be disgusted or "turned off" by her sagging stomach. Many older women are acutely aware of their sagging skin, wrinkles, and diminished pubic hair. They may fear that their lovers will perceive them as unattractive or undesirable. This reality struck close to home recently as I listened to the tall, thin, and attractive 70-year-old woman that my father has recently developed a relationship with lament the need to watch her weight for fear that she is getting "fat" and her stomach is beginning to show.

Older women may need assistance to accept their changing bodies. Counselors can help women learn to appreciate that their bodies have served them well. They may have carried and nurtured their children. They certainly have carried them through long and rich lives. As Nickerson (1992) notes, "We need to give ourselves permission to be what we are. It is imprudent to punish the body to reach some mythical measurement. Our bodies, respected and cared for, are what we need them to be at this stage of life" (p. 77). Counselors can ask women to engage in an appreciation exercise in which they are encouraged to identify their physical "badges of honor." These include the physical characteristics that are important markers of the significant accomplishments in their lives. This is not the same as identifying characteristics that women like about their appearance (e.g., the color of their eyes, their hair, the shape of their hands). Rather, the characteristics that are targeted in this exercise are those that are frequently viewed by the beauty brokers, and by women themselves, as sources of shame (e.g., wrinkles, stretch marks). For example, Posin (1991) chose to perceive her wrinkles not as signs of her failure to age well or take proper care of herself, but rather as "a sign of [her] deepening into [her] own aging, mellowing process" (p. 144). Similarly, rather than being viewed as ugly and disfiguring, the stretch marks that a woman carries on her belly can be reframed as symbols of a body that gave life to others. Like the proudly worn scars of men who were speared while running with the bulls in Pamplona, Spain, women's perceptions of their bodies may be much more accepting if they are able to view the stretch marks on their breasts and belly as "honorable" scars earned in the creation of their children (Nickerson, 1992). As I write this, I am reminded of the scene from *Shirley Valentine,* when, to Shirley's amazement, her Greek lover kissed her stretch marks, referring to them as symbols of beauty.

In reframing those characteristics that have been earned throughout their lives as symbols of their success, rather than as the inevitable and unattractive signs of aging, self-acceptance and esteem are reinforced. Such self-acceptance is important if women are to be comfortable in sharing their bodies with another. As noted in several other chapters, the use of mirrors can also be a helpful adjunct for those women who are comfortable in examining their own bodies in the privacy of their homes. The importance of self-nurturing and self-care should be underscored in helping women to become more loving with, and accepting of, their bodies. Rather than trying to eliminate their wrinkles with anti-aging creams, older women can be encourage to cream their skin and take luxurious bubble baths for their own sensory pleasure.

Women may also benefit from receiving feedback from others (including counselors) regarding those characteristics that others find attractive and appealing about them. It can be quite a gift for a woman to realize that others see strength, character, and beauty in her face, when she herself sees only a wrinkled and aging version of the young woman she once was.

Hags and Heroes

According to Nickerson (1992), older women are the "repositories of the experience and wisdom of our time." They are "the Elders" (p. 22). Recognition of the value of women's wisdom and authority is apparent in many native tribes and in some other cultures in the world. In some cultures, age bestows upon women a certain respect and authority. Within these cultures,

> honored elders are respected for wisdom born of memory and long life experience. The faces are strong and kindly. They make no apology for appearance, no false attempt at beauty. The elder is valued for her age. She is the traditional Crone, a present-day manifestation of the ancient mother goddess who appears as the Trinity of Maid, Mother *and* Crone. (p. 74)

Yet in our culture and in particular, in white, North American culture, there is no value placed on being old. There is no honored role for the older woman. Women spend years being the caretakers to, and nurturers of, others. Women serve as the peacekeepers and social bridges between the generations (Stevens-Long & Commons, 1992). Despite their wealth of accumulated wisdom and knowledge, however, older women are discarded and culturally denied the dignity and respect that they deserve.

Nickerson (1992) notes how "when women ignore the value of their lives, . . . they neglect their own inner resources and are caught short by the aging process" (p. 75). She suggests that there is an absence of both respect and ritual to mark women's passing into this important life stage. As such, it can be especially important for counselors to support women into this "unscripted adventure into age" (p. 87). We can encourage older women to identify other elders who serve as role models of creative and satisfying aging. Nickerson and others (e.g., Greer, 1991; Sang et al., 1991; Sheehy, 1992) return to the goddess literature in holding up the "Crone" as the most prominent historical figure who represents the power and wisdom of aging for women. She was the old wise woman who in early times was the "healer and dispenser of justice" (p. 96). These authors refer to the importance of creating a "rite-of-passage" or "ritual" to mark women's transition into their "Cronehood." For example, in her book, *Old and Smart,* Nickerson shares her experience of the power and validation that resulted from a now annual gathering of women, affectionately referred to as the "Amazing Grays." These women come together to celebrate their ritual passage into "Cronehood." This ritual involves laughter, song, and dance, in celebration and acknowledgment of each woman's "hard-earned growth and wisdom" (p. 16). Gentry and Seifert (1991) similarly present several examples of women's Croning celebrations. They suggest that women make this a public rite of passage in which they proudly claim their age and wisdom. In these public ceremonies, women share their visions for the future with other women who can affirm their choices and witness their transition into the next phase of their lives. These authors quote one "Crone's" words during her celebration: "this . . . has been/is about choices—the ones I've made and the ones I have ahead of me. I feel a sense of urgency that's new to me. I feel that I must be wise and even judicious in my choices from now on because the clock . . . really is ticking. But how it ticks, to whose rhythms and reasons it ticks are my decisions" (p. 231).

The creation of rituals and sharing of experiences with other women can be an important marker to validate the gifts that women bring with them—physical, mental, and spiritual—into this stage in their lives. Counselors can encourage women to seek out, participate in, and create personally meaningful rituals. They should be encouraged to include their sexual selves as a significant part of this transition. However, it is important to remember that some older women will not find the Crone and goddess imagery to be of comfort. Some will not be able to relate to this ideology. Instead, they may explore other ways to acknowledge this important transition in their lives that are more consistent with their spiritual beliefs. What seems to be most important in the creation of these rituals is having other women to bear witness to the transition; being a part of a community of women (Nickerson, 1992, p. 87).

Finding Your Bliss

As women move into the next stage of their lives, they do not leave their sexual selves behind. Whether they are actively involved in a sexual relationship, whether they are having orgasms or intercourse, or choose to express themselves in any other way that is typically defined as "sexual" in our culture, their sexuality is always with them. It is that part of them that is their sexual energy and vitality. It is a part of their history. It is embedded in their physical and mental memories, in their eyes and faces, in the lines of their bodies, and in the sensations of their skin.

Some women will wish to continue to pursue the pleasures of the body, alone or in the company of another. They may need both validation for, and assistance in, making this choice possible. Others already have, or will, happily let go of genital sexual expression and the pursuit of the physiological release of orgasm. They may be content to live with the warm memories of moments of pleasure and connection. This choice must also be supported by counselors. In reference to herself and her "age mates" Nickerson (1992) notes how "in our maturity we have the freedom to experience our sexuality fully, creatively, with the wisdom and compassion of our years" (p. 214). Reinforcing this freedom is an important part of working with older women.

Counselors also need to help women explore the many ways that they have in the past, and can continue to, express and enjoy their sexuality through their diverse passionate interests and pursuits. The exercises discussed in Chapter 14 may be helpful in this regard. Through guided fantasy and movement, women can also be assisted to get in touch with the erotic energy within themselves. They can explore the ways this energy is expressed in their enjoyment of gardening, flowers, clothes, food, perfume, movement, yoga, fantasy, physical activity, touch, and connection with others. In "finding their bliss," women can be encouraged to nurture this important part of themselves and their lives by committing themselves to those activities and relationships that provide satisfaction and renewal. Referring to her discussion with a group of women in their 60s and 70s, Sheehy (1992) notes how, for each

> there came a point, sometime in their fifties, when they had to let go of—or at least had to stop trying to hang on to—their youthful image. Although it was painful at the time, they had all found a source of new vitality and exhilaration—a "kicker." As each one described her personal struggle, a common denominator emerged and the group hit upon something profound: The source of continuing aliveness was to find your passion and pursue it, with whole heart and single mind. It is essential to . . . find this new source of aliveness and meaning that will make the years ahead even more precious than those past. (p. 140)

Older women should be encouraged to continue the sexual adventure that they embarked on in their youth. They should be supported in their explorations of new and satisfying ways to nurture and express their erotic life force. This is a "creative energy" (Lorde, 1984, p. 55) that is empowered by knowledge and wisdom. Women should be supported in rejecting the injunctions of a culture that discounts and limits their sexual power, desirability, and vitality. They should be encouraged to view the years ahead as another part of the sexual adventure they began in their youth.

EPILOGUE

It has been a daunting, sometimes frustrating, and always illuminating task to write about the changes in the sexual self-conceptions and experiences of girls and women as their bodies, like the seasons, change and develop over a lifetime. Despite the length of this book, the literature on women's sexual experience and expression is sparse. The one exception is the literature related to fertility and reproductive functioning. Unfortunately, much of this research is biased and flawed.

In sifting through the available literature, I have attempted to identify the source of women's difficulties in living comfortably in their bodies and in developing and maintaining a sense of sexual agency and entitlement throughout life. What has been most striking in this effort have been the voices of women themselves that cry out that something is indeed "rotten in the state of Denmark." These voices—voices of feminist theorists, researchers, and clinicians, voices of poets and writers, and voices of "ordinary" women—continue to resist the imposition of definitions and meanings that would serve to quell and repress women's erotic life force.

It is still impossible, as yet, to imagine a world in which women can freely claim their sexuality. A world does not yet exist in which women truly can experience "a body free for expression, a mind free for decision, and a soul free for enjoyment" (Bagley & King, 1990, p. 38). However, as mental health professionals, we can play an important role in honoring women's voices. We can encourage women to listen to that part of themselves that intuitively knows there is something deeper, richer, and more vital to women's sexuality than the dichotomous, paradoxical, and limiting images that are promoted in our culture. In our work with women, we can help move them "away from danger and oppression . . . toward pleasure, agency, and self-definition" (Vance, 1984, p. 24). We can help women reclaim the erotic life force "in our language, our history, our dancing, our loving, our work, our lives" (Lorde, 1984, p. 55). As Ussher (1989) suggests, we can

> use the voices of women ourselves, piece together the different parts of our lives, to help towards the realization that, although we are often

burdened with the definitions of womanhood which position us in order to constrain and control us, *we* can take control, change the definitions, and move towards a positive image of self. Psychology, within a feminist framework, can contribute to our knowledge about ourselves, our bodies, and our reproductive abilities, leading to the possibility of our reclaiming them with new power. (p. 142)

Appendix A

The Sexual Development of Children and Adolescents

EDUCATIONAL BOOKS FOR PARENTS AND THEIR CHILDREN

Bell, R. (1987). *Changing bodies, changing lives: A book for teens on sex and relationships* (rev. ed.). New York: Random House.

Bourgeois, F., & Wolfish, M. (1994). *Changes in you and me.* Toronto: Somerville.

Calderone, M., & Johnson, E. (1981). *The family book about sexuality.* New York: Harper & Row.

Calderone, M., & Ramey, J. (1982). *Talking with your child about sex.* New York: Random House.

Carrera, M. (1981). *Sex, the facts, the acts and your feelings.* New York: Lansdowne.

Cassell, C. (1987). *Straight from the heart: How to talk to your teenagers about love and sex.* New York: Simon & Schuster.

Clarke, J. I., & Dawson, C. (1989). *Growing up again: Parenting ourselves, parenting our children.* San Francisco: Harper & Row.

Gardner-Loulan, J. (1991). *Period.* Volcano, CA: Volcano Press.

Girard, L. W. (1984). *My body is private.* Niles, IL: Albert Whitman.

Goldman, R., & Goldman, J. (1988). *Show me yours: Understanding children's sexuality* (2nd ed.). New York: Penguin.

Gravelle, K., & Gravelle, J. (1996). *The period book: Everything you don't want to ask (but need to know).* New York: Walker.

Harris, R. H., & Emberley, M. (1994). *It's perfectly normal.* Cambridge, MA: Candlewick Press.

Hindman, J. (1985). *A very touching book: For little people and for big people.* Durkee, OR: McClure–Hindman.

Kaufman, M. (1995). *Easy for you to say: Q & A's for teens living with chronic illness or disability.* Toronto: Key Porter Books.

Madaras, L., & Madaras, A. (1983). *What's happening to my body?: A growing up guide for mothers and daughters.* New York: Newmarket Press.

Mayle, P. (1975). *What's happening to me?: The answers to some of the world's most embarrassing questions.* London: Macmillan.

Mayle, P. (1978). *Will I like it?* London: Allen.

Mayle, P., & Robins, A. (1978). *Where did I come from?: The facts of life without any nonsenses and with illustrations* (2nd ed.). London: Macmillan.
Meredith, S. (1987). *Understanding the facts of life*. London: Usborne.
McCoy, K., & Wibbelsman, C. (1986). *Growing and changing: A handbook for preteens*. New York: Perigee Books.
Riddell, E., & Smallman, C. (1986). *Outside in*. Hauppauge, NY: Barron's.
Schoen, M. (1990). *Belly buttons are navels*. Buffalo, NY: Prometheus.
Smallman, C., & Riddell, E. (1988). *See how you grow*. Hauppauge, NY: Barron's.

BOOKS FOR COUNSELORS WORKING WITH SEXUALLY ABUSED CHILDREN AND ADOLESCENTS

Bagley, C., & King, K. (1990). *Child sexual abuse: The search for healing*. London and New York: Routledge.
Davis, N. (1990). *Once upon a time: Therapeutic stories to heal abused children* (rev. ed.). Oxon Hill, MD: Psychological Associates of Oxon Hill.
Donovan, D. M., & McIntrye, D. (1990). *Healing the hurt child: A developmental–contextual approach*. New York: Norton.
Eth, S., & Pynoos, R. (Eds.). (1985). *Post-traumatic stress disorder in children*. Washington, DC: American Psychiatric Association Press.
Everstine, D. S., & Everstine, L. (1989). *Sexual trauma in children and adolescents: Dynamics and treatment*. New York: Brunner/Mazel.
Friedrich, W. N. (1990) *Psychotherapy of sexually abused children and their families*. New York: Norton.
Gil, E. (1991). *The healing power of play: Working with abused children*. New York: Guilford Press.
Gil, E., & Cavanaugh, J. (1993). *Sexualized children: Assessment and treatment of sexualized children and children who molest*. New York: Guilford Press.
Granger, B. (1991). *I think I see a rainbow: Group treatment for sexually abused girls*. Richmond, BC: Blue Heron.
Hudson, P. S. (1991). *Ritual child abuse: Discovery, diagnosis, and treatment*. Saratoga, CA: R&E Publishers.
Kaufman, B., & Wohl, A. (1992). *Casualties of childhood: A developmental perspective on sexual abuse using projective drawings*. New York: Brunner/Mazel.
Kehoe, P. (1988). *Helping abused children: A book for those who work with sexually abused children*. Seattle, WA: Parenting Press.
MacFarlane, K., & Waterman, J. (1986). *Sexual abuse of young children: Evaluation and treatment*. New York: Guilford Press.
Mandel, J. G., & Damon, L. (1989). *Group treatment for sexually abused children*. New York: Guilford Press.
Mather, C. L., & Debye, K. E. (1994). *How long does it hurt? A guide to recovering from incest and sexual abuse for teenagers, their friends and their families*. San Francisco: Jossey-Bass.
Miller, A. (1990). *Thou shalt not be aware: Society's betrayal of the child* (2nd ed.). New York: Meridian.
Miller, A. (1990). *The untouched key: Tracing childhood trauma in creativity and destructiveness*. New York: Doubleday.

Russell, D. (1986). *The secret trauma: Incest in the lives of girls and women.* New York: Basic Books.

Sgroi, S. M. (1983). *Handbook for clinical intervention in child sexual abuse.* Lexington, MA: Lexington Books.

Sgroi, S. M. (Ed.). (1988). *Vulnerable populations: Evaluation and treatment of sexually abused children and adult survivors* (Vol. 1). Lexington, MA: D.C. Heath.

Wohl, A., & Kaufman, B. (1985). *Silent screams and hidden cries: An interpretation of artwork by children from violent homes.* New York: Brunner/Mazel.

BOOKS FOR PARENTS AND THEIR ABUSED CHILDREN

Ashley, S. (1992). *The missing voice: Writings by mothers of incest victims.* Dubuque, IA: Kendall/Hunt.

Hillman, D., & Solek-Tefft, J. (1988). *Spiders and flies: Help for parents and teachers of sexually abused children.* Lexington, MA: Lexington Books.

Johnson, J. T. (1992). *Mothers of incest survivors: Another side of the story.* Bloomington: Indiana University Presss.

Johnson, K. (1986). *The trouble with secrets.* Seattle, WA: Parenting Press.

Johnson, T. C. (1989). *Human sexuality: Curriculum for parents and children in troubled families.* Los Angeles: Children's Institute International.

Kehoe, P. (1987). *Something happened and I'm scared to tell: A book for young victims of abuse.* Seattle, WA: Parenting Press.

Matsakis, A. (1991). *When the bough breaks: A guide for parents of sexually abused children.* Oakland, CA: New Harbinger.

Ovaris, W. (1991). *After the nightmare: The treatment of non-offending mothers of sexually abused children.* Holmes Beach, FL: Learning Publications.

Sanford, D. (1986). *I can't talk about it: A child's book about sexual abuse.* Portland, OR: Multnomah Press.

Appendix B

Body Image and Struggles with Weight

BOOKS FOR CLIENTS

Bell, R. (1987). *Changing bodies, changing lives.* New York: Random House.

Borysenko, J. (1988). *Minding the body, mending the mind.* New York: Bantam Books.

Bruch, H. (1978). *The golden cage: The enigma of anorexia nervosa.* London: Open Books.

Bruch, H., Czyzewski, D., & Suhr, M. A. (Eds.). (1988). *Conversations with anorexics.* New York: Basic Books.

Cash, T. F. (1991). *Body image therapy: A program for self-directed change.* New York: Guilford Press.

Chernin, K. (1983). *The tyranny of slenderness.* London: Women's Press.

Chernin, K. (1986). *The hungry self: Women, eating and identity.* London: Virago Press.

Crook, M. (1991). *The body image trap: Understanding and rejecting body image myths.* North Vancouver, BC: Self-Counsel Press.

Debold, E., Wilson, M., & Malave, I. (1993). *Mother–daughter revolution: From betrayal to power.* New York: Addison-Wesley.

Erdman, C. K. (1995). *Nothing to lose: A guide to sane living in a large body.* San Francisco: Harper San Francisco.

Freedman, R. (1988). *Bodylove: Learning to like out looks—ourselves.* New York: Harper & Row.

Greaves, K. (1990). *Big and beautiful.* London: Grafton Books.

Hancock, E. (1989). *The girl within.* New York: Dutton.

Hirschmann, J. R., & Munter, C. H. (1995). *When women stop hating their bodies: Freeing yourself from food and weight obsession.* New York: Fawcett Columbine.

Hutchinson, M. G. (1985). *Transforming body image: Learning to love the body you have.* Freedom, CA: Crossing Press.

Kano, S. (1989). *Making peace with food: A step-by-step guide to freedom from diet/weight conflict.* New York: Harper & Row.

Koffinke, C., & Jordon, J. (1993). *Mom, you don't understand: A daughter and mother share their views.* Minneapolis: Deaconess Press.

Madaras, L. (1983). *What's happening to my body?: Book for girls.* New York: Newmarket Press.
Madaras, L. (1993). *My feelings, myself.* New York: Newmarket Press.
Maine, M. (1991). *Father hunger: Fathers, daughters and food.* Carlsbad, CA: Gurze Books.
Melamed, E. (1983). *Mirror, mirror: The terror of not being young.* New York: Simon & Schuster.
Northrup, C. (1994). *Women's bodies, women's wisdom: Creating physical and emotional health and healing.* New York: Bantam Books.
Orbach, S. (1978). *Fat is a feminist issue.* New York: Paddington Press.
Orbach, S. (1983). *Fat is a feminist issue: Part II.* New York: Berkley Press.
Roberts, N. (1987). *Breaking all the rules: Feeling good and looking great no matter what your size.* New York: Penguin Books.
Roth, G. (1982). *Feeding the hungry heart.* New York: Signet.
Schoenfielder, L., & Weiser, B. (Eds.). (1983). *Shadows on a tightrope: Writings by women on fat oppression.* San Francisco: Spinsters/Aunt Lute Press.
Seid, R. P. (1989). *Never too thin: Why women are at war with their bodies.* New York: Prentice-Hall.
Siegel, M., Brisman, J., & Weinshel, M. (1988). *Surviving an eating disorder: Strategies for families and friends.* New York: Harper Perennial.
Thompson, B. W. (1994). *A hunger so wide and so deep: American women speak out on eating problems.* Minneapolis: University of Minnesota Press.

BOOKS FOR HELPING PROFESSIONALS

Bloom, C., Gitter, A., Gutwill, S., Kogel, L., & Zaphiropoulos, L. (1996). *Eating problems: A feminist psychoanalytic treatment model.* New York: Basic Books.
Brown, C., & Jasper, K. (Eds.). (1993). *Consuming passions: Feminist approaches to weight preoccupation and eating disorders.* Toronto: Second Story Press.
Brown, L., & Rothblum, E. (Eds.). (1989). *Overcoming fear of fat.* New York: Harrington Park Press.
Brumberg, J. J. (1989). *Fasting girls: The emergence of anorexia nervosa as a modern disease.* Cambridge, MA: Harvard University Press.
Fallon, P., Katzman, M. A., & Wooley, S. C. (Eds.). (1994). *Feminist perspectives on eating disorders.* New York: Guilford Press.
Friedman, S. S. (1994). *Girls in the 90's: Facilitators manual.* Vancouver, BC: Salal Books.
Jacobus, M., Keller, E. F., & Shuttleworth, S. (Eds.). (1990). *Body/politics: Women and the discourses of science.* New York: Routledge.
Meadow, R. M., & Weiss, L. (1992). *Women's conflicts about eating and sexuality: The relationship between food and sex.* New York: Harrington Park Press.
Orbach, S. (1985). *Hunger strike.* London: Faber & Faber.
Rodin, J. (1992). *Body traps.* New York: Quill, William Morrow.
Thorne, R. R. (1997). *Fat: A fate worse than death?* New York: Haworth Press.

Appendix C

The Aftermath of Sexual Violence

BOOKS FOR COUNSELORS AND FOR WOMEN SURVIVORS OF SEXUAL VIOLENCE

Angelou, M. (1983). *I know why the caged bird sings.* London: Virago.

Armstrong, L. (1987). *Kiss daddy goodnight: Ten years later.* New York: Simon & Schuster.

Bart, P., & O'Brien, P. (1985). *Stopping rape: Successful survival strategies.* Elmsford, NY: Pergamon Press.

Bass, E., & Davis, L. (1988). *The courage to heal: A guide for women survivors of sexual abuse.* New York: Harper & Row.

Blume, S. E. (1991). *Secret survivors: Uncovering incest and its aftereffects in women.* New York: Ballantine Books.

Brady, M. (1991). *Daybreak: Meditations for women survivors of sexual abuse.* New York: HarperCollins/Hazelden.

Briere, J. (1989). *Therapy for adults molested as children: Beyond survival.* New York: Springer.

Briere, J. (1992). *Child abuse trauma: Theory and treatment of the lasting effects.* Newbury Park, CA: Sage.

Brownmiller, S. (1975). *Against our will: Men, women and rape.* New York: Simon & Schuster.

Butler, S. (1985). *Conspiracy of silence: The trauma of incest.* Volcano, CA: Volcano Press.

Courtois, C. A. (1988). *Healing the incest wound: Adult survivors in therapy.* New York: Norton.

Davis, A. (1988). *Violence against women and the ongoing challenge to racism.* New York: Women of Color Press.

Davis, L. (1990). *The courage to heal workbook for women and men survivors of child sexual abuse.* New York: Harper & Row.

Davis, L. (1991). *Allies in healing: When the person you love was sexually abused as a child.* New York: HarperCollins.

Estrich, S. (1987). *Real rape.* Cambridge, MA: Harvard University Press.

Finney, L. (1990). *Reach for the rainbow: Advanced healing for survivors of sexual abuse.* Malibu, CA: Changes Publishing.

Gil, E. (1990). *Treatment of adult survivors of childhood abuse.* Walnut Creek, CA: Launch Press.

Herman, J. L. (1981). *Father–daughter incest*. Cambridge, MA: Harvard University Press.

Herman, J. L. (1992). *Trauma and recovery: The aftermath of violence—from domestic abuse to political terror*. New York: Basic Books.

Jehu, D., in association with Gazan, M., & Klassen, C. (1988). *Beyond sexual abuse: Therapy with women who were childhood victims*. New York: Wiley.

Katz, J. (1984). *No fairy godmothers, no magic wands: The healing process after rape*. Saratoga, CA: R&E Publishers.

Koss, M. P., & Harvey, M. R. (1991). *The rape victim: Clinical and community interventions* (2nd ed.). Newbury Park, CA: Sage.

Laidlaw, T. A., & Malmo, C. (Eds.). (1990). *Healing voices: Feminist approaches to therapy with women*. San Francisco: Jossey-Bass.

Ledray, L. (1986). *Recovering from rape*. New York: Henry Holt.

Levy, B. (1991). *Dating violence: Young women in danger*. Seattle, WA: Seal Press.

Lobel, K. (Ed.). (1986). *Naming the violence: Speaking out about lesbian battering*. Seattle, WA: Seal Press.

Maltz, W. (1991). *The sexual healing journey*. New York: HarperCollins.

Maltz, W., & Holman, B. (1987). *Incest and sexuality: A guide to understanding and healing*. Lexington, MA: D.C. Heath/Lexington Books.

Marshall, W., Laws, D., & Barbaree, H. (1990). *Handbook of sexual assault*. New York: Plenum.

McClure, M. (1990). *Reclaiming the heart: A handbook of help and hope for survivors of incest*. New York: Warner Books.

Roberts, C. (1989). *Women and rape*. New York: New York University Press.

Russell, D. E. (1984). *The politics of rape: The victim's perspective*. New York: Stein & Day.

Russell, D. E. (1986). *The secret trauma: Incest in the lives of girls and women*. New York: Basic Books.

Sanderson, C. (1995). *Counselling adult survivors of child sexual abuse* (2nd ed.). London: Jessica Kingsley.

Sanford, L. T. (1990). *Strong at the broken places: Overcoming the trauma of childhood abuse*. New York: Random House.

Simonds, S. L. (1994). *Bridging the silence: Nonverbal modalities in the treatment of adult survivors of childhood sexual abuse*. New York: Norton.

Waites, E. (1993). *Trauma and survival: Post-traumatic and dissociative disorders in women*. New York: Norton.

Walker, A. (1988). *You can't keep a good woman down*. San Diego: Harvest.

Warshaw, R. (1988). *I never called it rape: The Ms. report on recognizing, fighting and surviving date and acquaintance rape*. New York: Harper & Row.

Westerlund, E. (1992). *Women's sexuality after childhood incest*. New York: Norton.

Wiehe, V. R., & Richards, A. L. (1995). *Intimate betrayal: Understanding and responding to the trauma of acquaintance rape*. Thousand Oaks, CA: Sage.

Appendix D

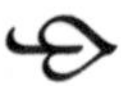

Lesbian Identity and Sexual Orientation

BOOKS AND ARTICLES FOR CLIENTS AND COUNSELORS

Adelman, M. (Ed.). (1986). *Long time passing: Lives of older lesbians*. Boston: Alyson.

Allen, J. (Ed.). (1990). *Lesbian philosophies and cultures*. Albany, New York: State University of New York Press.

American Friends Service Committee. (1989). *Bridges of respect: Creating support for lesbian and gay youth*. Philadelphia: American Friends Service Committee.

Baetz, R. (1988). *Lesbian crossroads: Personal stories of lesbian struggles and triumphs*. Tallahassee, FL: Naiad Press.

Balka, C., & Rose, A. (Eds.). (1989). *Twice blessed: On being lesbian, gay, and Jewish*. Boston: Beacon Press.

Berzon, B. (1988). *Permanent partnerships: Building gay and lesbian relationships that last*. New York: E.P. Dutton.

Blumenfeld, W., & Raymond, D. (1989). *Looking at gay and lesbian life*. Boston: Beacon Press.

Borhek, M.V. (1988). *Coming out to parents: A two-way survival guide for lesbians and gay men and their parents*. Cleveland, OH: Pilgrim Press.

Boston Lesbian Psychologies Collective (Ed.). (1987). *Lesbian psychologies: Explorations and challenges*. Urbana and Chicago: University of Illinois Press.

Burch, B. (1993). *On intimate terms: The psychology of difference in lesbian relationships*. Urbana: University of Illinois Press.

Clark, D. (1977). *Loving someone gay: A gay therapist offers sensitive, intelligent guidance to gay people and those who care about them*. New York: New American Library.

Cruikshank, M. (Ed.). (1985). *The lesbian path: Women loving women* (rev. ed.). San Francisco: Grey Fox.

Federman, L. (1990). *Old girls and twighlight lovers: A history of lesbian life in 20th century America*. New York: Columbia University Press.

Gagnon, J., & Simon, W. (1973). *Sexual conduct*. New York: Aldine.

Garnets, L., & Kimmel, D. (1993). *Psychological perspectives on lesbian and gay male experiences*. New York: Columbia University Press.

Gay and Lesbian Speakers' Bureau of Boston. (1987). *Gay/lesbian curriculum*. Boston: Author.

Golden, C. (1987). Diversity and variability in lesbian identities. In Boston Lesbian

Psychologies Collective (Ed.), *Lesbian psychologies: Explorations and challenges* (pp. 18–34). Chicago: University of Illinois Press.

Griffin, C. W. , Wirth, M. J., & Wirth, A. G. (1986). *Beyond acceptance: Parents of lesbians and gays talk about their experiences*. New York: St. Martin's Press.

Heron, A. (1983). *One teenager in ten: Testimony of gay and lesbian youth*. Boston: Alyson.

Herdt, G. (Ed). (1989). *Gay and lesbian youth*. New York: Harrington Park, Press.

Herdt, G., & Boxer, A. (1993). *Children of Horizons: How gay and lesbian teens are leading a new way out of the closet*. Boston: Beacon Press.

Hoagland, S., & Penelope, J. (Eds.). (1988). *For lesbians only: A separatist anthology* London: Onlywoman Press.

Human Rights Foundation, Inc. (1984). *Demystifying homosexuality: A teaching guide about lesbian and gay men for teachers and parents*. New York: Irvington Press.

Hutchins, L., & Ka'ahumanu, L. (1991). *Bi any other name: Bisexual people speak out*. Boston: Alyson.

Johnson, S. (1990). *Staying power: Long-term lesbian couples*. Tallahassee, FL: Naiad Press.

Kitzinger, C. (1987). *The social construction of lesbianism*. London: Sage.

Kitzinger, S., & Kitzinger, C. (1989). *Tough questions*. Cambridge, MA: Harvard Common Press.

Lorde, A. (1984). *Sister outsider*. Freedom: Crossing Press.

Loulan, J. (1987). *Lesbian passion: Loving ourselves and each other*. San Francisco: Spinsters/Aunt Lute.

Loulan, J. (1990). *The lesbian erotic dance: Butch, femme, androgyny, and other rhythms*. San Francisco, CA: Spinsters.

Maggiore, D. J. (1992). *Lesbianism: An annotated bibliography and guide to the literature, 1976–1991*. Metuchen, NJ: Scarecrow Press.

McCarn, S. R., & Fassinger, R. E. (1996). Revisioning sexual minority identity formation: A new model of lesbian identity and its implications for counseling and research. *The Counseling Psychologist, 24*, 508–534.

Onlywoman Press. (Ed.). (1981). *Love your enemy: The debate between heterosexual feminism and political lesbianism*. London: Onlywoman Press.

Patterson, C. J. (Ed.). (1995). *Lesbian, gay and bisexual identities across the lifespan*. New York: Oxford University Press.

Penelope, J., & Valentine, S. (Eds.). (1990). *Finding the lesbians: Personal accounts from around the world*. Freedom, CA: Crossing Press.

Penelope, J., & Wolfe, S. (1990). *The original coming out stories*. Freedom, CA: Crossing Press.

Pharr, S. (1988). *Homophobia: A weapon of sexism*. Little Rock, AR: Chardon Press.

Price, M. (1989). *Shattered mirrors: Our search for identity and community in the era of AIDS*. Cambridge, MA: Harvard University Press.

Rich, A. (1980). Compulsory heterosexuality and lesbian existence. *Signs, 5*, 631–660.

Rothblum, E. D., & Brehony, K. A. (Eds.). (1993). *Boston marriages: Romantic but asexual relationships among contemporary lesbians*. Amherst: University of Massachusetts Press.

Rothblum, E. D., & Cole, E. (Eds.). (1989). *Loving boldly: Issues facing lesbians.* New York: Harrington Park Press.
Saffron, L. (1994). *Challenging conceptions: Planning a family by self-insemination.* London: Cassell.
Sang, B., Warshow, J., & Smith, A. J. (1991). *Lesbians at midlife: The creative transition.* San Francisco: Spinsters.
Savin-Williams, R. (1990). *Gay and lesbian youth: Expressions of identity.* Bristol, PA: Hemisphere.
Silvera, M. (Ed.). (1991). *Piece of my heart: A lesbian of color anthology.* Toronto, Ontario: Sister Vision.
Tasker, F. L., & Golombok, S. (1997). *Growing up in a lesbian family: Effects on child development.* New York: Guilford Press.
Tee, C. (Ed.). (1989). *Intricate passions: A collection of erotic short fiction.* Austin, TX: Banned Books/Edward–William.
Weston, K. (1991). *Families we choose: Lesbian and gay kinship.* New York: Columbia University Press.
Whitlock, K. (1988). *Bridges of respect: Creating support for lesbian and gay youth.* Philadelphia: American Friends Service Committee.
Women and Therapy, (1988). *Lesbianism: Affirming nontraditional roles [Special issue] Vol. 8.*
Zulu, N. S. (1996). Sex, race, and the stained-glass window. *Women and Therapy* [Special Issue: Sexualities], *19*, 27–35.

FICTION AND NONFICTION BOOKS

Alyson, S. (Ed.). (1985). *Young, gay and proud.* Boston: Alyson.
Flagg, F. (1997). *Fried green tomatoes at the whistle stop cafe.* New York: Fawcette Columbine.
Garden, N. (1982). *Annie on my mind.* Toronto: McGraw-Hill.
Levy, M. (1990). *Rumors and whispers.* New York: Ballantine.
Nestle, J., & Holoch, N. (Eds.). (1990). *Women on women: An anthology of American lesbian short fiction.* New York: Penguin.

Appendix E

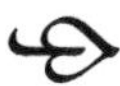

Reproductive Health and Decision Making

BOOKS AND JOURNAL ARTICLES ON PARENTHOOD DECISION MAKING AND REPRODUCTIVE CHOICE

Bombardieri, M. (1981). *The baby decision: How to make the most important choice of your life*. New York: Rawson, Wade.

Dagg, P. (1991). The psychological sequelae of therapeutic abortion. *American Journal of Psychiatry, 148*, 578–585.

Elvenstar, D. C. (1982). *Children: To have or have not?: A guide to making and living with your decision*. San Francisco: Harbor.

Gerson, K. (1985). *Hard choices: How women decide about work, career, and motherhood*. Berkeley: University of California Press.

Gordon, L. (1990). *Woman's body, woman's right: Birth control in America* (rev. ed.). New York: Penguin.

Kushner, E. (1997). *Experiencing abortion: A weaving of women's words*. New York: Haworth Press.

Lemkau, J. P. (1988). Emotional sequelae of abortion: Implications for clinical practice. *Psychology of Women Quarterly*, 7, 313–328.

Luker, K. (1984). *Abortion and the politics of motherhood*. Berkeley: University of California Press.

McDonnell, K. (1984). *Not an easy choice: A feminist re-examines abortion*. Boston: South End Press.

Radl, S. L. (1989). *Over our live bodies: Preserving choice in America*. Dallas: Steve Davis.

Whelan, E. (1980). *A baby? . . . Maybe: A guide to making the most fateful decision of your life* (rev. ed.). New York: Bobbs–Merrill.

Wilk, C. (1986). *Career women and childbearing: A psychological analysis of the decision process*. New York: Van Nostrand Reinhold.

BOOKS, CHAPTERS, AND JOURNAL ARTICLES ON MOTHERHOOD

American Psychological Association. (1995). *Lesbian and gay parenting: A resource for psychologists*. Washington, DC: Author.

Apfel, R.J., & Handel, M.H. (1992). *Madness and loss of motherhood: Sexuality, reproduction, and long-term mental illness*. Washington, DC: American Psychiatric Association Press.

Bergum, V. (1989). *Woman to mother: A transformation*. Granby, MA: Bergin & Garvey.

Block, J. (1990). *Motherhood as metamorphosis: Change and continuity in the life of a new mother*. New York: Plume.

Boston Women's Health Collective. (1978). *Ourselves and our children*. New York: Random House.

Boulton, M. G. (1983). *On being a mother: A study of women with pre-school children*. London: Tavistock.

Bozett, F. W. (Ed.). (1987). *Gay and lesbian parents*. New York: Praeger.

Brown, S. E., Conners, D., & Stern, N. (Eds.). (1985). *With the power of each breath: A disabled woman's anthology*. San Francisco: Cleiss Press.

Caplan, P. J. (1989). *Don't blame mother: Mending the mother–daughter relationship*. New York: Harper & Row.

Chesler, L. (Ed.). (1989). *Cradle and all*. Boston: Faber & Faber.

Chesler, P. (1979). *With child: A diary of motherhood*. New York: Thomas Y. Crowell.

Chodorow, N. (1978). *The reproduction of mothering: Psychoanalysis and the sociology of gender*. Berkeley: University of California Press.

Chodorow, N., & Contratto, S. (1992). The fantasy of the perfect mother. In B. Thorne & M. Yalom (Eds.), *Rethinking the family: Some feminist questions* (pp. 191–214). New York: Longman.

Clubb, A. (1988). *Love in the blended family: Falling in love with a package deal*. Toronto: NC Press.

Cole, J. B. (Ed.). (1986). *All American women: Lines that divide, ties that bind*. New York: Macmillan.

Collins, P. H. (1987). The meaning of motherhood in black culture and black mother–daughter relationships. *Sage: A Scholarly Journal on Black Women, 4*, 3–10.

Crawford, S. (1987). Lesbian families: Psychosocial stress and the family-building process. In Boston Lesbian Psychologies Collective (Eds.), *Lesbian psychologies: Explorations and challenges* (pp. 195–214). Chicago: University of Illinois Press.

Dally, A. (1982). *Inventing motherhood: The consequences of an ideal*. London: Burnett Books.

Dinkmeyer, D., McKay, G. D., & McKay, J. L. (1987). *New beginnings: Skills for single parents and stepfamily parents*. Champaign, IL: Research Press.

Dragu, M., Sheard, S., & Swan, S. (1991). *Mothers talk back*. Toronto: Coach House Press.

Genevie, L., & Margolies, E. (1987). *The motherhood report: How women feel about being mothers*. New York: McGraw-Hill.

Gieve, K. (1989). *Balancing acts: On being a mother*. London: Virago.

Glazer, E. (1990). *The long awaited stork: A guide to parenting after infertility*. Lexington, MA: Lexington Books.

Hall, N. L. (1984). *The true story of a single mother*. Boston: South End Press.

Heffner, E. (1978). *Mothering: The emotional experience of motherhood after Freud and feminism*. New York: Doubleday.

Hochschild, A. (1989). *The second shift*. New York: Avon.

Kaplan, M. M. (1992). *Mothers' images of motherhood*. London: Routledge.

Kitzinger, S. (1974). *The experience of childbirth*. New York: Penguin Press.

Kitzinger, S. (1978). *Women as mothers.* Oxford: Martin Robertson & Co.
Kitzinger, S. (1992). *Ourselves as mothers: The universal experience of motherhood.* Reading, MA: Addison-Wesley.
Kitzinger, S. (1994). *The year after childbirth: Surviving and enjoying the first year of motherhood.* New York: HarperCollins.
Kleiman, K., & Raskin, V. (1994). *This isn't what I expected: Recognizing and recovering from depression and anxiety after childbirth.* Toronto: Bantam Books.
Knowles, J. P., & Cole, E. (Eds.). (1990). *Woman-defined motherhood.* New York: Harrington Park Press.
Llewelyn, S., & Osborne, K. (1990). *Women's lives.* London: Routledge.
Mattes, J. (1997). *Single mothers by choice.* New York: Random House.
McBride, A. B. (1973). *The growth and development of mothers.* New York: Harper & Row.
McMahon, M. (1995). *Engendering motherhood: Identity and self-transformation in women's lives.* New York: Guilford Press.
Mercer, R. T. (1986). *First-time motherhood.* New York: Springer.
Mercer, R. T., Nichols, E. G., & Doyle, G. C. (1989). *Transitions in a woman's life: Major life events in developmental context.* New York: Springer.
Nicolson, P. (1989). Counselling women with post natal depression: Implications from recent qualitative research. *Counselling Psychology Quarterly, 2,* 123–132.
O'Barr, J. F., Pope, D., & Wyer, M. (Eds.). (1990). *Ties that bind: Essays on mothering and patriarchy.* Chicago: University of Chicago Press.
O'Donnell, L. N. (1985). *The unheralded majority: Contemporary women as mothers.* Toronto: Lexington Books.
Phoenix, A., Woollett, A., & Lloyd, E. (Eds.). (1991). *Motherhood: Meanings, practise, and ideologies.* London: Sage.
Pollack, S., & Vaughn, J. (Eds.). (1987). *Politics of the heart: A lesbian parenting anthology.* Ithaca, NY: Firebrand Books.
Price, J. (1988). *Motherhood: What it does to your mind.* London: Pandora.
Rafkin, L. (Ed.). (1987). *Different daughters: A book by mothers of lesbians.* San Francisco: Cleis Press.
Rafkin, L. (Ed.). (1990). *Different mothers: Sons and daughters of lesbians talk about their lives.* San Francisco: Cleis Press.
Rich, A. (1976). *Of woman born: Motherhood as experience and institution.* New York: Norton.
Ridington, J. (1985). Single-parenting in a wheelchair: What do you do with a sick kid when you can't afford an ambulance and you can't walk. *Women and Disabilities (Special Issue: Resources for Feminist Research), 14,* Toronto: Ontario Institute for Studies in Education.
Ruble, D. N., Brooks-Gunn, J., Fleming, A. S., Fitzmaurice, G., Stangor, C., & Deutsch, F. (1990). Transition to motherhood and the self: Measurement, stability, and change. *Journal of Personality and Social Psychology, 58,* 450–463.
Ruddick, S. (1989). *Maternal thinking: Toward a politics of peace.* New York: Macmillan.
Saffron, L. (1994). *Challenging conceptions: Planning a family by self-insemination.* London: Cassell.
Sheppard, T. (1989). *Motherhood.* London: Angus & Robertson.

Swigart, J. (1991). *The myth of the bad mother: The emotional realities of mothering*. New York: Doubleday.
Ussher, J. (1989). *The psychology of the female body*. London: Routledge.

BOOKS AND JOURNAL ARTICLES ON INFERTILITY AND REPRODUCTIVE LOSSES

Anton, L. H. (1992). *Never to be a mother: A guide for all women who didn't—or couldn't—have children*. San Francisco: Harper San Francisco.
Becker, G. (1990). *Healing the infertile family*. New York: Bantam.
Borg, S., & Lasker, J. (1981). *When pregnancy fails: Families coping with miscarriage, stillbirth, and infant death*. Boston: Beacon.
Carter, J., & Carter, M. (1989). *Sweet grapes: How to stop being infertile and start living again*. Indianapolis: Perspectives Press.
Cooper, S., & Glazer, E. (1994). *Beyond infertility: New paths to parenthood*. Lexington, MA: Lexington Books.
Daniluk, J. C. (1991). Strategies for counseling infertile couples. *Journal of Counseling and Development, 69*, 317–320.
DeCherney, A., & Polan, M. L. (1988). *Decision making in infertility*. Philadelphia: Decker.
Fleming, A. T. (1994). *Motherhood deferred: A woman's journey*. New York: Fawcett Columbine.
Friedman, R. M. D., & Gradstein, B. (1982). *Surviving pregnancy loss*. Boston: Little, Brown.
Gilman, L. (1988). *The adoption resource book*. New York: Harper & Row.
Glazer, E. S., & Cooper, S. L. (1988). *Without child: Experiencing and resolving infertility*. Lexington, MA: Lexington Books.
Greil, A. L. (1991). *Not yet pregnant: Infertile couples in contemporary America*. London: Rutgers University Press.
Johnson, P. I. (1994). *Taking charge of infertility.* Indianapolis: Perspectives Press.
Lasker, J., & Borg, S. (1987). *In search of parenthood*. Boston: Beacon Press.
Leiblum, S. R. (Ed.). (1997). *Infertility: Psychological issues and counseling strategies*. New York: Wiley.
Melina, L. (1989). *Making sense of adoption*. New York: Harper & Row.
Menning, B. E. (1988). *Infertility: A guide for the childless couple* (2nd ed.). New York: Prentice-Hall.
Mullens, A. (1990). *Missed conceptions: Overcoming infertility*. Toronto: McGraw-Hill Ryerson.
Panuthos, C., & Romeo, C. (1984). *Ended beginnings: Healing childbearing losses*. New York: Warner Books.
Robinson, S. (1985). *Having a baby without a man: A woman's guide to alternative insemination*. Boston: Simon & Schuster.
Rothman, B. (1989). *Re-inventing motherhood*. New York: Norton.
Salzer, L. P. (1991). *Surviving infertility: A compassionate guide through the emotional crisis of infertility* (rev. ed.). New York: Harper Perennial.
Sandelowski, M. (1994). *With child in mind: Studies of the personal encounter with infertility*. Philadelphia: University of Pennsylvania Press.

Schwartz, L. L. (1991). *Alternatives to infertility: Is surrogacy the answer?* New York: Brunner/Mazel.

Shapiro, C. H. (1988). *Infertility and pregnancy loss: A guide for helping professionals.* San Francisco: Jossey-Bass.

Shapiro, C. H. (1993). *When part of the self is lost: Helping clients heal after sexual and reproductive losses.* San Francisco: Jossey-Bass.

Stanton, A., & Dunkel-Schetter, C. (1991). *Infertility: Perspectives from stress and coping research.* New York: Plenum.

Vercollone, C. F., Moss, H., & Moss, R. (1997). *Helping the stork: The choices and challenges of donor insemination.* New York: Macmillan.

Zolbrod, A. P. (1993). *Men, women, and infertility: Intervention and treatment strategies.* New York: Lexington Books.

BOOKS, CHAPTERS, AND JOURNAL ARTICLES ON NONPARENTHOOD

Boyd, R. (1989). Racial differences in childlessness: A centennial review. *Sociological Perspective, 32,* 183–199.

Bram, S. (1984). Voluntarily childless women: Traditional or nontraditional? *Sex Roles, 10,* 195–206.

Bram, S. (1986). Childlessness revisited: A longitudinal study of voluntarily childless couples, delayed parents, and parents. *Lifestyles: A Journal of Changing Patterns, 3,* 46–65.

English, J. (1989). *Childlessness transformed: Stories of alternative parenting.* Mount Shasta, CA: Earth Heart.

Faux, M. (1984). *Childlessness by choice.* New York: Anchor Press.

Greer, G. (1984). *Sex and destiny: The politics of human fertility.* New York: Harper & Row.

Houseknecht, S. (1987). Voluntary childlessness. In M. B. Sussman & S. K. Steinmetz (Eds.), *Handbook of marriage and family* (pp. 369–395). New York: Plenum.

Ireland, M. S. (1993). *Reconceiving women: Separating motherhood from female identity.* New York: Guilford Press.

Lisle, L. (1996). *Without child: Challenging the stigma of childlessness.* New York: Ballantine.

Morell, C. (1994). *Unwomanly conduct: The challenges of intentional childlessness.* New York: Routledge.

Safer, J. (1996). *Beyond motherhood: Choosing a life without children.* New York: Pocketbooks.

Veevers, J. (1980). *Childless by choice.* Toronto: Butterworth.

Appendix F

Disability and Illness

BOOKS FOR CLIENTS WITH DISABILITIES AND CHRONIC ILLNESS

Ayrault, E.W. (1981). *Sex, love, and the physically handicapped*. New York: Continuum.

Brown, S. E, Connors, D., & Stein, N. (Eds.). (1985). *With the power of each breath: A disabled women's anthology*. San Francisco: Cleis Press.

Bullard, D. G., & Knight, S. E. (Ed.). (1981). *Sexuality and physical disability: Personal perspectives*. St. Louis: Mosby.

Campling, J. (Ed.). (1981). *Images of ourselves: Women with disabilities talking*. London: Routledge & Kegan Paul.

Corbette, K., Cupolo, A., & Lewis, V. (1982). *No more stares: A role model book for disabled teenage girls*. Berkeley, CA: Disability Rights Education Defense Fund.

Fine, M., & Asch, A. (Eds.). (1988). *Women with disabilities: Essays in psychology, culture and politics*. Philadelphia: Temple University Press.

Kaufman, M. (1995). *Easy for you to say: Questions and answers for teens living with chronic illness or disability*. Toronto: Key Porter Books.

National Clearinghouse on Women and Girls with Disabilities. (1990). *Bridging the gap: A national directory of services for women and girls with disabilities*. New York: Educational Equity Concepts.

Neistadt, M. E., & Freda, M. (1987). *Choices: A guide to sex counselling with physically disabled adults*. Malabar, FL: Krieger.

Sandelowski, C. (1989). *Sexual concerns when illness or disability strikes*. Springfield, IL: Charles C Thomas.

Saxton, M., & Howe, F. (Eds.). (1987). *With wings: An anthology of literature by and about women with disabilities*. New York: Feminist Press.

Schover, L., & Jensen, S. (1988). *Sexuality and chronic illness*. New York: Guilford Press.

Tallmer, M., De Sanctis, P. D., Bullard, D. G., Kutscher, A. H., Roberts, M. S., & Patterson, P. R. (1984). *Sexuality and life-threatening illness*. Springfield, IL: Charles C. Thomas.

BOOKS AND JOURNAL ARTICLES FOR CLIENTS AND COUNSELORS ON CANCER, HYSTERECTOMY, AND MASTECTOMY

Andersen, B. L., & Elliot, M. (1993). Sexuality for women with cancer: Assessment, therapy and treatment. *Sexuality and Disability, 11*, 7–37.

Baum, M., Saunders, C., & Merideth, S. (1994). *Breast cancer: A guide for every woman.* New York: Oxford University Press.

Brady, J. (Ed.). (1991). *1 in 3: Women with cancer confront an epidemic.* Pittsburgh: Cleis Press.

Butler, S., & Rosenblum, B. (1991). *Cancer in two voices.* San Francisco: Spinsters.

Canadian Journal of Human Sexuality, 3, (1994). Sexuality and cancer treatment [Special Issue].

Conti, J. V. (1989). *Counseling persons with cancer.* Springfield, IL: Charles C Thomas.

Cox, K., & Schwartz, J. (1990). *The well-informed patient's guide to hysterectomy.* New York: Dell.

Cunningham, A. J. (1992). *The healing journey: Overcoming the crisis of cancer.* Toronto: Key Porter Books.

Cutler, W. B. (1988). *Hysterectomy: Before and after—A comprehensive guide to preventing, preparing for, and maximizing health after hysterectomy.* New York: Harper & Row.

Dackman, L. (1990). *Up front: Sex and the post-mastectomy woman.* Markam, ON: Penguin.

Dally, A. (1992). *Women under the knife.* New York: Routledge.

Darty, T. E., & Potter, S. J. (1984). Social work with challenged women: Sexism, sexuality, and the female cancer experience. *Journal of Social Work and Human Sexuality*, 2, 83–100.

Dollinger, M., Rosenbaum, E. H., & Cable, G. (1991). *Everyone's guide to cancer therapy.* Toronto: Somerville House.

Drummond, J., & Field, P. A. (1984). Emotional and sexual sequelae following hysterectomy. *Health Care for Women International, 5*, 261–271.

Goldfarb, H. A., & Greif, J. (1990). *The no-hysterectomy option: Your body—your choice.* New York: Wiley.

Gross, A., & Ito, D. (1990). *Women talk about breast surgery: From diagnosis to recovery.* New York: Clarkson Potter.

Gross, A., & Ito, D. (1992). *Women talk about gynecological surgery: From diagnosis to recovery.* New York: Harper Perennial.

Hass, A., & Puretz, S. L. (1995). *The woman's guide to hysterectomy: Expectations and Options.* Berkeley, CA: Celestial Arts.

Hufnagel, V., & Golant, S. K. (1989). *No more hysterectomies.* New York: New American Library.

Johnson, J. (1987). *Intimacy: Living as a woman after cancer.* Toronto: NC Press.

Kelly, P. T. (1991). *Understanding breast cancer risk.* Philadelphia: Temple University Press.

Lorde, A. (1980). *The cancer journals.* San Francisco: Spinsters.

Loulan, J. (1996). Our breasts, ourselves. *Women and Therapy* [Special Issue: Sexualities] *19*, 95–98.

Love, S. (1990). *Dr. Susan Love's breast book*. Reading, MA: Addison-Wesley.
MacPhee, R. (1994). *Picasso's woman*. Vancouver, BC: Douglas & McIntyre.
McGinn, K. (1991). *Keeping abreast: Breast changes that are not cancer*. Palo Alto, CA: Bull.
Morgan, S. (1985). *Coping with a hysterectomy: Your own choice, your own solutions*. New York: Signet Books.
Payer, L. (1987). *How to avoid a hysterectomy: An indispensable guide to exploring all your options—before you consent to a hysterectomy*. New York: Pantheon Books.
Potts, E., & Morra, M. (1990). *Getting back to normal when you have cancer*. New York: Avon Books.
Rollin, B. (1977). *First you cry*. New York: New American Library.
Sandelowski, M. (1981). *Women, health, and choice*. Englewood Cliffs, NJ: Prentice-Hall.
Schover, L. (1988). *Sexuality and cancer: For the woman who has cancer and her partner*. New York: American Cancer Society.
Seltzer, V. (1987). *Every woman's guide to breast cancer*. New York: Penguin.
Stocker, M. (Ed.). (1991). *Cancer as a women's issue*. Chicago: Third Side Press.
Stokes, N. M. (1986). *The castrated woman: What your doctor won't tell you about hysterectomy*. New York: Franklin Watts.
Vaeth, J. M. (Ed.). (1986). *Body image, self-esteem and sexuality in cancer patients*. Basel, Switzerland: Karger.
Walsh, J. (1993). Healing the hidden scars: Sex after breast cancer. *Health*, 7, 94–97.
West, S., & Dranov, P. (1994). *The hysterectomy hoax*. Toronto: Doubleday.

JOURNALS AND ORGANIZATIONS

American Cancer Society. 19 West 56th Street, New York, NY 10019; (212) 586–8700.

Abilities: Canada's Lifestyle Magazine for People with Disabilities. Toronto, ON: Canadian Abilities Foundation.

Breast Cancer Action. P.O. Box 460185, San Francisco, CA 94146; (415) 922–8279.

Hysterectomy Educational Resources and Services (HERS). 422 Bryn Mawr Avenue, Bala Cynwyd, PA 19004; (215) 667–7757.

National Cancer Institute. Office of Cancer Communications, Building 31, 9000 Rockville Pike, Bethesda, MD 20892; Hotline: (800) 4-CANCER.

Appendix G

Issues for Women in the Middle and Later Years

BOOKS FOR CLIENTS AND COUNSELORS DEALING WITH MENOPAUSE

Andrews, L. (1993). *Woman at the edge of two worlds: The spiritual journal of menopause.* New York: Harper Perennial.

Barbach, L. (1993). *The pause: Positive approaches to menopause.* New York: Dutton.

Borton, J. C. (1992). *Drawing from the women's well: Reflections from the life passage of menopause.* San Diego: LuraMedia.

Cobb, J. O. (1993). *Understanding menopause: Answers and advice for women in the prime of life.* New York: Penguin.

Coney, S. (1991). *The menopause industry: A guide to medicine's "discovery" of the mid-life woman.* New York: Penguin Books.

Cutler, W. B., & Garcia, C. R. (1990). *Menopause: A guide for women and the men who love them.* New York: Norton.

Datan, N., Antonovsky, A., & Maoz, B. (1981). *A time to reap.* Baltimore: Johns Hopkins University Press.

Dickson, A., & Henriques, N. (1988). *Women on menopause: A practical guide to a positive transition.* New York: Harper & Row.

Doress, P. B., Siegal, D. L., & the Midlife and Older Women Book Project. (Eds.). (1987). *Ourselves, growing older: Women aging with knowledge and power.* New York: Simon & Schuster.

Downing, C. (1987). *Journey through menopause: A personal rite of passage.* New York: Crossroad.

Formanek, R. (1990). *The meanings of menopause: Historical, medical and clinical perspectives.* Hillsdale, NJ: Analytic Press.

Gannon, L. R. (1985). *Menstrual disorders and menopause.* New York: Praeger.

Gerson, M. (1990). *Menopause: A well woman book.* Toronto: Montreal Health Press.

Goldsworthy, J. (Ed.). (1993). *A certain age: Reflecting on the menopause.* New York: Columbia University Press.

Golub, S. (1992). *Periods: From menarche to menopause.* Newbury Park, CA: Sage.

Greenwood, S. (1992). *Updated menopause naturally: Preparing for the second half of life.* Volcano, CA: Volcano Press.

Greer, G. (1991). *The change: Women, aging and the menopause.* New York: Fawcett Columbine.

Hunter, M. (1990). *Your menopause: Prepare now for a positive future*. London: Pandora.

Kahn, A., & Holt, L. (1987). *Menopause: The best years of your life?* London: Bloomsbury.

Kenton, L. (1995). *Passage to power: Natural menopause revolution*. London: Ebury Press.

Lark, S. (1984). *Premenstrual syndrome self-help book*. Los Altos, CA: PMS Self-Help Center.

Lewin, E., & Olesen, V. (Eds.). (1985). *Women, health and healing: Toward a new perspective*. New York: Tavistock.

McCain, M. V. E. (1991). *Transformation through menopause*. New York: Bergin & Garvey.

Mahdi, L. C., Foster, S., & Little, M. (Eds.) (1987). *Betwixt and between: Patterns of masculine and feminine initiation*. La Salle, IL: Open Court.

Martin, E. (1987). *The woman in the body*. Boston: Beacon Press.

Ojeda, L. (1989). *Menopause without medicine*. Alameda, CA: Hunter House.

Page, L. (1993). *Menopause and emotions: Making sense of your feelings when your feelings make no sense*. Vancouver, BC: Primavera Press.

Reitz, R. (1979). *Menopause: A positive approach*. New York: Penguin.

Sand, G. (1993). *Is it hot in here or is it me?* New York: Random House.

Sheehy, G. (1992). *The silent passage: Menopause*. New York: Random House.

Stewart, G., & Hatcher, R. (1987). *Understanding your body: Every woman's guide to gynecology and health*. New York: Bantam Books.

Stoppard, M. (1994). *Menopause*. Toronto: Random House.

Taetzsch, L. (Ed.). (1995). *Hot flashes: Women writers on the change of life*. Boston: Faber & Faber.

Taylor, D., & Sumrall, A. (Eds.). (1991). *Women of the 14th moon: Writings on menopause*. Freedom, CA: Crossing Press.

Voda, A. M. (1997). *Menopause, me and you: The sound of women pausing*. New York: Haworth Press.

Voda, A. M., Dinnerstein, M., & O'Donnell, S. R. (Eds.). (1982). *Changing perspectives on menopause*. Austin: University of Texas Press.

Weed, S. S. (1992). *Menopausal years: The wise woman way—alternative approaches for women 30–90*. New York: Ash Tree.

Weideger, P. (1978). *Female cycles*. London: Women's Press.

Wolfe, H. L. (1990). *Second spring: A guide to healthy menopause through traditional Chinese medicine*. Boulder, CO: Blue Poppy Press.

BOOKS ON BODY IMAGE AND AGING

Chopra, D. (1993). *Ageless body, timeless mind: The quantum alternative to growing old*. New York: Harmony Books.

Cohen, L. (1984). *Small expectations: Society's betrayal of older women*. Toronto: McClellan & Stewart.

Copper, B. (1988). *Over the hill: Reflections on ageism between women*. Freedom, CA: Crossing Press.

Doress, P. B., & Siegal, D. L. (Eds.). (1987). *Ourselves, growing older: Women aging with knowledge and power*. New York: Simon & Schuster.

Downing, C. (1995). *Red, hot mammas: Coming into our own at fifty*. New York: Bantam Books.

Friedan, B. (1993). *The fountain of age*. New York: Simon & Schuster.

Hen Co-op Staff. (1994). *Growing old disgracefully: New ideas for getting the most out of life*. Freedom, CA: Crossing Press.

Markson, E. (Ed.). (1983). *Older women: Issues and prospects*. Lexington, MA: Lexington Press.

Nickerson, B. (1995). *Old and smart: Women and the adventure of aging*. Maderia Park, BC: Harbour.

Porcino, J. (1983). *Growing older, getting better: A handbook for women in the second half of life*. Reading, MA: Addison-Wesley.

Rubin, L. (1979). *Women of a certain age: The midlife search for self*. New York: Harper & Row.

Shapiro, B. (1991). *The big squeeze: Balancing the needs of aging parents, dependent children, and you*. Bedford, MA: Mills & Sanderson.

Turner, B. F., & Troll, L. E. (Eds.). (1993). *Women growing older: Psychological perspectives*. Thousand Oaks, CA: Sage.

Walker, B. G. (1985). *The crone: Women of age, wisdom, and power*. San Francisco: Harper & Row.

BOOKS ON SEXUALITY AND INTIMACY

Anderson, C. M., & Stewart, S. (1994). *Flying solo: Single women in midlife*. New York: Norton.

Banner, L. (1992). *In full flower: Aging women, power, and sexuality*. New York: Knopf.

Barbach, L. (1985). *Pleasures: Women write erotica*. New York: HarperCollins.

Barbach, L. (1987). *Erotic interludes: Tales told by women*. New York: HarperCollins.

Cline, S. (1993). *Women, passion and celibacy*. New York: Carol Southern.

Griffin, K. (1996). *After the change: Older women talk about sex and relationships after the menopause*. London: Vermilion.

Ogden, G. (1994). *Women who love sex*. New York: Pocket Books.

Sang, B., Warshow, J., & Smith, A. J. (Eds.). (1991). *Lesbians at midlife: The creative transition*. San Francisco: Spinsters.

Schwartzberg, N., Berliner, K., & Jacob, K. (1995). *Single in a married world: A life cycle framework for working with the unmarried adult*. New York: Norton.

Tallmer, M. (1996). *Questions & answers about sex in later life*. Philadelphia: Charles Press.

Weg, R. B. (Ed.). (1983). *Sexuality in the later years: Roles and behavior*. New York: Academic Press.

NEWSLETTERS

A Friend Indeed: A Newsletter for Women in the Prime of Life. P.O. Box 1710, Camplain, NY 12929-1710; in Canada: P.O. Box 515, Place du Parc Station, Montreal, Quebec H2W 2P1, Canada.

Hot Flash: Newsletter for Midlife and Older Women. Box 816, Stony Brook, NY 11790-0609.

REFERENCES

Abbey, A., Andrews, F. M., & Halman, L. J. (1991). Gender's role in responses to infertility. *Psychology of Women Quarterly, 15,* 295–316.

Achterberg, J. (1985). *Imagery in healing: Shamanism and modern medicine.* Boston: Shambhala.

Adams, C. G., & Turner, B. F. (1985). Reported change in sexuality from young adulthood to old age. *Journal of Sex Research, 21,* 126–141.

Adler, B. (1994). Postnatal sexuality. In P. Y. L. Choi & P. Nicolson (Eds.), *Female sexuality: Psychology, biology and social context* (pp. 83–99). New York: Harvester/Wheatsheaf.

Agell, G., & Rothblum, E. (1991). Effects of clients' obesity and gender on the therapy judgments of psychologists. *Professional Psychology: Research and Practice, 22,* 223–229.

Ahsen, A. (1996). Menopause: Imagery interventions and therpeutics. *Journal of Mental Imagery, 20,* 1–40.

Alberti, R. E., & Emmons, M. L. (1995). *Your perfect right: A guide to assertive living.* San Luis Obispo, CA: Impact.

Allen, P. (1986). *The sacred hoop.* Boston: Beacon Press.

Amann-Gainotti, M. (1986). Sexual socialization during early adolescence: The menarche. *Adolescence, 83,* 703–710.

Ambrogne-O'Toole, C. A. (1988). Exploring female sexuality through the expressive therapies. *The Arts in Psychotherapy, 15,* 109–117.

American Psychological Association. (1996). *Research agenda for psychosocial and behavioral factors in women's health* (Recommendations from the Advisory Committee of the Psychosocial and Behavioral Factors in Women's Health: Creating an Agenda for the 21st Century Conference). Washington, DC: Author.

Andersen, B. L., & Cyranowski, J. M. (1994). Women's sexual self-schema. *Journal of Personality and Social Psychology, 67,* 1079–1100.

Andersen, B. L., & Cyranowski, J. M. (1995). Women's sexuality: Behaviors, responses, and individual differences. *Journal of Consulting and Clinical Psychology, 63,* 891–906.

Anderson, C. M., & Stewart, S. (1994). *Flying solo: Single women in midlife.* New York: Norton.

Andre, T., Dietsch, C., & Cheng, Y. (1991). Sources of sex education as a function of sex, coital activity and type of information. *Contemporary Educational Psychology, 16,* 215–240.

Anthony, E. J., & Benedek, T. (1970). *Parenthood: Its psychology and psychopathology.* Boston: Little, Brown.

Anton, L. H. (1992). *Never to be a mother: A guide for all women who didn't—or couldn't— have children.* San Francisco: Harper San Francisco.

Apter, T. (1995). *Secret paths: Women in the new midlife.* New York: Norton.

Arditti, R., Klein, R. D., & Minden, S. (Eds.). (1984). *Test-tube women: What future for motherhood?* London: Pandora Press.

Attie, I., & Brooks-Gunn, J. (1989). The development of eating problems in adolescent girls: A longitudinal study. *Developmental Psychology, 25,* 70–79.

Bagley, C., & King, K. (1990). *Child sexual abuse: The search for healing.* London and New York: Routledge.

Baird-Carlsen, M. (1988). *Meaning-making: Therapeutic processes in adult development.* New York: Norton.

Banner, L. W. (1992). *In full flower: Aging women, power, and sexuality.* New York: Knopf.

Barbach, L. (1976). *For yourself: The fulfillment of female sexuality.* New York: Anchor Books.

Barbach, L. (1984). *For each other: Sharing sexual intimacy.* New York: New American Library.

Barbach, L. (1988). *Erotic interludes.* London: Futura.

Barbach, L. (1993). *The pause: Positive approaches to menopause.* New York: Dutton.

Bareford, C. G. (1991). An investigation of the nature of the menopausal experience: Attitude toward menopause, recent life change, coping method, and number and frequency of symptoms in menopausal women. In D. L. Taylor & N. F. Woods (Eds.), *Menstruation, health, and illness* (pp. 223–236). New York: Hemisphere.

Bartky, S. L. (1990). *Femininity and domination.* London: Routledge.

Baruch, G. K. (1984). The psychological well-being of women in the middle years. In G. Baruch & J. Brooks-Gunn (Eds.), *Women in midlife* (pp. 161–180). New York: Plenum.

Baruch, G., Barnett, R., & Rivers, C. (1983). *Lifeprints: New patterns of love and work for today's women.* New York: New American Library.

Bateman, A. J. (1948). Intra-sexual selection in Drosophila. *Heredity, 2,* 349–368.

Bazzini, D. G., McIntosh, W. D., & Harris, C. (1997). The aging woman in popular film: Underrepresented, unattractive, unfriendly, and unintelligent. *Sex Roles, 36,* 531–544.

Belenky, M. F., Clinchy, B. M., Goldberger, N. R., & Tarule, J. M. (1986). *Women's ways of knowing: The development of self, voice, and mind.* New York: Basic Books.

Bell, I. P. (1989). The double standard: Age. In J. Freeman (Ed.), *Women: A feminist perspective* (4th ed., pp. 236–244). Mountain View, CA: Mayfield.

Bell, R. (1987). *Changing bodies, changing lives: A book for teens on sex and relationships* (rev. ed.). New York: Random House.

Benedek, T. (1952). Infertility as a psychosomatic defense. *Fertility and Sterility, 3,* 527–538.

Benjamin, J. (1988). *The bonds of love: Psychoanalysis, feminism, and the problem of domination.* New York: Pantheon.

Bennett, P., & Rosario, V. A. (Eds.). (1995). *Solitary pleasures: The historical literary, and artistic discourses of eroticism.* New York: Routledge.

Beren, S. E., Hayden, H. A., Wilfley, D. E., & Striegel-Moore, R. H. (1997). Body dissatisfaction among lesbian college students: The conflict of straddling mainstream and lesbian cultures. *Psychology of Women Quarterly, 21,* 431–445.

Bereska, T. M. (1994). Adolescent sexuality and the changing romance novel market. *Canadian Journal of Human Sexuality, 3,* 35–44.

Berg, J. B., & Wilson, J. F. (1991) Psychological functioning across stages of infertility. *Journal of Behavioral Medicine, 14,* 11–26.

Berg, J. B., Wilson, J. F., & Weingartner, P. J. (1991). Psychological sequelae of infertility treatment: The role of gender- and sex-role identification. *Social Sciences and Medicine, 33,* 1071–1080.

Bergum, V. (1989). *Woman to mother: A transformation.* Granby, MA: Bergin & Garvey.

Bernhard, L. A. (1992). Consequences of hysterectomy in the lives of women. *Health Care for Women International, 13,* 281–291.

Bielay, G., & Herold, E. S. (1995). Popular magazines as a source of sexual information for university women. *Canadian Journal of Human Sexuality, 4,* 247–262.

Birren, J. E. (1987, May). The best of all stories. *Psychology Today,* pp. 74–75.

Blood, S. K. (1996). The dieting dilemma: Factors influencing women's decision to give up dieting. *Women and Therapy, 18,* 109–118.

Bloom, C., Gitter, A., Gutwill, S., Kogel, L., & Zaphiropoulos, L. (1994). *Eating problems: A feminist psychoanalytic treatment model.* New York: Basic Books.

Blumer, H. (1969). *Symbolic interactionism: Perspective and method.* Englewood Cliffs, NJ: Prentice-Hall.

Blumstein, P., & Schwartz, P. (1976). Bisexuality in women. *Archives of Sexual Behavior, 5,* 171–181.

Blyth, D. A., Simmons, R. G., & Zakin, D. F. (1985). Satisfaction with body image for early adolescent females: The impact of pubertal timing within different school environments. *Journal of Youth and Adolescence, 14,* 207–223.

Bombardieri, M. (1981). *The baby decision: How to make the most important choice of your life.* New York: Rawson, Wade.

Bordo, S. (1993). *Unbearable weight: Feminism, Western culture and the body.* Berkeley: University of California Press.

Borysenko, J. (1988). *Minding the body, Mending the mind.* New York: Bantam Books.

Boskind-White, M., & White, W. C. (1983). *Bulimarexia: The binge/purge cycle.* New York: Norton.

Boston Lesbian Psychologies Collective. (Ed.). (1987). *Lesbian psychologies: Explorations and challenges.* Chicago: University of Illinois.

Boston Women's Health Book Collective. (1992). *The new our bodies, ourselves: A book by and for women.* New York: Simon & Schuster.

Bowles, C. L. (1986). Measure of attitude toward menopause using the semantic differential model. *Nursing Research, 35,* 81–85.

Brand, P. A., Rothblum, E. D., & Solomon, L. J. (1992). A comparison of lesbians, gay men, and heterosexuals on weight and restrained eating. *International Journal of Eating Disorders, 11,* 253–259.

Braverman, A. M. (1997). When is enough, enough?; Abandoning medical treatment for infertility. In S. R. Leiblum (Ed.). *Infertility: Medical, ethical, and psychological perspectives* (pp. 209–229). New York: Wiley.

Brigman, B. (1994). Four generations of women: Our bodies and lives. In P. Fallon, M. A. Katzman, & S. C. Wooley (Eds.), *Feminist perspectives on eating disorders* (pp. 115–131). New York: Guilford Press.

Brockington, I. F. (1996). *Motherhood and mental illness.* New York: Oxford University Press.

Brockington, I. F., & Kumar, R. (1982). *Motherhood and mental illness.* New York: Grune & Stratton.

Brooks-Gunn, J. (1988). Antecedents and consequences of variations in girls' maturational timing. *Journal of Adolescent Health Care, 9,* 365–373.

Brooks-Gunn, J., & Ruble, D. N. (1983). Dysmenorrhea in adolescence. In S. Golub (Ed.), *Menarche: The transition from girl to woman* (pp. 251–261). Lexington, MA: Lexington Books.

Brooks-Gunn, J., & Warren, M. P. (1988). The psychological significance of secondary sexual characteristics in nine- to eleven-year-old girls. *Child Development, 59,* 1061–1069.

Brouwers, M. (1994). Bulimia and the relationship with food: A letters-to-food technique. *Journal of Counseling and Development, 73,* 220–222.

Brown, C., & Jasper, K. (Eds.). (1993). *Consuming passions: Feminist approaches to weight preoccupation and eating disorders.* Toronto: Second Story Press.

Brown, L., & Rothblum, E. (Eds.). (1989). *Overcoming fear of fat.* New York: Harrington Park Press.

Brown, L. S. (1987). Women, weight, and power: Feminist theoretical and therapeutic issues. *Women and Therapy, 4,* 61–71.

Brownmiller, S. (1984). *Femininity.* New York: Fawcett Columbine.

Brumberg, J. J. (1989). *Fasting girls: The emergence of anorexia nervosa as a modern disease.* Cambridge, MA: Harvard University Press.

Buchbinder, H., Burstyn, V., Forbes, D., & Steedman, M. (1987). *Who's on top?: The politics of heterosexuality.* Toronto: Garamond Press/Network Basics Books.

Buckley, T., & Gottlieb, A. (Eds.). (1988). *Blood magic: The anthropology of menstruation.* Berkeley: University of California Press.

Bullard, D. B., & Knight, S. E. (Ed.). (1981). *Sexual and physical disability: Personal perspectives.* St. Louis: Mosby.

Burgard, D., & Lyons, P. (1994). Alternatives in obesity treatment: Focusing on health for fat women. In P. Fallon, M. A. Katzman, & S. C. Wooley (Eds.), *Feminist perspectives on eating disorders* (pp. 212–230). New York: Guilford Press.

Butler, S. (1978). *Conspiracy of silence: The trauma of incest.* New York: Bantam Books.

Cairns, K. (1990). The greening of sexuality and intimacy. *Sieccan Journal, 25,* 1–10.

Caldwell, J. (1994). Afterword. In R. MacPhee, *Picasso's woman.* Vancouver, BC: Douglas & McIntyre.

Campling, J. (Ed.). (1981). *Images of ourselves: Women with disabilities talking.* London: Routledge & Kegan Paul.

Capacchione, L. (1985). *The creative journal: The art of finding yourself.* Athens, OH: Swallow Press.

Caplan, A. P. (Ed.). (1987). *The cultural construction of sexuality.* London and New York: Tavistock.

Caplan, P. J. (1989). *Don't blame mother: Mending the mother–daughter relationship*. New York: Harper & Row.

Carolan, M. T. (1994). Beyond deficiency: Broadening the view of menopause. *Journal of Applied Gerontology, 13,* 193–205.

Cash, T. (1990). Body, self, and society: The development of body images. In T. Cash & T. Pruzinsky (Eds.), *Body images: Development, deviance and change* (pp. 51–79). New York: Guilford Press.

Cassell, C. (1984). *Swept away: Why women fear their own sexuality.* New York: Simon & Schuster.

Chapman, B. E., & Brannock, J. C. (1987). Proposed model of lesbian identity development: An empirical examination. *Journal of Homosexuality, 14,* 69–80.

Chernin, K. (1986). *The hungry self: Women, eating and identity.* London: Virago Press.

Chodorow, N. J. (1978). *The reproduction of mothering: Psychoanalysis and the sociology of gender.* Berkeley: University of California Press.

Chodorow, N. J. (1994). *Femininities, masculinities, sexualities: Freud and beyond.* Lexington: University Press of Kentucky.

Chodorow, N., & Contratto, S. (1992). The fantasy of the perfect mother. In B. Thorne & M. Yalom (Eds.), *Rethinking the family: Some feminist questions* (pp. 191–214). Boston: Northeastern University Press.

Choi, M. W. (1995). The menopausal transition: Change, loss, and adaptation. *Holistic Nursing Practice, 9,* 53–62.

Choi, P. Y. L. (1994). Women's raging hormones. In P. Y. L. Choi & P. Nicolson, (Eds.), *Female sexuality: Psychology, biology and social context* (pp. 128–147). New York: Harvester/Wheatsheaf.

Christina, G. (1992). Are we having sex now or what? In D. Steinberg (Ed.), *The erotic impulse: Honoring the sensual self* (pp. 24–29). New York: Jeremy P. Tarcher.

Christopher, F. S. (1988). An initial investigation into a continuum of premarital sexual pressure. *Journal of Sex Research, 25,* 255–266.

Clare, A. W. (1983). The relationship between psychopathology and the menstrual cycle. *Women and Health, 8,* 125–136.

Cline, S. (1993). *Women, passion and celibacy.* New York: Carol Southern.

Cobb, J. O. (1988). *Understanding menopause.* Toronto: Key Porter.

Cobb, J. O. (1993). *Understanding menopause: Answers and advice for women in the prime of life.* New York: Penguin.

Cole E. (1988). Sex at menopause: Each in her own way. *Women and Therapy, 7,* 159–168.

Cole, E., & Rothblum, E. D. (1990). Commentary on "sexuality and the midlife woman." *Psychology of Women Quarterly, 14,* 509–512.

Cole, E., & Rothblum, E. D. (1991). Lesbian sex at menopause: As good as or better than ever. In B. Sang, J. Warshow, & A. J. Smith (Eds.), *Lesbians at midlife: The creative transition* (pp. 184–193). San Francisco: Spinsters.

Coleman, E. (1985). Developmental stages of the coming-out process. In J. C. Bonsisrek (Ed.), *A guide to psychotherapy with gay and lesbian clients* (pp. 31–43). New York: Haworth Press.

Collins, P. H. (1987). The meaning of motherhood in black culture and black mother–daughter relationships. *Sage: A Scholarly Journal on Black Women, 4,* 3–10.

Corea, G. (1985). *The mother machine: Reproductive technologies from artificial insemination to artificial wombs.* New York: Harper & Row.

Courtois, C. A. (1988). *Healing the incest wound: Adult survivors in therapy.* New York: Norton.

Covington, S. (1991). *Awakening your sexuality: A guide for recovering women.* San Francisco: HarperCollins.

Cowan, C. P., & Cowan, P. A. (1992). *When partners become parents: The big life change for couples.* New York: Basic Books.

Crawford, J., Kippax, S., & Waldby, C. (1994). Women's sex talk and men's sex talk: Different worlds. *Feminism and Psychology, 4,* 571–587.

Crawford, S. (1987). Lesbian families: Psychosocial stress and the family-building process. In Boston Lesbian Psychologies Collective (Ed.), *Lesbian psychologies: Explorations and challenges* (pp. 195–214). Chicago: University of Illinois Press.

Crenshaw, T. L., & Goldberg, J. P. (1996). *Sexual pharmacology: Drugs that affect sexual functioning.* New York: Norton.

Crockett, L.J., & Petersen, A.C. (1987). Pubertal status and psychosocial development: Findings from the early development study. In R. M. Lerner & T. T. Foch (Eds.), *Biological–psychosocial interactions in early adolescence: A life-span perspective* (pp. 173–188). Hillsdale, NJ: Erlbaum.

Crosbie, L. (Ed.). (1993). *The girl wants to.* Toronto: Coach House Press.

Crosthwaite, J. (1992, April). *Reproductive technologies: A problem for feminists.* Paper presented at New Birth Technologies—Women's Perspective Conference, University of Otago, Dunedin, New Zealand.

Cunningham, A. J. (1992). *The healing journey: Overcoming the crisis of cancer.* Toronto: Key Porter.

Currie, D. H. (1997). Decoding femininity: Advertisements and their teenage readers. *Sex Roles, 11,* 453–477.

Currie, D., & Raoul, V. (1992). *The anatomy of gender: Women's struggle for the body.* Ottawa: Carlton University Press.

Cutler, W.B., Garcia, C.R., & McCoy, N. (1987). Perimenopausal sexuality. *Archives of Sexual Behavior, 16,* 255–234.

Dackman, L. (1990). *Up front: Sex and the post-mastectomy woman.* Markam, Ontario: Penguin.

Dagg, P. (1991). The psychological sequelae of therapeutic abortion. *American Journal of Psychiatry, 148,* 578–585.

Daly, M. (1978). *Gyn-ecology.* Boston: Beacon Press.

Daniluk, J. C. (1988). Infertility: Intrapersonal and interpersonal impact. *Fertility and Sterility, 49,* 982–990.

Daniluk, J. C. (1991a). Strategies for counseling infertile couples. *Journal of Counseling and Development, 69,* 317–320.

Daniluk, J. C. (1991b). Female sexuality: An enigma. *Canadian Journal of Counselling, 25,* 433–446.

Daniluk, J. C. (1993). The meaning and experience of female sexuality: A phenomenological analysis. *Psychology of Women Quarterly, 17,* 53–69.

Daniluk, J. C. (1996). When treatment fails: The transition to biological childlessness for infertile women. *Women and Therapy, 19,* 81–98.

Daniluk, J. C. (1997). Gender and infertility. In S. Leiblum (Ed.), *Infertility: Psychological issues and counseling strategies* (pp. 103–125). New York: Wiley.

Daniluk, J. C., & Fluker, M. (1995). Fertility drugs and the reproductive imperative: Assisting the infertile woman. *Women and Therapy, 16,* 31–47).

Daniluk, J. C., Taylor, P. J., & Pattinson, A. T. (1996). *Reconstructing a life: The transition to biological childlessness for infertile couples. Health Canada: National Health Research and Development Program.*

Darling, C. A., & Davidson, J. K. (1987). Guilt: A factor in sexual satisfaction. *Sociological Inquiry, 57,* 251–271.

Datan, N., Antonovsky, A., & Maoz, B. (1981). *A time to reap.* Baltimore: Johns Hopkins University Press.

Davidson, J. K., & Darling, C. A. (1993). Masturbatory guilt and sexual responsiveness among post-college-age women: Sexual satisfaction revisited. *Journal of Sex and Marital Therapy, 19,* 289–300.

Davies, E., & Furnham, A. (1986). Body satisfaction in adolescent girls. *British Journal of Medical Psychology, 59,* 279–287.

Dayee, F. S. (1982). *Private zone.* Edmonds, WA: Franklin Press.

de Beauvoir, S. (1982). *When things of the spirit come first: Five early tales.* New York: Pantheon Books.

de Beauvoir, S. (1989). *The second sex* (1952 reprint). New York: Vintage Books.

Debold, E. (1991). The body at play. In C. Gilligan, A. Rogers, & D. Tolman (Eds.), *Women, girls, and psychotherapy: Reframing resistance* (pp. 169–183). New York: Haworth Press.

Debold, E., Wilson, M., & Malave, I. (1993). *Mother–daughter revolution: From betrayal to power.* Reading, MA: Addison-Wesley.

Delaney, J., Lupton, M. J., & Toth, E. (1988). *The curse: A cultural history of menstruation* (2nd ed.). Chicago: University of Illinois Press.

Denfeld, R. (1995). *The new Victorians: A young woman's challenge to the old feminist order.* New York: Warner Books.

Desey, J. (1986). The princess who stood on her own two feet. In J. Zipes (Ed.), *Don't bet on the prince: Contemporary feminist fairy tales in North America and England* (pp. 39–47). New York: Methuen.

Deutsch, J. (1945). *The psychology of women: Motherhood* (Vol. II). New York: Grune & Stratton.

de Vries, B., Birren, J.E., & Deutchman, D.E. (1990). Adult development through guided autobiography: The family context. *Family Relations, 39,* 3–7.

Dickson, G.L. (1990). A feminist poststructuralist analysis of the knowledge of menopause. *Advances in Nursing Science, 12,* 15–31.

Dionne, M., Davis, C., Fox, J., & Gurevich, M. (1995). Feminist ideology as a predictor of body dissatisfaction in women. *Sex Roles, 33,* 277–287.

Dolan, B. (1991). Cross-cultural aspects of anorexia nervosa and bulimia: A review. *International Journal of Eating Disorders, 10,* 67–78.

Dowling, C. (1996). *Red hot mamas: Coming into our own at fifty.* New York: Bantam Books.

Drake, S. M. (1992). Personal transformation: A guide for the female hero. *Women and Therapy, 12,* 51–65.

Dworkin, A. (1983). *Pornography: Men possessing women.* New York: Perigee.

Dyer, G., & Tiggemann, M. (1996). The effect of school environment on body concerns in adolescent women. *Sex Roles, 34,* 127–138.

Ehrenreich, B., & English, D. (1978). *For her own good: 150 years of the experts' advice to women.* New York: Anchor/Doubleday.

Ehrenreich, B., Hess, E., & Jacobs, G. (1986). *Remaking love: The feminization of sex*. New York: Doubleday.

Eichenbaum, L., & Orbach, S. (1983). *Understanding women: A feminist psychoanalytical approach*. New York: Viking.

Eisler, R. (1988). *The chalice and the blade: Our history, our future*. San Francisco: HarperCollins.

Ellis, H. (1942). *Studies in the psychology of sex: Vol. 1. The sexual impulse in women*. New York: Random House.

Ellis, J. (1990). The therapeutic journey: A guide for travelers. In T. A. Laidlaw & C. Malmo (Eds.), *Healing voices: Feminist approaches to therapy with women* (pp. 243–271). San Francisco: Jossey-Bass.

Ellis, K. (1990). Essay: Fatal attraction, or the post-modern prometheus. *Journal of Sex Research, 27,* 111–121.

Elvenstar, D. C. (1982). *Children: To have or have not?: A guide to making and living with your decision*. San Francisco: Harbor.

Erdman, C. K. (1995). *Nothing to lose: A guide to sane living in a large body*. San Francisco: Harper San Francisco.

Erikson, E. (1968). Womanhood and the inner space. In *Identity: Youth and crisis* (pp. 261–293). New York: Norton.

Estes, C. P. (1992). *Women who run with the wolves: Myths and stories of the wild woman archetype*. New York: Ballantine Books.

Estok, P. J., & O'Toole, R. (1991). The meanings of menopause. *Health Care for Women International, 12,* 27–39.

Ettorre, E. M. (Ed.). (1980). *Lesbians, women and society*. London: Routledge & Kegan Paul.

Evans, E. D., Ruthberg, J., Sather, C., & Turner, C. (1991). Content analysis of contemporary teen magazines for adolescent females. *Youth and Society, 23,* 99–120.

Fabian, L. J., & Thompson, J. K. (1989). Body image and eating disturbance in young females. *International Journal of Eating Disorders, 8,* 63–74.

Fallon, A. (1990). Culture in the mirror: Sociocultural determinants of body image. In T. Cash & T. Pruzinsky (Eds.), *Body images: Development, deviance, and change* (pp. 80–109). New York: Guilford Press.

Fallon, P., Katzman, M. A., & Wooley, S. C. (Eds.). (1994). *Feminist perspectives on eating disorders*. New York: Guilford Press.

Faludi, S. (1991). *Backlash: The undeclared war against American women*. New York: Anchor, Doubleday.

Ferguson, A. (1986). Motherhood and sexuality: Some feminist questions. *Hypatia, 1,* 3–22.

Fillion, K. (1996, February). This is the sexual revolution? *Saturday Night,* pp. 36–41.

Fine, M. (1988). Sexuality, schooling, and adolescent females: The missing discourse of desire. *Harvard Educational Review, 58,* 29–53.

Finkelhor, D., Hotaling, G., Lewis, I., & Smith, C. (1990). Sexual abuse in a national survey of adult men and women: Prevalence, characteristics and risk factors. *Child Abuse and Neglect, 14,* 19–28.

Firestein, B. A. (Ed.). (1996). *Bisexuality: The psychology and politics of an invisible minority*. Thousand Oaks, CA: Sage.

Fisher, S. (1986). *Development and structure of the body image* (Vols. 1 & 2). Hillsdale, NJ: Erlbaum.

Flagg, F. (1997). *Fried green tomatoes at the whistle stop cafe.* New York: Fawcett Columbine.

Flax, J. (1990). *Thinking fragments: Psychoanalysis, feminism, and postmodernism in the contemporary West.* Berkeley: University of California Press.

Flax, J. (1994). *Disputed subjects: Essays on psychoanalysis, politics, and philosophy.* London, New York: Routledge.

Flemming, A. T. (1994). *Motherhood deferred: A woman's journey.* New York: G. P. Putnam's Sons.

Flint, M. (1982). Male and female menopause: A cultural put-on. In A. M. Voda, M. Dinnerstein, & S. R. O'Donnell (Eds.), *Changing perspectives on menopause* (pp. 363–375). Austin: University of Texas Press.

Flint, M., & Samil, R. S. (1990). Cultural and subcultural meanings of the menopause. In M. Flint, F. Kronenberg, & W. Utian (Eds.), Multidisciplinary perspectives on menopause. *Annals of the New York Academy of Sciences, 592,* 134–155.

Foucault, M. (1978). *The history of sexuality: Vol. I. An introduction.* New York: Pantheon Books.

Fox, R. C. (1996) Bisexuality in perspective: A review of theory and research. In B. A. Firestein (Ed.), *Bisexuality: The psychology and politics of an invisible minority* (pp. 3–52). Thousand Oaks, CA: Sage.

Franzoi, S. L. (1995). The body-as-object versus the body-as-process: Gender differences and gender considerations. *Sex Roles, 33,* 417–437.

Fredrickson, B. L., & Roberts, T. I. (1997). Objectification theory: Toward understanding women's lived experiences and mental health risks. *Psychology of Women Quarterly, 21,* 173–206.

Freedman, R. (1988). *Body love: Learning to like our looks—and ourselves: A practical guide for women.* New York: Harper & Row.

Freeman, L. (1982). *It's my body.* Seattle, WA: Parenting Press.

Freud, S. (1948). Some psychological consequences of the anatomical distinction between the sexes. In *Collected papers* (Vol. 5, pp. 186–197). London: Hogarth.

Freud, S. (1969). Excerpts from "Anatomy is Destiny." In B. Roszak and T. Roszak (Eds.), *Masculine/feminine* (pp. 19–29). New York: Harper & Row.

Friday, N. (1973). *My secret garden.* New York: Simon & Schuster.

Friday, N. (1975). *Forbidden flowers.* New York: Pocket Books.

Friedan, B. (1993). *The fountain of age.* New York: Simon & Schuster.

Friedman, S. (1993). Decoding the "language of fat": Placing eating-disorder groups in a feminist framework. In C. Brown & K. Jasper (Eds.), *Consuming passions: Feminist approaches to weight preoccupation and eating disorders* (pp. 288–305). Toronto: Second Story Press.

Friedrich, W. M. (1990). *Psychotherapy of sexually abused children and their families.* New York: Norton.

Friedrich, W. N., Grambsch, P., Broughton, D., Kuiper, J., & Beilke, R. L. (1991). Normative sexual behavior in children. *Pediatrics, 88,* 456–464.

Gagnon, J. H. (1977). *Human sexualities.* Glenview, IL: Scott, Foresman.

Gagnon, J. H. (1985). Attitudes and responses of parents to pre-adolescent masturbation. *Archives of Sexual Behavior, 14,* 451–466.

Gagnon, J. H., & Parker, R. G. (1995). Conceiving sexuality. In R. G. Parker & J. H. Gagnon (Eds.), *Conceiving sexuality* (pp. 3–18). New York: Routledge.

Gagnon, J. H., & Simon, W. (1973). *Sexual conduct: The social sources of human sexuality.* Chicago: Aldine.

Gagnon, J. H., & Simon, W. (1982). Excerpts from sexual conduct: The social sources of human sexuality. In M. Brake (Ed.), *Human sexual relations: A reader in human sexuality* (pp. 197–222). New York: Penguin.

Gannon, L. (1985). *Menstrual disorders and menopause.* New York: Praeger.

Gannon, L. (1994). Sexuality and menopause. In P. Y. L. Choi & P. Nicolson (Eds.), *Female sexuality: Psychology, biology and social context* (pp. 100–124). New York: Harvester/Wheatsheaf.

Gardner-Loulan, J. (1991). *Period.* Volcano, CA: Volcano Press.

Garner, D., & Garfinkel, P. (1985). *Handbook of psychotherapy for anorexia nervosa and bulimia.* New York: Guilford Press.

Gartrell, N., & Mosbacher, D. (1984). Sex differences in the naming of children's genitalia. *Sex Roles, 10,* 869–876.

Gentry, J., & Seifert, F. (1991). A joyous passage: Becoming a crone. In B. Sang, J. Warshow, & A. Smith (Eds.), *Lesbians at midlife: The creative transition* (pp. 225–236). San Francisco: Spinsters.

George, S. (1993). *Women and bisexuality.* London: Scarlet Press.

Gergen, K. J. (1985). The social constructionist movement in modern psychology. *American Psychologist, 40,* 266–275.

Gergen, M. M. (1990). Finished at 40: Women's development within patriarchy. *Psychology of Women Quarterly, 14,* 471–493.

Gerson, M. J., Alpert, J. L., & Richardson, M. S. (1990). Mothering: The view from psychological research. In J. F. O'Barr, D. Pope, & Mary Wyer (Eds.), *Ties that bind: Essays on mothering and patriarchy* (pp. 15–34). Chicago: University of Chicago Press.

Gieve, K. (1989). *Balancing acts: On being a mother.* London: Virago.

Gil, V. E. (1990). Sexual fantasy experiences and guilt among conservative Christians: An exploratory study. *Journal of Sex Research, 27,* 629–638.

Gil, E., & Johnson, T. C. (1993). *Sexualized children: Assessment and treatment of sexualized children and children who molest.* Rockville, MD: Launch Press.

Gilfoyle, J., Wilson, J., & Brown (1993). Sex, organs and audiotape: A discourse analytic approach to talking about heterosexual sex and relationships. In S. Wilkinson & C. Kitzinger (Eds.), *Heterosexuality: A feminism and psychology reader* (pp. 181–202). London: Sage.

Gillespie, R. (1996). Women, the body and brand extension in medicine: Cosmetic surgery and the paradox of choice. *Women and Health, 24,* 69–85.

Gilligan, C. (1991). Women's psychological development: Implications for psychotherapy. In C. Gilligan, A. Rogers, & D. Tolman (Eds.), *Women, girls and psychotherapy: Reframing resistance* (pp. 5–31). New York: Harrington Park Press.

Gilligan, C. (1982). *In a different voice: Psychological theory and women's development.* Cambridge, MA: Harvard University Press.

Gilligan, C., & Brown, L. M. (1992). *Meeting at the crossroads: Women's psychology and girls' development.* Cambridge, MA: Harvard University Press.

Gilligan, C., Rogers, A., & Tolman, D. (Eds.). (1991). *Women, girls and psychotherapy: Reframing resistance.* New York: Haworth Press.

Gilman, C. (1973). *The yellow wallpaper* (Afterword by E. R. Hedges). New York: Feminist Press.

Gimbutas, M. (1989). *The language of the goddess.* San Francisco: Harper & Row.

Girard, L. W. (1984). *My body is private.* Niles, IL: A. Whitman.

Glazer, E. S., & Cooper, S. L. (1988). *Without child: Experiencing and resolving infertility.* New York: Lexington Books.

Glazer, G., & Rozman, A.S. (1991). Marital adjustment, life stress, attitudes toward menopause, and menopausal symptoms in premenopausal, menopausal, and postmenopausal women. In D. L. Taylor, & N. F. Woods (Eds.), *Menstruation, health, and illness* (pp. 237–244). New York: Hemisphere.

Goddess remembered. (1990). Los Angeles: Direct Cinema Ltd.

Golden, C. (1987). Diversity and variability in women's sexual identities. In Boston Lesbian Psychologies Collective (Ed.), *Lesbian psychologies* (pp. 18–34). Urbana: University of Illinois Press.

Golden, G. H. (1988). The theory of sexual relativity: Female reality/male myth. *Women and Therapy, 7,* 77–85.

Goldenberg, N. (1990). *Returning words to flesh: Feminism, psychoanalysis, and the resurrection of the body.* Boston: Beacon Press.

Golding, J. M. (1996). Sexual assault history and women's reproductive and sexual health. *Psychology of Women Quarterly, 20,* 101–121.

Goldman, R., & Goldman, J. (1988). *Show me yours: Understanding children's sexuality* (2nd ed). New York: Penguin.

Goldner, V. (1987). Feminism and family therapy. *Family Process, 24,* 31–47.

Goldner, V. (1991). Sex, power, and gender: A feminist systemic analysis of the politics of passion. *Journal of Feminist Family Therapy, 3,* 63–83.

Goldsworthy, J. (Ed.). (1993). *A certain age: Reflecting on the menopause.* New York: Columbia University Press.

Golombeck, H., Marton, P., Stein, B., & Korenblum, M. (1987). Personality functioning status during early and middle adolescence. *Adolescent Psychiatry, 14,* 365–377.

Golub, S. (1983). Menarche: The beginning of menstrual life. *Women and Health, 8,* 17–36.

Golub, S. (1992). *Periods: From menarche to menopause.* Newbury Park, CA: Sage.

Golub, S., & Catalano, J. (1983). Recollections of menarche and women's subsequent experiences with menstruation. *Women and Health, 8,* 49–61.

Gottfried, A. E., & Gottfried, A. W. (1994) *Redefining families: Implications for children's development.* New York: Plenum.

Grambs, J. D. (1989). *Women over forty: Visions and realities.* New York: Springer.

Grant, L. (1994). *Sexing the millennium: Women and the sexual revolution.* New York: Grove Press.

Gravelle, K., & Gravelle, J. (1996). *The period book: Everything you don't want to ask (but need to know).* New York: Walker.

Gray, J. (1997). *Mars and Venus in the bedroom: A guide to lasting romance and passion.* New York: Harper Perennial.

Greaves, K. (1990). *Big and beautiful.* London: Grafton Books.

Greenspan, M. (1983). *A new approach to women and therapy.* Blue Ridge Summit, PA: Tab Books.

Greenwood, S. (1992). *Updated menopause naturally: Preparing for the second half of life.* Volcano, CA: Volcano Press.

Greer, G. (1971). *The female eunuch.* London: Paladin.

Greer, G. (1984). *Sex and destiny: The politics of human fertility.* New York: Harper & Row.

Greer, G. (1991). *The change: Women, aging and menopause.* New York: Fawcett Columbine.

Greil, A. L. (1991). *Not yet pregnant: Infertile couples in contemporary America.* New Brunswick, London: Rutgers University Press.

Grogan, S., Williams, Z., & Conner, M. (1996). The effects of viewing same-gender photographic models on body-esteem. *Psychology of Women Quarterly, 20,* 569–575.

Gross, A., & Ito, D. (1990). *Women talk about breast surgery: From diagnosis to recovery.* New York: Clarkson Potter.

Gross A., & Ito, D. (1992). *Women talk about gynecological surgery: From diagnosis to recovery.* New York: Harper Perennial.

Gruen, D. (1990). Postpartum depression: A debilitating yet often unassesed problem. *Health and Social Work, 15,* 261–270.

Hallstrom, R., & Samuelson, S. (1990). Changes in women's sexual desire in middle age: The longitudinal study of women in Gothenburg. *Archives of Sexual Behavior, 19,* 259–268.

Hancock, E. (1989). *The girl within: Recapture the childhood self, the key to female identity.* New York: Dutton.

Hare-Mustin, R., & Marecek, J. (Eds.). (1990). *Making a difference: Psychology and the construction of gender.* New Haven, CT: Yale University Press.

Harris, M. B. (1990). Is love seen as different for the obese? *Journal of Applied Social Psychology, 20,* 1209–1224.

Havens, B., & Swenson, I. (1988). Imagery associated with menstruation in advertising targeted to adolescent women. *Adolescence, 89,* 89–96.

Hawkins, M. (1990). Women's identity: Pregnancy, mothering and motherhood. In M. Walker (Ed.), *Women in therapy and counselling: Out of the shadows* (pp. 83–100). Philadelphia: Open University Press.

Hays, T. E. (1987). Menstrual expressions and menstrual attitudes. *Sex Roles, 16,* 605–614.

Heilburn, C. G. (1988). *Writing a woman's life.* New York: Norton.

Herdt, G., & Boxer, A. (1993). *Children of horizons: How gay and lesbian teens are leading a new way out of the closet.* Boston: Beacon Press.

Herman, J. L. (1992). *Trauma and recovery: The aftermath of violence—from domestic abuse to political terror.* New York: Basic Books.

Hesse-Biber, S. J. (1996). *Am I thin enough yet?: The cult of thinness and the commercialization of identity.* New York: Oxford University Press.

Heyward, C. (1989). *Coming out and relational empowerment: A lesbian feminist theological perspective* (The Stone Center: Work in Progress, 38). Wellesley, MA: Wellesley College.

Hill, J. P. (1988). Adapting to menarche: Familial control and conflict. In M. R. Gunnar & W. A. Collins (Eds.), *Development during the transition to adolescence: Minnesota Symposia on Child Development* (Vol. 21, pp. 43–77). Hillsdale, NJ: Erlbaum.

Hill, J. P., & Holmbeck, G. N. (1987). Familial adaptation to biological change during adolescence. In R. M. Lerner & T. T. Foch (Eds.), *Biological–psychosocial interactions in early adolescence* (pp. 207–223). Hillsdale, NJ: Erlbaum.

Hill, J. P., Holmbeck, G. N., Marlow, L., Green, T. M., & Lynch, M. E. (1985). Menarcheal status and parent–child relations in families of seventh-grade girls. *Journal of Youth and Adolescence, 14,* 301–315.

Hill, J. P., & Lynch, M. E. (1983). The intensification of gender-related role expectations during early adolescence. In J. Brooks-Gunn & A. C. Petersen (Eds.), *Girls at puberty* (pp. 201–228). New York: Plenum.

Hirschmann, J. R., & Munter, C. H. (1995). *When women stop hating their bodies: Freeing yourself from food and weight obsession.* New York: Fawcett Columbine.

Hite, S. (1981). *The Hite report: A nationwide study of female sexuality.* New York: Dell.

Hite, S. (1987). *Women and love: The Hite report.* New York: St. Martin's Press.

Hollway, W. (1984). Gender difference and the production of subjectivity. In J. Henriques, W. Hollway, C. Urwin, C. Venn, & V. Walkerdine (Eds.), *Changing the subject: Psychology, social regulation and subjectivity* (pp. 227–263). London: Metheun.

Hollway, W. (1989). *Subjectivity and method in psychology: Gender, meaning and science.* London: Sage.

Holmbeck, G. N., & Bale, P. (1988). Relations between instrumental and expressive personality traits and behaviors: A test of Spence and Helmreich's theory. *Journal of Research in Personality, 22,* 37–59.

Holmbeck, G. N., & Hill, J. P. (1986). A path-analytic approach to the relations between parental traits and acceptance and adolescent adjustment. *Sex Roles, 14,* 315–334.

Houseknecht, S. (1987). Voluntary childlessness. In M. B. Sussman & S. K. Steinmetz (Eds.), *Handbook of marriage and family* (pp. 369–395). New York: Plenum.

Howe, K. G. (1990). Daughters discover their mother through biographies and genograms: Educational and clinical parallels. In J. P. Knowles & E. Cole (Eds.), *Woman-defined motherhood* (pp. 31–40). New York: Harrington Park Press.

Hubbard, R. (1990). *The politics of women's biology.* New Brunswick, NJ: Rutgers University Press.

Hunter, M. (1990). *Your menopause: Prepare now for a positive future.* London: Pandora.

Hurcombe, L. (Ed.). (1987). *Sex and God: Some varieties of women's religious experience.* New York, London: Routledge & Kegan Paul.

Hutchins, L., & Ka'ahumanu, L. (1991). *Bi any other name: Bisexual people speak out.* Boston: Alyson.

Hutchinson, M. (1982). Transforming body image. *Women and Therapy, 1,* 59–67.

Hutchinson, M. (1985). *Transforming body image.* Freedom, CA: Crossing Press.

Hutchinson, M. G. (1994). Imagining ourselves whole: A feminist approach to treating body image disorders. In P. Fallon, M. A. Katzman, & S. C. Wooley (Eds.), *Feminist perspectives on eating disorders* (pp. 152–168). New York: Guilford Press.

Hyde, J. S. (1990). *Understanding human sexuality* (4th ed.). New York: McGraw-Hill.

Ireland, M. S. (1993). *Reconceiving women: Separating motherhood from female identity.* New York: Guilford Press.

Isberg, R. S., Hauser, S. T., Jacobson, A. M., Powers, S. I., Noam, G., Weis-Perry, B., & Follansbee, D. (1989). Parental contexts of adolescent self-esteem: A developmental perspective. *Journal of Youth and Adolescence, 18,* 1–23.

Jackson, L. A., Sullivan, L. A., & Hymes, J. (1987). Gender, gender role, and physical appearance. *Journal of Psychology, 121,* 151–156.

Jackson, L. A., Sullivan, L. A., & Rostker, R. (1988). Gender, gender role, and body image. *Sex Roles, 19,* 429–443.

Jacob, M. C. (1997). Concerns of single women and lesbian couples considering conception through assisted reproduction. In S. R. Leiblum (Ed.), *Infertility: Psychological issues and counseling strategies* (pp. 189–206). New York: Wiley.

Jacobus, M., Keller, E. F., & Shuttleworth, S. (Eds.). (1990). *Body/politics: Women and the discourses of science.* New York: Routledge.

Jaggar, A., & Bordo, S. (1989). *Gender/body/knowledge: Feminist reconstructions of being and knowing.* New Brunswick, NJ: Rutgers University Press.

Janeway, E. (1980). Who is Sylvia?: On the loss of sexual paradigms. In C. R. Stimpson & E. S. Person (Eds.), *Women: Sex and sexuality* (pp. 4–20). Chicago: University of Chicago Press.

Jeffreys, S. (1990). *Anticlimax: A feminist perspective on the sexual revolution.* London: Women's Press.

Johnson, J. (1987). *Intimacy: Living as a woman after cancer.* Toronto: NC Press.

Jordan, J. V. (1986). The meaning of mutuality. *Work in Progress.* Wellesley, MA: Stone Center for Developmental Services and Studies, Wellesley College.

Jordan, J. V. (1987). *Clarity in connection: Empathic knowing, desire and sexuality.* Wellesley, MA: Stone Center, Wellesley College.

Jordan, J., Kaplan, A. G., Baker-Miller, J., Stiver, I., & Surrey, J. (1991). *Women's growth in connection: Writings from the Stone Center.* New York: Guilford Press.

Kahn, A., & Holt, L. (1987). *Menopause: The best years of your life?* London: Bloomsbury.

Kamptner, L. N. (1988). Identity development in early adolescence: Causal modeling of social and familial influences. *Journal of Youth and Adolescence, 17,* 493–513.

Kaplan, B. J. (1986). A psychobiological review of depression during pregnancy. *Psychology of Women Quarterly, 10,* 35–38.

Kaplan, E. A. (1990). Sex, work and motherhood: The impossible triangle. *Journal of Sex Research, 27,* 409–425.

Kaplan, H. S. (1981). *The new sex therapy.* Hamondsworth, UK: Penguin.

Kaplan, M. M. (1992). *Mothers' images of motherhood.* London: Routledge.

Katz, S. A. (1987). New directions. In S. Martz (Ed.), *When I am an old woman I shall wear purple: An anthology of short stories and poetry* (2nd ed., p. 71). Watsonville, CA: Papier-Mache Press.

Karen, R. (1992, February). Shame. *The Atlantic Monthly,* pp. 40–70.

Kaschak, E. (1988). Limits and boundaries: Toward a complex psychology of women. *Women and Therapy,* 7(4), 109–123.

Kaschak, E. (1992). *Engendered lives: A new psychology of women's experience.* New York: Basic Books.

Kasl, C. D. (1989). *Women, sex, and addiction: A search for love and power.* New York: Harper & Row.

Katchadourian, H. (1977). *The biology of adolescence.* San Francisco: Freeman.

Kaufert, P. (1982). Anthropology and menopause: The development of a theoretical framework. *Maturitas, 4,* 181–193.

Kaufert, P. (1986). Menstruation and menstrual change: Women in midlife. *Health Care of Women International, 7,* 63–76.

Kaufman, B., & Wohl, A. (1992). *Casualties of childhood: A developmental perspective on sexual abuse using projective drawings.* New York: Brunner/Mazel.

Kegan, R. G. (1982). *The evolving self: Problem and process in human development.* Cambridge, MA: Harvard University Press.

Kellett, J. M. (1991). Sexuality and the elderly. *Sexual and Marital Therapy, 6,* 147–155.

Kilbourne, J. (1994). Still killing us softly: Advertising and the obsession with thinness. In P. Fallon, M. A. Katzman, & S. C. Wooley (Eds.), *Feminist perspectives on eating disorders* (pp. 395–418). New York: Guilford Press.

Kimlicka, T. M., Cross, T. H., & Tarhai, J. (1983). A comparison of androgynous, feminine, masculine, and undifferentiated women on self-esteem, body satisfaction, and sexual satisfaction. *Psychology of Women Quarterly, 7,* 291–294.

Kimmel, D. C. (1990). *Adulthood and aging: An interdisciplinary, developmental view* (3rd ed.). New York: Wiley.

Kinsey, A., Pomeroy, W., & Martin, C. (1948). *Sexual behavior in the human male.* Philadelphia: Saunders.

Kinsey, A., Pomeroy, W., Martin, C., & Gebhard, P. (1953). *Sexual behavior in the human female.* London: Saunders.

Kirkpatrick, M. (1982). *Women's sexual experience: Explorations of the dark continent.* New York: Plenum.

Kitzinger, C. (1987). *The social construction of lesbianism.* London: Sage.

Kitzinger, S. (1985). *Women's experience of sex.* New York: Penguin.

Kitzinger, S. (1992). *Ourselves as mothers: The universal experience of motherhood.* Reading, MA: Addison-Wesley.

Kitzinger, S. (1994). *The year after childbirth: Surviving and enjoying the first year of motherhood.* New York: HarperCollins.

Kjerulff, K., Langenberg, P., & Guzinski, G. (1993). The socioeconomic correlates of hysterectomies in the United States. *American Journal of Public Health, 83,* 106–108.

Kleiman, K., & Raskin, V. (1994). *This isn't what I expected: Recognizing and recovering from depression and anxiety after childbirth.* Toronto: Bantam Books.

Klein, F. (1993). *The bisexual option* (2nd ed.). New York: Harrington Park Press.

Klein, R., & Rowland, R. (1988). Women as test-sites for fertility drugs: Clomiphene citrate and hormonal cocktails. *Reproductive and Genetic Engineering, 1,* 251–273.

Kleinberg, L. (1986). *Coming home to self, going home to parents: Lesbian identity disclosure.* (The Stone Center: Work in Progress, 24). Wellesley, MA: Wellesley College.

Klohnen, E. C., Vandewater, E. A., & Young, A. (1996). Negotiating the middle years: Ego-resiliency and successful midlife adjustment in women. *Psychology and Aging, 11,* 431–442.

Knowles, J. P. (1990). Woman-defined motherhood. In J. P. Knowles & E. Cole (Eds.), *Woman-defined motherhood* (pp. 1–7). New York: Harrington Park Press.

Koeske, R. D. (1983). Lifting the curse of menstruation: Toward a feminist perspective on the menstrual cycle. *Women and Health, 8,* 1–16.

Koff, E., Rierdan, J., & Stubbs, M. L. (1990). Conceptions and misconceptions of the menstrual cycle. *Women and Health, 16,* 119–136.

Koss, M. P. (1990). The women's mental health research agenda: Violence against women. *American Psychologist, 45,* 374–380.

Koss, M. P. (1993). Rape: Scope, impact, interventions, and public policy responses. *American Psychologist, 48,* 1062–1069.

Koss, M. P., & Burkhart, B. R. (1989). A conceptual analysis of rape victimization. *Psychology of Women Quarterly, 13,* 27–40.

Koss, M. P., Gidycz, C. A., & Wisniewski, N. (1987). The scope of rape: Incidence and prevalence of sexual aggression and victimization in a national sample of higher education students. *Journal of Consulting and Clinical Psychology, 55,* 162–170.

Kraus, M., & Redman, E. (1986). Postpartum depression: An interactional view. *Journal of Marital and Family Therapy, 12,* 63–74.

Kronenberg, F. (1990). Hot flashes: Epidemiology and physiology. In M. Flint, F. Kronenberg, & W. Utian (Eds.), Multidisciplinary perspectives on menopause. *Annals of the New York Academy of Sciences, 592,* 52–86.

Kuhn, M. H. (1964). Major trends in symbolic interaction theory in the past twenty-five years. *Sociological Quarterly, 61*–84.

Kushner, E. (1997). *Experiencing abortion: A weaving of women's words.* New York: Haworth Press.

Laidlaw, T. A., & Malmo, C. (Eds.). (1990). *Healing voices: Feminist approaches to therapy with women.* San Francisco: Jossey-Bass.

Lamb, S., & Coakley, M. (1993). "Normal" childhood sexual play and games: Differentiating play from abuse. *Child Abuse and Neglect, 17,* 515–525.

Landa, A. (1990). No accident: The voices of woluntarily childless women—an essay on the social construction of fertility choices. In J. P. Knowles & E. Cole (Eds.), *Woman-defined motherhood* (pp. 139–158). New York: Harrington Park Press.

La Sorsa, V. A., & Fodor, I. G. (1990). Adolescent daughter/midlife mother dyad: A new look at separation and self-definition. *Psychology of Women Quarterly, 14,* 593–606.

Laws, J. L. (1980). Female sexuality through the life span. In P. B. Baltes & O. G. Brim, Jr. (Eds.), *Life-span development and behavior* (Vol. 3, pp. 207–252). New York: Academic Press.

Leader, A. S., Taylor, P. J., & Daniluk, J. D. (1984). Infertility: Clinical and psychological aspects. *Psychiatric Annals, 14,* 461–467.

Leaper, C., Hauser, S. T., Kremen, A., Powers, S. I., Jacobson, A. M., Noam, G. G., Weis-Perry, B., & Follansbee, D. (1989). Adolescent–parent interactions in relation to adolescents' gender and ego-development pathway: A longitudinal study. *Journal of Early Adolescence, 9,* 335–361.

Lear, D. (1997). *Sex and sexuality: Risk and relationships in the age of AIDS.* Thousand Oaks, CA: Sage.

LeCroy, C. W. (1988). Parent–adolescent intimacy: Impact on adolescent functioning. *Adolescence, 23,* 137–147.

Lees, S. (1986). *Losing out: Sexuality and adolescent girls.* Dover, NH: Hutchinson Education.

Leiblum, S. R. (1990). Sexuality and the midlife woman. *Psychology of Women Quarterly, 14,* 495–508.

Leiblum, S. R. (1994). The impact of infertility on marital and sexual satisfaction. *Annual Review of Sex Research, 4,* 99–120.

Leiblum, S. R. (1997) Love, sex, and infertility: The impact of infertility on couples. In S. R. Leiblum (Ed.), *Infertility: Psychological issues and counseling strategies* (pp. 149–166). New York: Wiley.

Leiblum, S. R., Palmer, M. G., & Spector, I. P. (1995). Non-traditional mothers: Single heterosexual/lesbian women and lesbian couples electing motherhhod via donor insemination. *Journal of Psychosomatic Obstetrics and Gynaecology, 16,* 11–20.

Leiblum, S. R., & Swartzman, L.C. (1986). Women's attitudes toward the menopause: An update. *Maturitas, 8,* 47–56.

Leigh, S. (1987). Growing old disgracefully. *Trouble and Strife, 10,* 20–22.

Lemkau, J. P. (1988). Emotional sequelae of abortion: Implications for clinical practice. *Psychology of Women Quarterly, 12,* 461–472.

Lerman, H. (1986). From Freud to feminist personality theory: Getting there from here. *Psychology of Women Quarterly, 10,* 1–18.

Leroy, M. (1993). *Pleasure: The truth about female sexuality.* London: HarperCollins.

Letson, D. (1987). Maid in God's image? *Sieccan Journal, 2,* 53–61.

Levine, E. M., & Kanin, E. J. (1987). Sexual violence among dates and acquaintances: Trends and their implications for marriage and family. *Journal of Family Violence, 2,* 55–65.

Lewis, M. I. (1980). The history of female sexuality in the United States. In M. Kirkpatrick (Ed.), *Women's sexual development: Explorations of inner space* (pp. 19–38). New York: Plenum.

Lindemann, C. (1983). Women's health/sexuality: The case of menopause. *Journal of Social Work and Human Sexuality, 2,* 101–112.

Lindgren, A. (1950). *Pippi Longstocking.* New York: Viking Press.

Ling, A. (1989). Chinamerican women writers: Four forerunners of Maxine Hong Kingston. In A. Jaggar & S. Bordo (Eds.), *Gender/body/knowledge: Feminist reconstructions of being and knowing* (pp. 309–324). New Brunswick, NJ: Rutgers University Press.

Lisle, L. (1996). *Without child: Challenging the stigma of childlessness.* New York: Ballantine Books.

Llewelyn, S., & Osborne, K. (1990). *Women's lives.* London: Routledge.

Loewenstein, S. F. (1985). On the diversity of love object orientations among women. *Journal of Social Work and Human Sexuality, 3,* 7–24.

Lorde, A. (1984). Uses of the erotic: The erotic as power. In *Sister outsider: Essays and speeches* (pp. 53–59). Freedom, CA: Crossing Press.

Loulan, J. (1984). *Lesbian sex.* San Francisco: Spinsters/Aunt Lute.

Loulan, J. (1987). *Lesbian passion: Loving ourselves and each other.* San Francisco: Spinsters/Aunt Lute.

Loulan, J., & Thomas, S. (1990). *The lesbian erotic dance: Butch, femme, androgyny, and other rhythms.* San Francisco: Spinsters.

Love, S. (1990). *Dr. Susan Love's breast book.* Reading, MA: Addison-Wesley.

MacPhee, R. (1994). *Picasso's woman.* Vancouver, BC: Douglas & McIntyre.

Madaras, L. (1993). *My body, myself.* New York: Newmarket Press.

Madaras, L., & Madaras, A. (1983). *What's happening to my body: A growing up guide for mothers and daughters.* New York: Newmarket Press.

Mahlstedt, P. P. (1985). The psychological component of infertility. *Fertility and Sterility, 43,* 335–346.

Malamuth, N. M., & Briere, J. (1986). Sexual violence in the media: Indirect effects on aggression against women. *Journal of Social Issues, 42,* 75–92.

Maltz, W. (1991). *The sexual healing journey.* New York: HarperCollins.

Maltz, W., & Holman, B. (1987). *Incest and sexuality: A guide to understanding and healing.* Lexington, MA: Lexington Books.

Mansfield, P. K. (1988). Midlife childbearing: Strategies for informed decision making. *Psychology of Women Quarterly, 12,* 445–460.

Mansfield, P. K., Theisen, C. S., & Boyer, B. (1992). Midlife women and menopause: A challenge for the mental health counselor. *Journal of Mental Health Counseling, 14,* 73–83.

Marin, P. (1983, July). A revolution's broken promises. *Psychology Today,* pp. 50–57.

Markus, H., & Cross, S. (1993). The interpersonal self. In D. K. Freedheim (Ed.), *History of psychotherapy: A century of change* (pp. 576–608). Washington, DC: American Psychological Association Press.

Martin, E. (1987). *The woman in the body: A cultural analysis of reproduction.* Boston: Beacon Press.

Martinson, F. M. (1991). Normal sexual development in infancy and childhood. In G. D. Ryan & S. L. Lane (Eds.), *Juvenile sexual offending: Causes, consequences and correction* (pp. 57–82). Lexington, MA: Lexington Books.

Masters, W. H., & Johnson, V. E. (1966). *Human sexual response.* Boston: Little, Brown.

Masters, W. H., & Johnson, V. E. (1970). *Human sexual inadequacy.* Boston: Little, Brown.

Mattes, J. (1997). *Single mothers by choice: A guidebook for single women who are considering or have chosen motherhood.* New York: Random House.

Matteson, D. R. (1996). Counseling and psychotherapy with bisexual and exploring clients. In B. A. Firestein (Ed.), *Bisexuality: The psychology and politics of an invisible minority* (pp. 185–213). Thousand Oaks, CA: Sage.

Mayle, P. (1975). *What's happening to me?: The answers to some of the world's most embarrassing questions.* London: Macmillan.

Mayle, P., & Robins, A. (1978). *Where did I come from?: The facts of life without any nonesense and with illustrations* (2nd ed.). London: Macmillan.

McCarn, S. R., & Fassinger, R. E. (1996). Revisioning sexual minority identity formation: A new model of lesbian identity and its implications for counseling and research. *Counseling Psychologist, 24,* 508–534.

McCormick, N. B. (1994). *Sexual salvation: Affirming women's sexual rights and pleasures.* Westport, CT: Praeger.

McCrea, F. B. (1983). The politics of menopause: The "discovery" of a deficiency disease. *Social Problems, 31,* 111–123.

McDermott, S. (1970). *Female sexuality: Its nature and conflicts.* New York: Simon & Schuster.

McGoldrick, M. (1989). Women through the family life cycle. In M. McGoldrick, C. M. Anderson, & F. Walsh (Eds.), *Women in families: A framework for family therapy* (pp. 200–226). New York: Norton.

McGrade, J. J., & Tolor, A. (1981). The reaction to infertility and the infertility investigation: A comparison of the responses of men and women. *Infertility, 4,* 7–27.

McKinlay, J. B., & McKinlay, S. M. (1987). Depression in middle-aged women: Social circumstances versus estrogen deficiency. In M. R. Walsh (Ed.), *The psychology of women: Ongoing debates* (pp. 157–161). New Haven and London: Yale University Press.

McKinley, N. M., & Hyde, J. S. (1996). The objectified body consciousness scale: Development and validation. *Psychology of Women Quarterly, 20,* 181–215.

McKinney, K., & Sprecher, S. (Eds.). (1989). *Human sexuality: The societal and interpersonal context.* Norwood, NJ: Ablex.

McMahon, K. (1990). The *Cosmopolitan* ideology and the management of desire. *Journal of Sex Research, 27,* 381–396.

McMahon, M. (1995). *Engendering motherhood: Identity and self-transformation in women's lives.* New York: Guilford Press.

McNeill, E. (1994). Blood, sex and hormones: A theoretical review of women's sexuality over the menstrual cycle. In P. Y. L. Choi & P. Nicolson (Eds.), *Female sexuality: Psychology, biology and social context* (pp. 56–82). New York: Harvester/Wheatsheaf.

Mead, G. H. (1934). *Mind, self, and society: From the standpoint of a social behaviorist* (Vol. 3). Chicago: University of Chicago Press.

Meador, B. D. (1986). The thesmophoria: A women's ritual. *Psychological Perspectives, 17,* 35–45.

Meadow, R. M., & Weiss, L. (1992). *Women's conflicts about eating and sexuality: The relationship between food and sex.* New York: Harrington Park Press.

Medical Research International, Society for Assisted Reproductive Technology (SART), The American Fertility Society. (1992). *In vitro* fertilization–embryo transfer (IVF-ET) in the United States: 1990 results from the IVF-ET registry. *Fertility and Sterility, 57,* 15–24.

Mendelsen, B. K., & White, D. R. (1985). Development of self-body esteem in overweight youngsters. *Developmental Psychology, 21,* 90–96.

Menning, B. E. (1988). *Infertility: A guide for the childless couple* (2nd ed.). New York: Prentice-Hall.

Mercer, R. T., Nichols, E. G., & Doyle, G. C. (1988). *Transitions in a woman's life.* Springer Series: Vol. 12. Focus on Women. New York: Springer.

Metts, S., & Cupach, W. R. (1989). Communication and sexuality. In K. McKinney & S. Sprecher (Eds.), *Human sexuality: The societal and interpersonal context* (pp. 139–161). Norwood, NJ: Ablex.

Miller, A. (1990). *Thou shalt not be aware: Society's betrayal of the child* (2nd ed.). New York: Meridian.

Miller, J. B. (1983). *The development of women's sense of self.* (The Stone Center: Work in Progress). Wellesley, MA: Wellesley College.

Miller, J. B. (1986). *Toward a new psychology of women* (2nd ed.). Boston: Beacon Press.

Miller P. Y., & Fowlkes, M. R. (1980). Social and behavioral constructions of female sexuality. In C. R. Stimpson & E. S. Person (Eds.), *Women: Sex and sexuality* (pp. 256–273). Chicago: University of Chicago Press.

Millman, M. (1980). *Such a pretty face: Being fat in America.* New York: Norton.

Minuk, L. (1995). *No regrets: The experiences of voluntarily childless women at midlife.* Unpublished master's thesis, University of British Columbia, Vancouver, BC.

Moen, P., Erickson, M. A., & Dempster-McClain, D. (1997). Their mother's daughters? The intergenerational transmission of gender attitudes in a world of changing roles. *Journal of Marriage and the Family, 59,* 281–293.

Money, J., & Ehrhardt, A. (1972). *Man and woman, boy and girl.* Baltimore: Johns Hopkins University Press.

Money, J., & Tucker, P. (1975). *Sexual signatures.* Boston: Little, Brown.

Moore, S. M., & Rosenthal, D. A. (1996). Young people assess their risk of sexually transmissible diseases. *Psychology and Health, 11,* 345–355.

Morell, C. (1994). *Unwomanly conduct: The challenges of intentional childlessness.* New York: Routledge.

Morokoff, P. J. (1988). Sexuality in perimenopausal and postmenopausal women. *Psychology of Women Quarterly, 12,* 489–511.

Morris, L. A. (1997). *The male heterosexual: Lust in his loins, sin in his soul?* Thousand Oaks, CA: Sage.

Mosher, W. D. (1988). Fecundity and infertility in the United States. *American Journal of Public Health, 78,* 181–182.

Muehlenhard, C.L. (1988). "Nice women" don't say yes and "real men" don't say no: How miscommunication and the double standard can cause sexual problems. *Women and Therapy, 7,* 95–108.

Muelenhard, C. L., & McCoy, M. L. (1991). Double standard/double bind: The sexual double standard and women's communication about sex. *Psychology of Women Quarterly, 15,* 447–461.

Munsch, R. (1982). *The paper bag princess* (3rd ed.). Toronto: Annick Press.

Nachtigall, R. D., Becker, G., & Wozny, M. (1992). The effects of gender-specific diagnosis on men's and women's response to infertility. *Fertility and Sterility, 57,* 113–121.

Nestle, J. (1991). Desire perfected: Sex after forty. In B. Sang, J. Warshow, & A. Smith (Eds.), *Lesbians at midlife: The creative transition* (pp. 180–183). San Francisco: Spinsters.

Neugarten, B. L., Wood, V., Kraines, R. J., & Loomis, B. (1968). Women's attitudes toward menopause. In B. L. Neugarten (Ed.), *Middle age and aging* (pp. 195–200). Chicago: University of Chicago Press.

Nickerson, B. (1992). *Old and smart: Women and the adventure of aging.* Madeira Park, BC: Harbour.

Nicolson, P. (1986). Developing a feminist approach to depression following childbirth. In S. Wilkinson (Ed.), *Feminist social psychology* (pp. 142–158). Milton Keynes: Open University Press.

Noble, K.D. (1990). The female hero: A quest for healing and wholeness. *Women and Therapy, 9,* 3–18.

Norwood, R. (1997). *Women who love too much: When you keep wishing and hoping he'll change.* New York: Pocket Books.

Oberman, Y., & Josselson, R. (1996). Matrix of tensions: A model of mothering. *Psychology of Women Quarterly, 20,* 341–359.

Ogden, G. (1985). Women and sexual ecstasy: How can therapists help? *Women and Therapy, 7,* 43–56.

Ogden, G. (1994). *Women who love sex.* New York: Pocket Books.

Omer-Hashi, K.H., & Entwistle, M. (1995). Female genital mutilation: Cultural and health issues and their implications for sexuality counselling in Canada. *Canadian Journal of Human Sexuality, 4,* 137–147.

Orbach, S. (1978). *Fat is a feminist issue.* New York: Paddington Books.

Orbach, S. (1986). *Hunger strike: The anorectic's struggle as a metaphor for our age.* New York: Norton.

Orbuch, T. L. (1989). Human sexuality education. In K. McKinney & S. Sprecher (Eds.), *Human sexuality: The societal and interpersonal context* (pp. 438–462). Norwood, NJ: Ablex.

Oyefeso, A., & Osinowo, H. O. (1990). The development of the attitudes towards menstruation questionnaire (ATMQ). *Indian Journal of Behavior, 14,* 60–63.

Page, L. (1993). *Menopause and emotions: Making sense of your feelings when your feelings make no sense.* Vancouver, BC: Primavera Press.

Palladino, D., & Stephenson, Y. (1990). Perceptions of the sexual self: Their impact on relationships between lesbian and heterosexual women. In L. S. Brown & M. P. Root (Eds.), *Diversity and complexity in feminist therapy* (pp. 231–253). New York: Haworth Press.

Parker, R. G., & Gagnon, J. H. (Eds.). (1995). *Conceiving sexuality: Approaches to sex research in a postmodern world.* New York: Routledge.

Parlee, M. B. (1987). Media treatment of premenstrual syndrome. In B. E. Ginsburg & B. F. Carter (Eds.), *Premenstrual syndrome: Ethical and legal implications in a biomedical perspective* (pp. 189–205). New York: Plenum.

Parrot, A. (1989). Acquaintance rape among adolescents: Identifying risk groups and intervention strategies. *Journal of Social Work and Human Sexuality, 8,* 47–61.

Partridge, K. (1996, September). Beyond the baby blues: Understanding postpartum depression. *Today's Parent,* pp. 84–89.

Patterson, E. T., & Hale, E. S. (1985). Making sure: Integrating menstrual care practices into activities of daily living. *Advances in Nursing Science, 7,* 18–31.

Penelope, J., & Wolfe, S. (1990). *The original coming out stories.* Freedom, CA: Crossing Press.

Schneider, K. S. (1996). Too fat? Too thin? How media images of celebrities teach kids to hate their bodies. *People, 45,* 64–74.

Perera, S. B. (1981). *Descent to the goddess: A way of initiation for women.* Toronto: Inner City Books.

Perrott, R. L., & Condit, C. M. (Eds.). (1996). *Evaluating women's health messages: A resource book.* Thousand Oaks, CA: Sage.

Person, E. S. (1980). Sexuality as the mainstay of identity: Psychoanalytic perspectives. In C. Stimpson & E. Person (Eds.), *Women: Sex and sexuality* (pp. 36–61). Chicago: University of Chicago Press.

Pettersen, A. C. (1983). Menarche: Meaning of measures and measuring meaning. In S. Golub (Ed.), *Menarche: The transition from girl to woman* (pp. 63–76). Lexington, MA: Lexington Books.

Petersen A. (1988). Adolescent development. *Annual Review of Psychology, 39,* 583–607.

Phoenix, A., Woollett, A., & Lloyd, E. (Eds.). (1991). *Motherhood: Meanings, practise, and ideologies.* London: Sage.

Piaget, J. (1950). *The psychology of intelligence.* New York: International Universities Press.

Pigott, C. (1991, December). They called me "chicken hips": Adding weight to an image of beauty. *The Optimist,* p. 17.

Pike, K., & Rodin, J. (1991). Mothers, daughters and disordered eating. *Journal of Abnormal Psychology, 100,* 198–204.

Pipher, M. (1994). *Reviving Ophelia: Saving the selves of adolescent girls.* New York: Ballantine.

Plaut, E. A., & Hutchinson, F. L. (1986). The role of puberty in female psychosexual development. *International Review of Psychoanalysis, 13,* 417–432.

Plous, S., & Neptune, D. (1997). Racial and gender biases in magazine advertising: A content-analytic study. *Psychology of Women Quarterly, 21,* 627–644.

Plummer, K. (1975). *Sexual stigma: An interactionist account.* London: Routledge.

Plummer, K. (1982). Symbolic interactionism and sexual conduct: An emergent perspective. In M. Brake (Ed.), *Human sexual relations: A reader in human sexuality* (pp. 223–241). New York: Penguin.

Plummer, K. (1991). Understanding childhood sexualities. *Journal of Homosexuality, 20,* 231–249.

Plummer, K. (1992). *Modern homosexualities: Fragments of lesbian and gay experience.* London, New York: Routledge.

Pollack, S. (1990). Lesbian parents: Claiming our visibility. In J. P. Knowles & E. Cole (Eds.), *Woman-defined motherhood.* New York: Harrington Park Press.

Pokras, R., & Hufnagel, V. G. (1988). Hysterectomy in the United States, 1965–84. *American Journal of Public Health, 78,* 852–853.

Ponse, B. (1980). Finding self in the lesbian community. In M. Kirkpatrick (Ed.), *Women's sexual development: Explorations of inner space* (pp. 181–200). New York: Plenum.

Porcino, J. (1983). *Growing older, getting better: A handbook for women in the second half of life.* Reading, MA: Addison-Wesley.

Posin, R. (1991). Ripening. In B. Sang, J. Warshow, & A. Smith (Eds.), *Lesbians at midlife: The creative transition* (pp. 143–146). San Francisco: Spinsters.

Price, J. (1988). *Motherhood: What it does to your mind.* London: Pandora.

Prusank, D. T., Duran, R. L., & DeLillo, D. A. (1993). Interpersonal relationships in women's magazines: Dating and relating in the 1970's and 1980's. *Journal of Social and Personal Relationships, 10,* 307–320.

Psychology Today. (1996, March/April). *29*(2). New York: Sussex.

Rabinor, J. R. (1994). Mothers, daughters, and eating disorders: Honoring the mother–daughter relationship. In P. Fallon, M. A. Katzman, & S. C. Wooley (Eds.), *Feminist perspectives on eating disorders* (pp. 272–286). New York: Guilford Press.

Raudenbush, B., & Zellner, D. A. (1997). Nobody's satisfied: Effects of abnormal eating behaviors and actual perceived weight status on body image satisfaction in males and females. *Journal of Social and Clinical Psychology, 16,* 95–104

Reid, A., & Deaux, K. (1996). Relationship between social and personal identities: Segregation or integration. *Journal of Personality and Social Psychology, 71,* 1084–1091.

Reinisch, J. M., Rosenblum, L. A., & Sanders, S. S. (Eds.). (1987). *Masculinity/femininity: Basic perspectives.* New York: Oxford University Press.

Rich, A. (1976). *Of woman born: Motherhood as experience and institution.* New York: Basic Books.

Rich, A. (1980). Compulsory heterosexuality and lesbian existence. In C. R. Stimpson & E. S. Person (Eds.), *Women: Sex and sexuality* (pp. 62–91). Chicago: University of Chicago Press.

Rice, A. (1990). *The witching hour.* New York: Ballantine Books.

Rierdan, J. (1983). Variations in the experience of menarche as a function of preparedness. In S. Golub (Ed.), *Menarche: The transition from girl to woman* (pp. 119–126). Lexington, MA: Lexington Books.

Rierdan, J., & Koff, E. (1980). The psychological impact of menarche: Integrative versus disruptive changes. *Journal of Youth and Adolescence, 9,* 49–58.
Rierdan, J., & Koff, E. (1985). Timing of menarche and initial menstrual experience. *Journal of Youth and Adolescence, 14,* 237–243.
Rierdan, J., Koff, E., & Flaherty, J. (1985). Conceptions and misconceptions of menstruation. *Women and Health, 10,* 33–45.
Rierdan, J., Koff, E., & Stubbs, M. L. (1989). Timing of menarche, preparation, and initial menstrual experience: Replication and further analyses in a prospective study. *Journal of Youth and Adolescence, 18,* 413–426.
Roberto, K. A. (Ed.). (1996). *Relationships between women in later life.* New York: Haworth Press.
Roberts, J., Chambers, L. F., Blake, J., & Webber, C. (1992). Psychosocial adjustment in post-menopausal women. *Canadian Journal of Nursing Research, 24,* 29–46.
Rodeheaver, D., & Stohs, J. (1991). The adaptive misperception of age in older women: Sociocultural images and psychological mechanisms of control. *Educational Gerontology, 17,* 141–156.
Rodin, J. (1992). *Body traps.* New York: Quill/William Morrow.
Rodin, J., Silberstein, L., & Striegel-Moore, R. (1984). Women and weight: A normative discontent. *Nebraska Symposium on Motivation, 32,* 267–307.
Roiphe, K. (1993). *The morning after: Sex, fear, and feminism on campus.* New York: Little, Brown.
Root, M. P. P. (1990). Disordered eating in women of color. *Sex Roles, 14,* 59–68.
Rosen, R. C., & Leiblum, S. R. (1995). Treatment of sexual disorders in the 1990's: An integrated approach. *Journal of Consulting and Clinical Psychology, 63,* 877–890.
Rostosky, S. S., & Travis, C. B. (1996). Menopausal research and the dominance of the biomedical model 1984–1994. *Psychology of Women Quarterly, 20,* 285–312.
Rotberg, A. R. (1987). An introduction to the study of women, aging, and sexuality. *Physical and Occupational Therapy in Geriatrics, 5,* 3–12.
Roth, G. (1982). *Feeding the hungry heart.* New York: Signet.
Rothbaum, B. O., & Jackson, J. (1990). Religious influence on menstrual attitudes and symptoms. *Women and Health, 16,* 63–78.
Rothblum, E. D. (1989). Introduction: Lesbianism as a model of a positive lifestyle for women. In E. D. Rothblum & E. Cole (Eds.), *Loving boldly: Issues facing lesbians* (pp. 1–12). New York: Harrington Park Press.
Rothblum, E. D. (1992). The stigma of women's weight: Social and economic realities. *Feminism and Psychology, 2,* 61–73.
Rothblum, E. D. (1994). Lesbians and physical appearance: Which model applies? In B. Greene & G. M. Herek (Eds.), *Psychological perspectives on lesbian and gay issues* (Vol. 1, pp. 84–97). Thousand Oaks, CA: Sage.
Rothblum, E. D., & Brehony, K. A. (1993). *Boston marriages: Romantic but asexual relationships among contemporary lesbians.* Amherst: University of Massachusetts Press.
Rothblum, E. D., & Cole, E. (1991). Lesbian sex at menopause: As good as or better than ever. In B. Sang, J. Warshow, & A. J. Smith (Eds.), *Lesbians at midlife: The creative transition* (pp. 184–193). San Francisco: Spinsters.
Rothman, B. K. (1989). The meanings of choice in reproductive technology. In R.

Arditti, R. D. Klein, & S. Minden (Eds.), *Test-tube women* (3rd ed., pp. 23–34). London: Pandora Press.

Ruben, D. (1969). *Everything you always wanted to know about sex but were afraid to ask.* New York: David McKay.

Rubin, L. B. (1979). *Women of a certain age: The midlife search for self.* New York: Harper & Row.

Rubin, L. B. (1984). *Intimate strangers: Men and women together.* New York: Harper & Row.

Rubin, L. B. (1990). *Erotic wars: What happened to the sexual revolution?* New York: Farrar, Straus & Giroux.

Rush, A. (1975). *Getting clear: Body work for women.* New York: Random House/Bookwords.

Russell, D. E. (1986). *The secret trauma: Incest in the lives of girls and women.* New York: Basic Books.

Russo, N. F. (1976). The motherhood mandate. *Journal of Social Issues, 32,* 143–154.

Russo, N. F. (1979). Overview: Sex roles, fertility, and the motherhood mandate. *Psychology of Women Quarterly, 4,* 7–15.

Rust, P. C. (1996). Managing multiple identities: Diversity among bisexual women and men. In B. A. Firestein (Ed.), *Bisexuality: The psychology and politics of an invisible minority* (pp. 53–83). Thousand Oaks, CA: Sage.

Safer, J. (1996). *Beyond motherhood: Choosing a life without children.* New York: Pocket Books.

Sand, G. (1993). *Is is hot in here or is it me?* New York: Random House.

Sandelowski, C. (1989). *Sexual concerns when illness or disability strikes.* Springfield, IL: Charles C Thomas.

Sandelowski, M. J. (1990a). Failures of volition: Female agency and infertility in historical perspective. In J. F. O'Barr, D. Pope, & Mary Wyer (Eds.), *Ties that bind: Essays on mothering and patriarchy* (pp. 35–60). Chicago: University of Chicago Press.

Sandelowski, M. J. (1990b). Fault lines: Infertility and imperiled sisterhood. *Feminist Studies, 16,* 33–51.

Sandelowski, M. J. (1993). *With child in mind.* Philadelphia: University of Pennsylvania Press.

Sang, B. (1991). Moving toward balance and integration. In B. Sang, J. Warshow, & A. Smith (Eds.), *Lesbians at midlife: The creative transition* (pp. 206–214). San Francisco: Spinsters.

Sang, B., Warshow, J., & Smith, A. (1991). *Lesbians at midlife: The creative transition.* San Francisco: Spinsters.

Savin-Williams, R. (1990). *Gay and lesbian youth: Expressions of identity.* Bristol, PA: Hemisphere.

Schnarch, D. M. (1991). *Constructing the sexual crucible: An integration of sexual and marital therapy.* New York: Norton.

Schnarch, D. M. (1997). *Passionate marriage: Sex, love and intimacy in emotionally committed relationships.* New York: Norton.

Schneider, K. S. (1996). Too fat? Too thin?: How media images of celebrities teach kids to hate their bodies. *People, 45,* 64–74.

Seid, R. P. (1989). *Never too thin: Why women are at war with their bodies.* Scarborough, ON: Prentice-Hall.

Seid, R. P. (1994). Too "close to the bone": The historical context for women's obsession with slenderness. In P. Fallon, M. A. Katzman & S. C. Wooley (Eds.), *Feminist perspectives on eating disorders* (pp. 3–15). New York: Guilford Press.

Sevely, J. L. (1987). *Eve's secrets: A new perspective on human sexuality.* London: Bloomsbury.

Shapiro, B. L., & Schwartz, C. (1997). Date rape: Its relationship to trauma symptoms and sexual self-esteem. *Journal of Interpersonal Violence, 12,* 407–415.

Shapiro, C. H. (1988). *Infertility and pregnancy loss: A guide for helping professionals.* San Francisco: Jossey-Bass.

Shapiro, C. H. (1993). *When part of the self is lost: Helping clients heal after sexual and reproductive losses.* San Francisco: Jossey-Bass.

Sheehy, G. (1992). *The silent passage: Menopause.* New York: Random House.

Sheinkin, L., & Golden, G. (1985). Therapy with women in the later stages of life: A symbolic quest. *Women and Therapy, 4,* 83–92.

Sherwin, B. B. (1988). A comparative analysis of the role of androgen in human male and female sexual behavior: Behavioral specificity, critical thresholds, and sensitivity. *Psychobiology, 16,* 416–425.

Sherwin, B. B., & Gelfand, M. M. (1987). The role of androgen in the maintenance of sexual functioning in oophorectomized women. *Psychosomatic Medicine, 48,* 397–409.

Sherwin, B., Gelfand, M., & Brender, W. (1985). Androgen enhances sexual motivation in females: A prospective crossover study of sex steroid administration in the surgical menopause. *Psychosomatic Medicine, 47,* 339–351.

Siegel, S. J. (1986). The effect of culture on how women experience menstruation: Jewish women and *mikvah. Women and Health, 10,* 63–74.

Simmons, R. G., & Blyth, D. A. (1987). *Moving into adolescence: The impact of pubertal change and school context.* New York: Aldine De Gruyter.

Simonds, S. L. (1994). *Bridging the silence: Nonverbal modalities in the treatment of adult survivors of childhood sexual abuse.* New York: Norton.

Skultans, V. (1988). Menstrual symbolism in South Wales. In T. Buckley & A. Gottlieb (Eds.), *Blood magic: The anthropology of menstruation* (pp. 133–160). Berkeley: University of California Press.

Smart, C., & Smart, B. (1978). Accounting for rape: Reality and myth in press reporting. In C. Smart & B. Smart (Eds.), *Women, sexuality and social control* (pp. 89–103). Chicago: Chicago University Press.

Smith, A. M., Rosenthal, D. A., & Reichler, H. (1996). High schoolers' masturbatory practices: Their relationship to sexual intercourse and personal characteristics. *Psychological Reports, 79,* 499–509.

Smith, V. (1990, January 13). Tens of thousands seek beauty under the knife. *Toronto Globe and Mail,* pp. A1, A13.

Snitow, A. (1980). The front line: Notes on sex in novels by women, 1969–1979. In C. Stimpson & E. Person (Eds.), *Women: Sex and sexuality* (pp. 158–174). Chicago: University of Chicago Press.

Snitow, A., Stansell, C., & Thompson, S. (Eds.). (1983). *Powers of desire: The politics of sexuality.* New York: Monthly Review Press.

Sommer, B. (1983). How does menstruation affect cognitive competence and psychophysiological response? *Women and Health, 8,* 53–90.

Sontag, S. (1979). The double standard of aging. In J. H. Williams (Ed.), *Psychology of women: Selected readings* (pp. 462–478). New York: Norton.

Sophie, J. (1985/1986). A critical examination of stage theories of lesbian identity development. *Journal of Homosexuality, 12,* 39–51.

Spalding, L. R. & Peplau, L. A. (1997). The unfaithful lover: Heterosexuals' perceptions of bisexuals and their relationships. *Psychology of Women Quarterly, 21*, 611–626.

Sprecher, S., & McKinney, K. (1993). *Sexuality.* New York: Sage.

Sprinkle, A. (1996). 101 uses for sex—or why sex is so important. *Women and Therapy* [Special Issue: Sexualities], *19,* 5–6.

Stanworth, M. (1987). Reproductive technologies and the deconstruction of motherhood. In M. Stanworth (Ed.), *Reproductive technologies: Gender, motherhood and medicine* (pp. 10–35). Minneapolis: University of Minnesota Press.

Starr, B. D., & Weiner, M. B. (1981). *The Starr–Weiner report on sex and sexuality in the mature years.* New York: Stein & Day.

Steinem, G. (1981). *Outrageous acts and everyday rebellions.* New York: Holt, Rinehart Winston.

Steinem, G. (1992). *Revolution from within: A book of self-esteem.* Boston: Little, Brown.

Steiner-Adair, C. (1986). The body politic: Normal female adolescent development and the development of eating disorders. *Journal of the American Academy of Psychoanalysis, 14,* 95–114.

Steiner-Adair, C. (1991). When the body speaks: Girls, eating disorders and psychotherapy. In C. Gilligan, A. Rogers, & D. Tolman (Eds.), *Women, girls, and psychotherapy: Reframing resistance* (pp. 253–266). New York: Haworth Press.

Stevens-Long, J., & Commons, M. L. (1992). *Adult life: Developmental processes* (4th ed). London: Mayfield.

Stiglitz, E. (1990). Caught between two worlds: The impact of a child on a lesbian couple's relationship. In J. P. Knowles & E. Cole (Eds.), *Woman-defined motherhood* (pp. 99–116). New York: Harrington Park Press.

Stock, W. (1988). Propping up the phallocracy: A feminist critique of sex therapy and research. *Women and Therapy* [Special Issue: Women and Sex Therapy], *7,* 23–41.

Stoltzman, S. M. (1986). Menstrual attitudes, beliefs and symptom experiences of adolescent females, their peers, and their mothers. *Health Care for Women International, 7,* 97–114.

Storz, N., & Greene, W. (1983). Body weight, body image and perception of fad diets in adolescent girls. *Journal of Nutritional Education, 15,* 15–18.

Striegel-Moore, R., Silberstein, R., & Rodin, J. (1986). Toward an understanding of risk factors for bulimia. *American Psychologist, 41,* 246–263.

Striegel-Moore, R., Tucker, N., & Hsu, J. (1990). Body image dissatisfaction and disordered eating in lesbian college students. *International Journal of Eating Disorders, 9,* 493–500.

Strober, M., & Yager, J. (1985). A developmental perspective on the treatment of anorexia nervosa in adolescents. In D. M. Garner & P. E. Garfinkel (Eds.), *Handbook of psychotherapy for anorexia nervosa and bulimia* (pp. 363–390). New York: Guilford Press.

Sweet, P. E. (1981). *Something happened to me.* Racine, WI: Mother Courage Press.

Symonds, D. (1979). *The evolution of human sexuality.* New York: Oxford University Press.

Taetzsch, L. (Ed.). (1995). *Hot flashes: Women writers on the change of life.* Boston: Faber & Faber.

Tannen, D. (1991). *You just don't understand: Women and men in conversation.* Milson's Point, NSW: Random House.

Tantleff-Dunn, S., & Thompson, J. K. (1995). Romantic partners and body image disturbance: Further evidence for the role of perceived-actual disparities. *Sex Roles, 33,* 589–605.

Tasker, F. L., & Golombok, S. (1997). *Growing up in a lesbian family: Effects on child development.* New York: Guilford Press.

Tavris, C. (1992). *The mismeasure of woman.* New York: Simon & Schuster.

Taylor, D. (1988). *Red flower: Rethinking menstruation.* Freedom, CA: Crossing Press.

Taylor, D. L., & Woods, N. F. (Eds.). (1991). *Menstruation, health, and illness.* New York: Hemisphere.

Thomas, C. L. (Ed.). (1989). *Taber's cyclopedic medical dictionary* (16th ed.). Philadelphia: F.A. Davis.

Thomas, V., & James, M. (1988). Body image, dieting tendencies, and sex role traits in urban black women. *Sex Roles, 18,* 523–529.

Thompson, B. (1992). "A way outa no way": Eating problems among African-American, Latina, & white women. *Gender and Society, 6,* 546–561.

Thompson, B. W. (1994). *A hunger so wide and so deep: American women speak out on eating problems.* Minneapolis: University of Minnesota Press.

Thompson, S. (1990). Putting a big thing into a little hole: Teenage girls' accounts of sexual initiation. *Journal of Sex Research, 27,* 341–361.

Thornton, C. E. (1981). Sexuality counseling of women with spinal cord injuries. In D. G. Bullard, & S. E. Knight (Eds.)., *Sexuality and physical disability: Personal perspectives* (pp. 156–168). St Louis: Mosby.

Tiefer, L. (1987). Social constructionism and the study of human sexuality. In P. Shaver & C. Hendrick (Eds.), *Sex and gender* (pp. 70–94). Newbury Park, CA: Sage.

Tiefer, L. (1988). A feminist critique of the sexual dysfunction nomenclature [Special Issue: Women and Sex Therapy]. *Women and Therapy, 7,* 5–21.

Tiefer, L. (1991). Historical, Scientific, clinical and feminist criticisms of "The Human Sexual Response Cycle" model. *Annual Review of Sex Research, 2,* 1–24.

Tiefer, L. (1995). *Sex is not a natural act and other essays.* Boulder, Co: Westview Press.

Tiefer, L. (1996). Towards a feminist sex therapy. *Women and Therapy* [Special Issue: Sexualities], *19,* 53–64.

Tiggeman, M., & Rothblum, E. D. (1997). Gender differences in internal beliefs about weight and negative attitudes towards self and others. *Psychology of Women Quarterly, 21,* 581–594.

Tolman, D. L. (1991). Adolescent girls, women and sexuality: Discerning dilemmas of desire. In C. Gilligan, A. Rogers, & D. Tolman (Eds.), *Women, girls, and psychotherapy: Reframing resistance* (pp. 55–69). New York: Haworth Press.

Tolman, D. L., & Debold, E. (1994). Conflicts of body and image: Female adolescents, desire, and the no-body body. In P. Fallon, M. A. Katzman, & S.

C. Wooley (Eds.), *Feminist perspectives on eating disorders* (pp. 301–317). New York: Guilford Press.

Toubia, N. (1993). *Female genital mutilation: A call for global action.* New York: Women, Ink.

Troll, L. E. (1994). Family connectedness of old women: Attachments in later life. In B. F. Turner & L. E. Troll (Eds.), *Women growing older: Psychological perspectives* (pp. 169–201). Thousand Oaks, CA: Sage.

Turner, J. (1990). Let my soul soar: Touch therapy. In T. A. Laidlaw & C. Malmo (Eds.), *Healing voices: Feminist approaches to therapy with women* (pp. 221–240). San Francisco: Jossey-Bass.

Udry, J. R., & Cliquet, R. L. (1982). A cross-cultural examination of the relationship between ages at menarche, marriage, and first birth. *Demography, 19,* 53–63.

Udry, J. R., Talbert, L., & Morris, N. M. (1986). Biosocial foundations for adolescent female sexuality. *Demography, 23,* 217–230.

Ulbrich, P. M., Coyle, A. T., & Llabre, M. M. (1990). Involuntary childlessness and marital adjustment: His and hers. *Journal of Sex and Marital Therapy, 16,* 147–158.

Unger, R., & Crawford, M. (1992). *Women and gender: A feminist psychology.* New York: McGraw-Hill.

Usmiani, S., & Daniluk, J.C. (1997). Mothers and their adolescent daughters: Relationship between self-esteem, gender role identity, and body image. *Journal of Youth and Adolescence, 26,* 45–55.

Ussher, J. (1997). *Fantasies of feminity: Reframing the boundaries of sex.* London: Penguin Press.

Ussher, J. M. (1989). *The psychology of the female body.* New York: Routledge.

Ussher, J. (1992a). Reproductive rhetoric and the blaming of the body. In P. Nicolson & J. Ussher (Eds.), *The psychology of women's health and health care* (pp. 31–61). London: Macmillan.

Ussher, J. (1992b). Research and theory related to female reproduction: Implications for clinical psychology. *British Journal of Clinical Psychology, 31,* 129–151.

Ussher, J. M. (1994). Theorizing female sexuality: Social constructionist and poststructuralist accounts. In P. Y. L. Choi & P. Nicolson (Eds.), *Female sexuality: Psychology, biology and social context* (pp. 148–175). New York: Harvester/Wheatsheaf.

Valentich, M. (1990). Talking sex: Implications for practice in the 1990's. *Sieccan Journal, 5,* 3–11.

Valverde, M. (1985). *Sex, power, and pleasure.* Toronto: Woman's Press.

Vance, C. S. (1984). Pleasure and danger: Toward a politics of sexuality. In C. S. Vance (Ed.), *Pleasure and danger: Exploring female sexuality* (pp. 1 –27). London: Routledge & Kegan Paul.

Vance, C. S. (Ed.). (1992). *Pleasure and danger: Exploring female sexuality* (2nd ed.). London: Pandora Press.

Vance, C. S., & Pollis, C. A. (1990). Introduction: A special issue on feminist perspectives on sexuality. *Journal of Sex Research, 27,* 1–5.

Veevers, J. (1980). *Childless by choice.* Toronto: Butterworth.

Villanueva, A. L. (1989). "Sassy." In J. Canan (Ed.), *She rises like the sun: Invocations of the goddess by contemporary American women poets* (pp. 171–172). Freedom, CA: Crossing Press.

Villanueva, A. L. (1989). "The object." In J. Canan (Ed.), *She rises like the sun:*

Invocations of the goddess by contemporary American women poets (pp. 171–172). Freedom, CA: Crossing Press.

Voda, A. M., & Eliasson, M. (1983). Menopause: The closure of menstrual life. In S. Golub (Ed.), *Lifting the curse of menstruation* (pp. 137–156). New York: Haworth Press.

Walker, G. (1992). *Women's sexuality from the inside out.* Workshop presentation at the Association of Women in Psychology National Feminist Psychology Conference, Long Beach, CA.

Walton, M. T., Fineman, R. M., & Walton, P. J. (1996). Why can't a woman be more like a man? A Renaissance perspective on the biological basis for female inferiority. *Women and Health, 24,* 87–95.

Ward, L. M., & Wyatt, G. E. (1994). The effects of childhood sexual messages on African-American and white women's adolescent sexual behavior. *Psychology of Women Quarterly, 18,* 183–201.

Waterman, C. K., Dawson, L. J., & Bologna, M. J. (1989). Sexual coercion in gay male and lesbian relationships: Predictions and implications for support services. *Journal of Sex Research, 26,* 118–124.

Weasel, L. H. (1996). Seeing between the lines: Bisexual women and therapy. *Women and Therapy, 19,* 5–16.

Webster, D. (1988). Tensions, dilemmas and possibilities for understanding women's sexuality. *Women and Therapy* [Special Issue: Women and Sex Therapy], *7,* 295–299.

Weed, S. S. (1992). *Menopausal years: The wise woman way—alternative approaches for women 30–90.* New York: Ash Tree.

Weeks, J. (1981). *Sex, politics and society: The regulation of sexuality since 1800.* London: Longman.

Weeks, J. (1985). *Sexuality and its discontents: Meanings, myths, and modern sexualities.* London: Routledge & Kegan Paul.

Weeks, J. (1987). Questions of identity. In A. P. Caplan (Ed.), *The cultural construction of sexuality* (pp. 31–51). London, New York: Tavistock.

Weeks, J. (1995). History, desire, and identities. In R. G. Parker & J. H. Gagnon (Eds.), *Conceiving sexuality* (pp. 33–50). New York: Routledge.

Weideger, P. (1978). *Female cycles.* London: Women's Press.

Weise, E. R. (Ed.). (1992). *Closer to home: Bisexuality and feminism.* Seattle, WA: Seal Press.

Weiser, J. (1990). More than meets the eye: Using ordinary snapshots as tools for therapy. In T. A. Laidlaw, & C. Malmo (Eds.), *Healing voices: Feminist approaches to therapy with women* (pp. 83–117). San Francisco: Jossey-Bass.

Westerlund, E. (1992). *Women's sexuality after childhood incest.* New York: Norton.

Whelan, E. (1980). *A baby? . . . maybe?: A guide to making the most fateful decision of your life* (rev. ed.). New York: Bobbs–Merrill.

White, J. W., & Humphrey, J. A. (1991). Young people's attitudes toward rape. In A Parrot & L. Bechhofer (Eds.), *Acquaintance rape: The hidden crime* (pp. 43–56). New York: Wiley.

Wilbur, J. E., Miller, A., & Montgomery, A. (1995). The influence of demographic characteristics, menopausal status, and symptoms on women's attitudes toward menopause. *Women and Health, 23,* 19–39.

Wilson, E. O. (1978). *On human nature.* Cambridge, MA: Harvard University Press.

Wohl, A., & Kaufman, B. (1985). *Silent screams and hidden cries: An interpretation of artwork by children from violent homes.* New York: Brunner/Mazel.

Wolf, N. (1991). *The beauty myth.* Toronto: Vintage Books.

Wolf, N. (1997). *Promiscuities: The secret struggle for womanhood.* New York, Toronto: Random House.

Wooley, O. W. (1994). . . . And man created "woman": Representations of women's bodies in Western culture. In P. Fallon, M. A. Katzman, & S. C. Wooley (Eds.), *Feminist perspectives on eating disorders* (pp. 17–52). New York: Guilford Press.

Wooley, S. C., & Wooley, O. W. (1980). Eating disorders: Obesity and anorexia. In A. M. Brodsky & R. Hare-Mustin (Eds.), *Women and psychotherapy* (pp. 135–158). New York: Guilford Press.

Wooley, S. C., & Wooley, O. W. (1984, February). Feeling fat in a thin society. *Glamour,* pp. 198–252.

Wooley, S. C., & Wooley, O. W. (1985). Intensive outpatient and residential treatment for bulimia. In D. M. Garner & P. E. Garfinkel (Eds.), *Handbook of psychotherapy for anorexia nervosa and bulimia* (pp. 391–430). New York: Guilford Press.

Woollett, A. (1991). Having children: Accounts of childless women and women with reproductive problems. In A. Phoenix, A. Woollett, & E. Lloyd (Eds.), *Motherhood: Meanings, practices and ideologies* (pp. 47–65). London: Sage.

Wright, J., Allard, M., Lecours, A., & Sabourin, S. (1989). Psychosocial distress and infertility: A review of controlled research. *International Journal of Fertility, 34,* 126–142.

Wyatt, G. E., & Dunn, K. M. (1991). Examining predictors of sex guilt in multiethnic samples of women. *Archives of Sexual Behavior, 20,* 471–485.

Wyatt, G. E., Peters, S. D., & Guthrie, D. (1988a). Kinsey revisited: Part I. Comparisons of the sexual socialization and sexual behavior of white women over 33 years. *Archives of Sexual Behavior, 17,* 201–239.

Wyatt, G. E., Peters, S. D., & Guthrie, D. (1988b). Kinsey revisited: Part II. Comparisons of the sexual socialization and sexual behavior of black women over 33 years. *Archives of Sexual Behavior, 17,* 289–332.

Wyatt, G. E., & Riederle, M. H. (1994). Reconceptualizing issues that affect women's sexual decision-making and sexual functioning. *Psychology of Women Quarterly, 18,* 611–625.

Yalom, M., Estler, S., & Brewster, W. (1982). Changes in female sexuality: A study of mother/daughter communication and generational differences. *Psychology of Women Quarterly, 7,* 141–154.

Yates, W. (1987). Human sexuality: Dualistic and holistic paradigms. *Sieccan Journal, 2*(2), 2–12.

Zilbergeld, B. (1993). *The new male sexuality.* New York: Bantam.

Zipes, J. (Ed.). (1986). *Don't bet on the prince: Contemporary feminist fairy tales in North America and England.* New York: Methuen.

INDEX